MW00674061

Health Psychology and Behavioral Medicine

James J. Snyder
THE WICHITA STATE UNIVERSITY

Health Psychology and Behavioral Medicine

PRENTICE HALL, Englewood Cliffs, New Jersey 07632

Library of Congress Cataloging-in-Publication Data

Snyder, James J.
Health psychology and behavioral medicine / James J. Snyder.
p. cm.
Includes bibliographies and index.
ISBN 0-13-385550-3
1. Clinical health psychology. 2. Medicine and psychology.
I. Title.
[DNLM: 1. Behavioral Medicine. 2. Psychology, Medical.
3. Psychophysiologic Disorders. WM 90 S675h]
R726.7.S68 1989
616'.0019--dc19
DNLM/DLC
for Library of Congress 88-39079
CIP

Editorial / production supervision and interior design: P. M. Gordon Associates
Cover design: Lundgren Graphics, Ltd.
Manufacturing buyer: Ray Keating

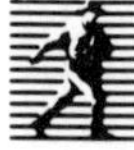

Printed in the United States of America
10 9 8 7 6 5 4 3 2 1

ISBN 0-13-385550-3

Prentice-Hall International (UK) Limited, *London*
Prentice-Hall of Australia Pty. Limited, *Sydney*
Prentice-Hall Canada, Inc., *Toronto*
Prentice-Hall Hispanoamericana, S.A., *Mexico*
Prentice-Hall of India Private Limited, *New Delhi*
Prentice-Hall of Japan, Inc., *Tokyo*
Simon & Schuster Asia Pte. Ltd., *Singapore*
Editora Prentice-Hall do Brasil, Ltda., *Rio de Janeiro*

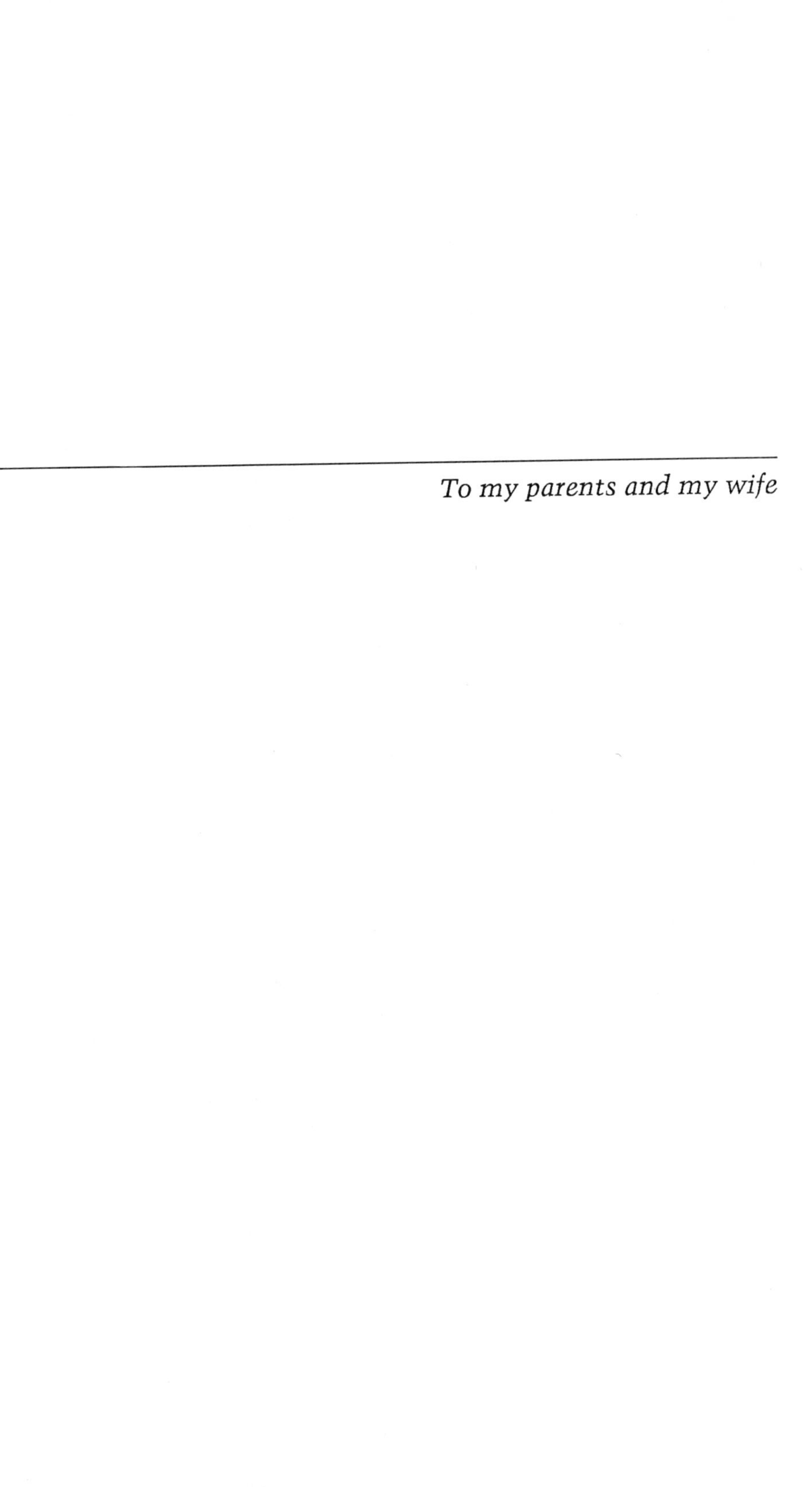

To my parents and my wife

Contents

Preface xiii

Acknowledgments xv

PART I The Relationship Between Behavior and Health Status 1

1. **Paradigms of Health and Medicine** 1

The Nature of Paradigms 1
The Biomedical Paradigm 2
The Medical Paradigm of Helping 3
Historical Development of Current Paradigms in Medicine 5
Evaluation of the Biomedical Paradigm and the Medical Paradigm of Helping 8
Alternate Paradigms 14
Summary 23
References 23

2. Health, Illness, and Behavior 25

Introduction 25
Direct Links Between Behavior and Health: Biomedical and Systems Paradigms 26
Direct Health-Behavior Link: Helping Perspectives 28
Health-Impairing and Health-Promoting Behaviors 31
Eating and Obesity 33
Food Preferences and Nutrition 37
Exercise 41
Smoking 42
Summary 44
References 45

3. Illness-Related Decisions and Actions 48

Introduction 48
Symptom Recognition 48
Symptom Interpretation 50
Actions in Response to Illness 51
Client-Health Provider Interaction and Communication 54
Adherence to Treatment Recommendations 57
Summary 62
References 62

4. Stress 65

Introduction 65
Definitions of Stress 65
Stress: A Systems View 70
The Physiology of Stress 78
Stress as a Process 88
Adaptational Outcomes 89
Summary 92
References 92

5. Health and Illness: A Systems View 96

Introduction 96
Biological and Genetic Factors in Health and Illness 97
Health and Disease:
A Systems Perspective 100

The Systems Paradigm of Health and Disease: Implications for Intervention 110
Summary 111
References 112

PART II Prevalent Diseases: Etiology, Symptoms, Course, and Prognosis 113

6. **Coronary Artery Disease 113**

Introduction 113
Cardiovascular Anatomy and Physiology 114
Coronary Artery Disease: A Definition 115
Causes of Coronary Artery Disease 116
Illness-Related Decisions and Actions in Coronary Artery Disease 130
Summary 136
References 136

7. **Infectious Diseases 140**

Introduction 140
The Immune System 141
Immune, Nervous, and Endocrine System Relationships 145
Psychoneuroimmunology 147
Contact with Infectious Agents: The Role of Behavioral and Environmental Variables 153
Infectious Diseases: Impact and Coping 157
Summary 158
References 159

8. **Cancer 161**

Introduction 161
What Is Cancer? 162
Who Gets Cancer? 162
Behavioral and Psychological Factors in the Etiology of Cancer 164
The Effect of Cancer on the Person 174
Summary 184
References 185

9. Pain 188

Introduction 188
Pain as a Multidimensional Process 189
The Biomedical Paradigm of Pain 189
Psychosocial Aspects of Pain 197
Pain Behavior 201
A Systems Conceptualization of Pain 203
Clinical Pain 204
Summary 210
References 210

PART III Principles of Cognitive and Behavioral Interventions 213

10. Basic Behavioral Interventions: Operant, Respondent, and Observational Learning 213

Introduction 213
Operant Conditioning 214
Respondent Conditioning 227
Observational Learning 231
Summary 234
References 234

11. Self-Control and Cognitive Therapy 236

Introduction 236
Self-Control 237
Cognitive Therapy 248
Health Enhancement and Education 255
Summary 256
References 257

12. Biofeedback and Relaxation Training 258

Introduction 258
Biofeedback 259
The Effectiveness of Biofeedback 270
Relaxation Training 274
Summary 279
References 280

PART IV Applications of Behavior Change Principles to Specific Health Problems 282

13. Health- and Illness-Related Behaviors: Clinical and Preventative Interventions 282

Introduction 282
Smoking 283
Obesity, Eating, and Exercise 289
Enhancing Adherence to Treatment Recommendations 297
Summary 302
References 303

14. Stress Management: Clinical and Preventative Applications 306

Introduction 306
Coping Skills Interventions: General Guidelines 307
Targets of Coping Skills Training 310
Stress Management: Altering the Environment 314
Stress Management: Applications 318
Summary 323
References 324

15. Coronary Artery Disease and Cancer: Preventative and Clinical Interventions 327

Introduction 327
Coronary Artery Disease 329
Cancer 340
References 354

16. Pain and Infectious Diseases: Preventative and Clinical Interventions 358

Introduction 358
Pain 359
Pain: A Summary 378
Behavioral, Psychosocial, and Environmental Interventions in Infectious Diseases 378

Behavioral, Psychosocial, and Environmental Interventions in Infectious Diseases: A Summary 387
References 388

17. Behavioral Health and Medicine: Current Status and Future Directions 391

Introduction 391
Conceptual Issues in Behavioral Health and Medicine 392
Biobehavioral Relationships: Variations on Three Themes 393
Current Status and Future Directions in Behavioral Health and Medicine 394
Summary 398
References 399

Index 401

Preface

In the past twenty years, the empirical, theoretical, and clinical applications of psychological principles to health care have undergone explosive growth. This explosion has moved the field from the status of a stepchild traditionally labeled "psychosomatic medicine" to that of an adolescent experiencing rapid growth, excitement, and promise but still searching for a firm identity. There are many books on behavioral medicine, behavioral health, health psychology, and medical psychology. Why is another needed? Most works in the field are highly specialized, edited volumes that focus on one area of application. Others attempt an encyclopedic coverage of all applications. In both cases, the development of an integrative perspective that explicitly unifies and extends this seemingly disparate information is often lacking.

This book has three goals. The first aim is to provide the reader with the means to conceptualize the interaction of psychological and biological processes in an integrative manner that leads to more effective prevention and treatment. To accomplish this goal, existing paradigms of health and helping are examined and critically evaluated. A systems paradigm of helping and a compensatory model of helping are offered as optimal. The second goal is to describe the principles by which behavior, cognition, affect, and the social and physical environment influence health as well as the basic behavior change methods relevant to preventative and clinical health care. The third goal is to describe and evaluate the applications of these paradigms, principles, and methods to four major health problems: heart disease, infectious diseases, cancer, and pain. Preventative as well as clinical interventions targeting these problems are described.

This book is intended for use in upper division undergraduate courses, but may also be helpful in introductory graduate courses in behavioral health and medicine and for health care professionals who want to integrate psychological principles and methods into their practice. The book presumes completion of introductory courses in psychology and human biology. Comprehension is relatively easier as additional background courses are available in both areas.

The text is not a comprehensive review of all relevant fields in behavioral health and medicine. Rather, four basic health-related problems are used as exemplars and considered in detail. The material can be supplemented by outside, independent readings on other health problems, for it provides a theoretical framework that is widely applicable to these concerns. The book is divided into four parts. The first explains how psychosocial processes play an important role in health and illness, and develops a theoretical perspective for understanding the interaction of psychosocial and biological processes. Part II examines the role of psychosocial variables in the development of specific medical problems and in responses to these problems. Basic behavior change principles relevant to disease prevention, health promotion, and clinical intervention are described in Part III. Part IV details and evaluates the application of these principles in changing the health-related behaviors detailed in Part I and in addressing the health problems considered in Part II.

Acknowledgments

A number of persons provided the intellectual impetus for this book. Students who have taken my course in the psychology of health and illness over the past seven years motivated me to formulate my thoughts and to write by asking challenging questions and consistently seeking more information. Early formative influences on my thinking about the interaction of psychological and biological processes were Robert A. Levitt, Donald Shoemaker, and Richard Depue.

At a more practical level, numerous persons have provided me with the encouragement, time, and support for this work: Gerald Patterson, who has served as a mentor and model; the faculty in the Psychology Department at The Wichita State University; and the editors and staff of Prentice Hall. Perhaps most importantly, I want to thank my wife and children for tolerating my compulsiveness.

Health Psychology and Behavioral Medicine

PART I

The Relationship Between Behavior and Health Status

1 Paradigms of Health and Medicine

The first five chapters provide basic information about the relationship between psychological variables and health. In Chapter 1, basic paradigms, or models, of health and health care are described and evaluated. This discussion provides an introductory structure of the role of thinking, affect, and behavior in health and health care. Chapters 2 through 4 detail the theory and research on the principle modes by which thinking, affect, and behavior influence health: health-impairing and health-promoting behavior, illness-related decisions and actions, and stress and coping. In Chapter 5, paradigms of health and health care are again considered to provide an integrated perspective on the interaction of socioenvironmental, psychological, physiological, and genetic determinants of health and on the implications of these interactions for health care delivery.

THE NATURE OF PARADIGMS

Suppose you were given a jigsaw puzzle to complete. You would quickly attempt to fit the pieces together with their plain side down in an interlocking fashion based on shape, color, and pattern. You would not scatter the pieces haphazardly or sort them according to color, although these solutions may result in aesthetically pleasing or conceptually reasonable outcomes. You would also assume that the pieces you were given would be from one puzzle and not parts of two or three puzzles, for that would seem unfair.

In working on a puzzle or some other task, certain rules or organizing principles define what types of information are relevant, what kinds of solutions are acceptable, and the steps by which those solutions are to be obtained. We make assumptions and develop rules when trying to solve a problem. In science, these assumptions and rules are called paradigms. The type of paradigm that is adopted to solve a problem is somewhat arbitrary. Paradigms are not, a priori, right or wrong. However, because a paradigm is arbitrary does not mean that it is unimportant. Without rules or organizing principles, our attempts to solve a problem would be confused and unsystematic. We would not know how to select information, how to extract meaning, or what actions to take. The type of paradigm adopted is also important because all paradigms do not lead to similar or equally useful solutions. A paradigm is selected because it is more successful than competing paradigms in solving a problem (Kuhn, 1970).

The more socially disruptive and individually distressing the problem, the greater is the need to devise some way to explain and deal with it. Disease is a distressing problem that demands explanation and action. It is person-centered, harmful, and associated with pain and impairment (Engel, 1977). Medicine has adopted a set of rules, or a paradigm, for seeking an explanation and a solution for disease. Historically, the most widely accepted set of rules and assumptions about disease in Western society is called the biomedical paradigm. Because medicine is an applied discipline, it involves a transaction between a health provider and a patient. Within this helping relationship, a set of rules and expectations governs the roles and responsibilities of both the provider and the patient. In Western history, the most widely accepted set of these roles and responsibilities is called the medical paradigm of helping.

In this chapter, the nature of the biomedical paradigm of disease and of the medical paradigm of helping will be outlined, and their usefulness in promoting health will be evaluated. Alternate paradigms of disease and of helping relationships will also be explored.

THE BIOMEDICAL PARADIGM

The biomedical paradigm is characterized by two assumptions: materialism and reductionism. Materialism regards persons as physical beings whose existence and functions can be examined, explained and altered using the principles of anatomy, physiology, biochemistry, and physics. Reductionism asserts that persons can be understood by examining their constituent parts. From this viewpoint, the only conceptual tools needed to study human beings are physical and chemical in nature (Engel, 1977).

According to the biomedical paradigm, people are biological organisms. Disease is a measurable disruption in or deviation from the biological norm caused by some identifiable physical or chemical event. Thus, for example, when health teams were called in during the outbreak of Legionnaires' Disease in Philadelphia, they looked for the presence of some pathogenic substance in the ventilation system of the hotel to account for the disease. Medical treatment involves the use of physical or chemical agents to correct the disruption or deviation. Thus, if a person has a fever and a high white blood cell count due to contact with an infectious agent, an antibiotic is prescribed to combat that agent.

The biomedical paradigm has not only been promulgated by health-care providers but has also been the prevailing lay view of disease and medical treatment in Western society (Fabrega, 1974). For example, if you sought the services of a physician because of an intense, persistent pain in your knee, you would expect the physician to palpate your knee and take x-rays. You might then expect to receive some medication to reduce the pain or a physical device to immobilize your knee to promote healing. You would be surprised (and probably less than enthusiastic) if the physician cut open a chicken, studied its entrails, and did an incantation to diagnose and treat your painful knee. Culturally, we share the biomedical paradigm. In fact, it has been so common and unquestioned that it has taken on the status of a dogma.

In summary, the biomedical paradigm defines disease as a disruption in or deviation from biological norms caused by some physical or chemical factor. Intervention involves the introduction of a corrective physical or chemical agent. Complaints for which there is no evidence of structural or functional deviation are irrelevant or outside the province of medicine. Those interventions that do not involve physical or chemical manipulations are not medical. The biomedical paradigm takes a relatively circumscribed view of people, since it leaves no room within its framework for social, psychological, and behavioral dimensions of humans.

THE MEDICAL PARADIGM OF HELPING

When individuals notice a physical problem that is not self-limiting and that is beyond their ability to remedy, they seek the aid of an expert who has the knowledge and skills to solve the problem. The roles and responsibilities of persons seeking health care and of professionals providing that care have a relatively consistent set of characteristics that in Western culture has been called the medical paradigm of helping. In this paradigm, patients are not held responsible for either the origin or the solution of their problem. They are instead seen as ill or incapacitated and are expected to accept that designation which exempts them from ordinary social obligations but imposes a responsibility to seek help and to cooperate in getting well. The health provider is responsible for identifying the problem and providing an effective solution.

The patients' role in the helping relationship is largely passive and dependent. They are to seek help for a problem, to describe their experience with the problem, and to comply with the recommendations of the health provider. The health provider is an active agent who is expected to possess the skills and knowledge needed to achieve an effective solution and who is responsible for bringing about a return to a nondiseased state. The patient is seen as a collection of organs that can malfunction and thus demand treatment; the patient as a whole person is generally ignored. Implicit in these roles and expectations is the patient's dependence on the provider (Brickman et al., 1983).

In the medical paradigm of helping, the health provider is given and assumes a powerful position, whereas the patient is in the role of a supplicant. The nature of the rules and roles of the health provider and seeker in this model are congruent with cultural expectations and stereotypes. On television, the skill and expertise of physicians (e.g., "Trapper" John and "Hawkeye" Pierce) are emphasized and reinforced. Persons who fail to engage in a patient role when ill or who engage in the patient role when not ill are pejoratively labeled as malingerers or medical management problems. The lack of individual responsibility for health and the ascendancy of experts are consistent with the general "fix it" and "technology can solve it" ethos in our culture. Now not only the Ford and Frigidaire but also our organs can be replaced.

The biomedical paradigm and the medical paradigm of helping are congruent and complimentary. The focus on people as organs or organ systems that may malfunction and require physical or chemical treatment logically produces a relationship in which the health provider works on a passive, cooperative subject. In both paradigms, the psychosocial and behavioral aspects of persons are minimized. The emphasis is rather on the workings within the skin of a person. In this sense, the paradigms are highly circumscribed and limited. The effect is similar to looking through a powerful pair of binoculars: What is seen is powerfully magnified with excellent resolution, but only a small area of the total is in view.

HISTORICAL DEVELOPMENT OF CURRENT PARADIGMS IN MEDICINE

The Biomedical Paradigm

To gain another perspective on these paradigms and to appreciate their relativity, it is useful to examine their historical context and development. The materialistic, reductionistic principles characteristic of the biomedical paradigm represent only one way to look at humans and their health. In Western history, a competing paradigm that emphasizes the spiritual nature of people is called animism. Animism views a soul or spirit as necessary for life. Health and illness are attributable to nonmaterial forces. Curative intervention involves influencing those forces.

The animistic paradigm of disease and medicine may seem nonsensical. However, it merely involves the choice of a different set of rules about the nature of persons, disease, and treatment. It is not inherently wrong, even though it may be less useful than a more materialistic approach. If the assumptions or rules of the paradigm are accepted, beliefs and actions based on them are quite logical and consistent.

Prior to 1700, animism was the dominant paradigm of persons, health, and medicine. Christianity was ascendant and emphasized the spiritual nature of individuals. The body was seen as an imperfect vessel of the soul until it was transferred from this world to the next. Disease was viewed as inherent in the imperfection of the body and a result of punishment for collective or personal wrongdoing. Treatment of disease involved either spiritual intervention by some person with special power or mitigation by prayer (Walker, 1955).

Materialism appeared in Western Europe in the twelfth and thirteenth centuries. This led to an interest in natural observation and materialistic explanations of phenomena in contrast to reliance on Christian dogma. Knowledge of anatomy and physiology was expanded using scientific methods. This new materialistic approach and the established animisitic approach were often in competition and conflict. Efforts to obtain information via empirical observation or to draw conclusions from those observations that were in opposition to established Christian teachings often resulted in censure. Dissection of a human body, for example, was considered a grave sin and forbidden by the church. To an extent, this debate between materialism and animisim is still with us; a contemporary example is the competition between evolutionary and creationist points of view.

In the first half of the seventeenth century, the conflict between materialism and animism was defused by René Descartes, who proposed that persons consist of two parts, or natures: the body and the mind (soul). He argued that the body, or material person, was subject to scientific scrutiny and understanding, whereas mind, or soul, was beyond the bounds of science. The body and mind were subject to different laws of causality. This solution was successful in that it fit with the Christian view of the body as unimportant and imperfect and protected the church's domain over persons' mind and behavior. This dualism fostered the growth of science, including anatomy and physiology, by freeing it from religious constraints. But it also resulted in the notions of the body as a machine, disease as a breakdown of the machine, and medicine as the repair of the machine (Blair, 1961). The dualistic base of medicine also led to the fractionating of persons into seemingly independent parts. People are thus seen as a collection of organs rather than as an active organism living in and acting on the environment. Dualism is quite evident in current medical language. Complaints by patients that have a biological basis are considered real, while those that have no identifiable biological basis are viewed as existing only in the person's head.

The Medical Paradigm of Helping

The history of the art of healing and of the healer-patient relationship is more difficult to document. The experience of disease has always elicited uncertainty and emotionality. The changes in physical appearance and function that mark the onset of disease frighten and puzzle the individual. These feelings are conducive to beliefs that ascribe special powers to the healer. The belief that there is an expert who has special skills and knowledge provides reassurance and hope for the patient. Throughout history, healers have been viewed as part-priest, part-technician, and part-counselor. The exact nature of the powers assigned to the healer depends upon the prevailing cultural ethos. To be effective, health providers must engage in behaviors and methods that enhance their credibility.

The attribution of special powers to healers occurs both in animistic and materialistic approaches to medicine. The Azande, a tribe in southern Sudan, provides a good example of this within an animistic paradigm. They believe severe illness is caused by the malevolent influence of another person. The sick person thus consults an oracle, whose task is to identify the party responsible for the disease. The oracle then confronts this party and deflects the pathogenic influence by performing a complex set of rituals using special materials. These rituals are closely observed by the tribe and are congruent with their expectations and beliefs. The oracle is seen as having special powers and skills, and his actions augment that view (Miller, 1978). If the specifics in this example are changed (oracle to physician, malevolent influence to biological toxin, chanting to drugs, etc.), we can see a strong parallel between the attribution of power to the oracle and to the modern-day physician. Both healers engage in actions that are congruent with societal beliefs and reinforce their expertise.

The ascription of special powers and knowledge to healers is also evident in materialistic models of disease. The ancient Greek physiologist and physician Galen, for example, was reportedly flamboyant and self-serving in his practice. He noted, in an account of treating the Roman emperor Marcus Aurelius, that the ruler described "'me as the first of physicians and the only philosopher, for he had tried many before who were not only lovers of money but also contentious, ambitious, envious and malignant.'" Hippocrates, in a different view, also emphasized the special responsibilities and characteristics of physicians: "'I will use my power to help the sick to the best of my ability and judgement. Whenever I go into a house, I will go to help the sick and never with the intention of doing harm or injury. I will be chaste and religious in my life and practice'" (quoted in Walker, 1955, p. 137).

Idealized views of physicians are also evident in more recent Western culture. This ideal was particularly apparent when individuals had a one-to-one relationship with a general practitioner. Prior to World War II, such a physician made house calls, carried most of his equipment in a black bag, and appeared indefatigable, compassionate, and committed. He stayed with the patient until the crisis had passed, earning the family's trust and gratitude. This picture appeals to one's sentiments, for it presents a warmth and concern that is reassuring. Individual attention, personal concern, continuity of care and dedication as well as high levels of technical knowledge and skills are the ideal characteristics of health providers. Currently, however, people express increasing dissatisfaction and criticism about physicians and other health providers (Ley, 1976). This dissatisfaction is the result of a number of changes both in the health care system and in our culture. Let us examine some of these changes.

The dramatic scientific and technological developments in medicine over the last forty years were not isolated phenomena but part of a broader cultural change. As health providers became more knowledgeable and skilled, their patients also became more sophisticated. Patients now experience less dependency and expect a more egalitarian relationship with their health providers. As persons become more educated and knowledgeable, they ask more questions and want to understand what is being done to them (Somers & Somers, 1977).

The amount of threat and fear experienced by the sick has decreased as a result of the success of modern medicine. As disease is experienced as less threatening, less mystique is ascribed to health providers. In fact, modern medicine is expected to find solutions for *all* health problems. In the popular press, articles commonly appear that describe new wonder drugs, surgical techniques, and diagnostic equipment that hold promise for dealing with formerly hopeless conditions. Fund-raising drives for research on disease suggest that if enough money is available, a cure can be found. We expect that anything can be done, and the failure of medicine to deliver solutions free of side effects tarnishes this idealized image.

More people have access to health care now than in the past. In fact, this access is increasingly seen as a basic human right that numerous government programs have been developed to insure. Most payment for services is made through third-party reimbursement such as health insurance, Medicaid, and Medicare. As a result, individuals feel comfortable asking for services and experience less gratitude toward providers of those services. Concurrently, the practice of medicine has become highly profitable. Health care providers have become increasingly managerial and business oriented. Because of increased demand, access, and profitability, the amount of time a healer spends with a patient has become shorter. This leaves little time for friendly conversation and the development of a personal relationship. It is not uncommon for a physician to see twenty to forty people per day at the office, or for a surgeon to make rounds on fifteen to twenty patients in a short period (Somers & Somers, 1977). This depersonalization of patients may have been amplified by the increased specialization and technological nature of recent developments in medicine.

The medical model of helping is beginning to strain as a result of the changes in society and in the health care system. Shifting roles and expectations promote more activity by the patient and less unquestioning respect and trust of the health provider. Simultaneously, the training of health providers and the characteristics of the health care system have fractionated and depersonalized patients even further.

EVALUATION OF THE BIOMEDICAL PARADIGM AND THE MEDICAL PARADIGM OF HELPING

The biomedical paradigm of disease and the medical paradigm of helping are insufficient descriptions of the current state of affairs in health care because of their inability to address adequately a number of health problems. This has led to the development of new paradigms of health and helping. Before describing these new models, let us examine the impetus for this paradigmatic change.

The Etiology of Disease

Over the last sixty years, there has been a dramatic shift in the types of diseases that are most life threatening (see Table 1-1). The percent of total mortalities caused by infectious agents has decreased, while the percent of deaths caused by chronically developing conditions like heart disease, stroke, and cancer has increased. Whereas infectious diseases appear to be tied to contact with a specific agent, chronic diseases have multiple behavioral and sociocultural as well as biological causes. These diseases are related to individuals' health habits; ability to adapt

Table 1-1 Death Rates from Ten Leading Causes of Death, 1900 and 1979

1900		1979	
Disease	Rate per 100,000 persons	Disease	Rate per 100,000 persons
1. Influenza and pneumonia	202.2	1. Heart disease	331.3
2. Tuberculosis	194.4	2. Cancer	183.5
3. Gastroenteritis	142.7	3. Cerebrovascular disease	76.9
4. Heart disease	137.4	4. Accidents	47.9
5. Cerebrovascular disease	106.9	5. Obstructive lung disease	22.7
6. Nephritis	81.0	6. Pneumonia and influenza	20.0
7. Accidents	72.3	7. Diabetes mellitus	15.0
8. Cancer	64.0	8. Liver disease, including cirrhosis	13.6
9. Diseases of infancy	62.6	9. Atherosclerosis	13.0
10. Diphtheria	40.3	10. Suicide	12.6

Note: From *Statistical Abstract of the United States* (79th ed.), 1979, Washington, DC: U.S. Government Printing Office.

to economic, social, and cultural demands (i.e., stress); and contact with biologically toxic agents.

For example, studies by Belloc and Breslow (1972) show that life expectancy and health are positively related to practicing the following health habits: (1) three meals a day at regular times with no snacks, (2) breakfast every day, (3) moderate exercise two or three times a week, (4) adequate sleep, (5) no smoking, (6) maintaining moderate body weight, and (7) no or moderate alcohol use. The health status of adults who practice all seven habits is similar to those thirty years younger who practice none.

The biomedical paradigm focuses mainly on the biological consequences of our misbehaviors and attempts, in a remedial fashion, to correct the resulting pathology. Heart attacks, for example, result from an occlusion of the coronary arteries. Treatment involves intervention to replace those arteries surgically (bypass operation) or to inhibit the occlusion mechanically (balloon catheterization) or chemically. There is recognition of the behavioral and environmental causes of heart disease (e.g., smoking and obesity), but these factors are inadequately and ineffectually addressed in the biomedical paradigm.

The medical paradigm of helping also constrains the development of effective interventions to deal with chronic disorders. The passive, irresponsible role assigned to patients makes the task of changing their behavior difficult. Persons need to accept responsibility and to participate in order to change in their own behavior.

The biomedical paradigm and the medical paradigm of helping both focus on clinical rather than preventative intervention. The greatest portion of our health care efforts, as measured in personnel, research, and insurance dollars, goes into after-the-fact medicine (Knowles, 1977). We expend our time and money fixing what goes wrong rather than preventing it from happening.

The Prevention of Disease

We could dramatically reduce the incidence of the diseases listed in Table 1-1 by focusing on a handful of behaviors: (1) tobacco use, (2) alcohol consumption, (3) dietary and caloric intake, (4) physical exercise, (5) seat belt use, and (6) handgun use. The biological consequences of these behaviors are well established. Factors that determine the acquisition and performance of these actions are not solely or primarily biological. Rather, these behaviors are strongly influenced by cultural, social, and psychological variables as well.

The biological emphasis of the biomedical paradigm precludes the effective consideration and manipulation of the social and psychological variables requisite to changing health-related behavior. Behavior change virtually requires the activity, responsibility, and participation of those persons whose behavior is targeted for change. The roles and responsibilities ascribed to patients in the medical paradigm of helping are also not congruent with these requirements.

Simply providing information about the consequences of health-destructive behavior is insufficient to effect change. Since the surgeon general's first report on the dangers of smoking in 1964, the per capita consumption by persons over eighteen years of age has decreased by less than 20%: from 4,200 to 3,400 cigarettes per year. Total sales have increased from 500 to 600 billion cigarettes per year during that same period.

Persons do not necessarily behave in a manner that promotes their biological self-interest. If we are to engender health-promoting behaviors in our children or to change health-destructive actions that have already been learned, we need paradigmatic alternatives to the biomedical model of health and the medical model of helping.

Promoting the Adherence to and Appropriate Use of Health Care

The efficacy of medical intervention is dependent on the timely use of services to promote and maintain health. Such actions include getting immunizations, receiving periodic dental and medical checkups, seeking treatment when a problem is not self-limiting, and adhering to prescribed treatment to ameliorate the problem. The mere availability of effective preventative and curative medical procedures does not insure effective medical intervention unless those procedures are sought and used in a timely fashion.

Persons' adherence to and use of health care may or may not be consistent with their health state. Illness and its seriousness are not easily defined by an individual. It has been estimated that 95% of people experience some type of physical symptom over any two-week period (Rachman & Phillips, 1980). These individuals have to evaluate the meaning and seriousness of their symptoms, but their evaluations may not be congruent with the actual biological threat they pose. For example, it has been estimated that 24 million Americans are hypertensive. But only one-half of those afflicted are aware of their condition, even though hypertension is the primary cause of around 50,000 deaths per year.

Nor are individuals' evaluations of their physical symptoms and their seriousness (which are much less objective measures of occurrence and severity) good predictors of the likelihood of seeking health care. Even though people know what *should* be done given certain symptoms, they report that they would not necessarily do so (Feldman, 1966). To continue with the hypertension example, only one-third of those who know that they are hypertensive seek and carry out adequate therapy. More broadly, it has been estimated that 70 to 90% of perceived illnesses are not treated within the health care system (Dingle, Badger & Jordan, 1964). Conversely, over one-half of the visits to physicians are related to patient-identified problems for which no discernible biological cause can be determined (Zola, 1966).

When an individual appropriately seeks treatment, that treatment is frequently implemented by the client. For example, the client self-administers drugs, changes health habits, and returns for new appointments. Averaging many studies, Sackett (1976) found that 50% of patients do not take prescribed medication in accordance with instructions, 20 to 40% do not obtain recommended immunizations, and 20 to 50% fail to keep treatment appointments.

The efficacy of treatment depends on the timely performance of such behaviors. These behaviors are complexly determined, and biological variables often have a minor influence. Many of the variables that influence adherence are not under the control of health providers. The emphasis of the medical paradigm of helping on the passivity, naïveté, and lack of responsibility of the individual does not promote periodical self evaluation of current health state, timely use of health care, or adherence to treatment recommendations.

Health and Disease

The manner in which disease is experienced and expressed by a person, and the overt manifestations of disease to outside observers are dependent on both biological and nonbiological variables. This has important implications for the diagnosis of disease and the evaluation of the effectiveness of intervention.

The clinical manifestations of disease are not solely dependent on the biochemical defect (Engel, 1977) and may vary depending on situational and behavioral factors. For example, the manifestations of diabetes depend on the person's diet, exercise, and stress. An individual may experience an uncomfortable allergic response, including rashes and labored breathing, when exposed to milk. These symptoms do not occur when dairy products are not ingested. Does the person have the disease when dairy products are not ingested? To understand and treat the problem, it is often necessary to move beyond a biochemical or physiological analysis to the relationship between the person and the environment. It is thus helpful to engage the client actively in the problem-solving process.

The effectiveness of medical treatment needs to be evaluated at behavioral and environmental levels. Restoration of a person to biological normality does not necessarily return that person to health. Someone whose broken leg has healed may be "doing well" at a biological level. But if that person fails to walk, he is not "doing well" at a behavioral level. Similarly, the degree to which a medical problem is ameliorated may depend on environmental factors. A certain level of recovery from a heart attack has a different meaning for a blue-collar worker whose job involves physical exertion than for a white-collar worker whose job is mainly sedentary. Not "doing well" at a behavioral level is often dismissed as a mental problem or given the label "compensation neurosis" in the biomedical paradigm. Situational and behavioral aspects of recovery are important, but do not fit comfortably within the biomedical framework. A most extreme example of this is the saying, "The operation was a success, but the patient died."

Medical Intervention

In the biomedical paradigm, the effectiveness of treatment is viewed as dependent on the specific action of the therapeutic agent or procedure. The effectiveness of an analgesic for pain, for example, depends upon its chemical activity. The effectiveness of radiation therapy for a cancer depends upon its physical destruction of cancer cells. While this view is not wrong in an absolute sense, it is quite limited. A broad array of factors in addition to the specific effects of therapeutic agents and procedures influence individuals' physiological and behavioral response to treatment. These factors are called the nonspecific effects of treatment.

A host of psychosocial stimuli influence a person's response to treatment. These stimuli include the physical and social setting in which the intervention takes place, the technology and instrumentation involved in the intervention, and the social milieu in which treatment occurs. Medical clients are not passive recipients. They actively process, interpret, and react to all of the stimuli involved in carrying out the intervention. They seek information about what is happening, attempt to anticipate what may occur, and make judgments about the efficacy, safety, and sensibleness of the whole process.

These nonspecific effects may powerfully influence a person's physiological and behavioral response to treatment. Information, predictability and coping skills have been found to enhance clients' postsurgical recovery and reduce their need for medication (Johnson, 1975), and the availability of coping strategies and the perception of control influence the prognosis of individuals who have cancer (Sklar & Anisman, 1981). Clients' expectations about the effectiveness of medical treatment likewise affect their biological and behavioral response to that treatment. Because such influences are not attributable to the direct physical or biochemical actions of the medical treatment, they are termed placebo effects. Placebo effects are not always short-lived, nor are they always positive (Rachman & Phillips, 1980). This nonspecific effect may enhance or diminish the biological procedure. Positive expectations may enhance the speed and degree of biological recovery. Conversely, the lack of hope may have a powerful negative impact, even to the point of hastening death (Engel, 1968; Kübler-Ross, 1969). Placebo effects thus do not fit well within the confines of the biomedical paradigm.

The roles and responsibilities of the patient and the health provider play an integral role in nonspecific effects. On one hand, the assignment of special powers, knowledge, and skills to the health provider may provide the patient with relief and hope. This assurance may function as a very powerful, positive placebo. On the other hand, the relatively passive and noninvolved role assigned to the patient in the medical paradigm may have a negative impact on both the health provider and the patient.

The medical paradigm of helping conveys not only power and authority to health providers but also immense responsibility. Health providers are in the position of having to "do all and be all." They are expected and expect themselves to succeed regardless of the patient or the problem. This results in chronic stress, which may play a part in their high incidence of drug abuse, suicide, and other disorders (Haan, 1979).

The passivity of the patient reduces the sources of information that are needed to promote feelings of predictability, knowledge, and control. The patient may be unable to develop and use adequate coping strategies to deal with the threats to life, body integrity, and comfort. As suggested above, this lack of control and inability to cope may negatively affect the person's biological recovery.

Other forms of helping relationships need to be explored. A relationship that provides more balance or symmetry between the patient and the health provider may be useful. This would not diminish the responsibility and expertise of the health provider (and the accompanying positive nonspecific effects), but would promote the patient's sense of involvement and control. This in turn may enhance biological recovery and reduce the patient's stress.

ALTERNATE PARADIGMS

The previous evaluation suggests that the biomedical paradigm of disease and the medical paradigm of helping are useful but have a limited scope that inadequately addresses several important problems. Alternative paradigms have been developed that incorporate useful aspects of the biomedical and medical paradigms but expand their scope by including psychosocial, behavioral, and biological variables.

The Systems Paradigm: An Alternative to the Biomedical Paradigm

Psychosocial, behavioral, biological, biochemical, and physical variables influence health. These factors are not independent; they are highly related. Any alternative to the biomedical paradigm needs to include all of these variables and to describe how they are related. The systems paradigm accomplishes this task.

Abstractly, a system is defined as a purposive set of elements arranged in a hierarchical manner. These elements interact such that a change in one element alters the others. Living organisms, including humans, can be conceptualized as very complex systems (Miller, 1975). They are all made of matter, which is composed of organic compounds that, when combined and differentiated, form cells, tissues, organs, and organ systems whose function is to sustain the life of the organism. Living organisms are open systems. They reside in a changing environment, and material and energy are exchanged across the organism-environment boundary. The various organs and organ systems maintain life by restoring physiological homeostasis and by adapting to the external environment.

Humans are not passive recipients of environmental stimuli. They actively interpret these stimuli and act on the environment to effect desired outcomes. Thus, the environment cannot be adequately described by the physical characteristics of the stimuli impinging on the person, but must also be understood in terms of their social and personal meaning to the individual. Our environment is strongly influenced by our behavior.

Let's consider the systems view of humans more concretely. People can be understood at many organizational levels: molecular, cellular, organ, organ system, psychological, behavioral, environmental, social, and so on. These levels are hierarchically arranged such that each lower level is nested within the next higher level. Each level is a component of higher levels and is composed of lower level components. Disturbances at one organizational level are communicated to superordinate and subordinate levels and affect their functioning (Reiser & Rosen, 1984).

We can easily think of many processes that require multilevel explanations. For example, when blood sugar levels are low, energy is taken out of body storage to return them to normal. We also feel hungry and seek food. The food we seek is not just any palatable substance but is chosen on the basis of learned preferences. Some foods that are highly nutritional, like liver, may be avoided, while less nutritionally desirable foods, like a candy bar, may be sought. Physiology influences behavior, but behavior also influences physiology. Such culturally relative stimuli as an attractive male or female, a patriotic song, and a failed test not only influence behavior but also result in physiological arousal. Changes at one level in the system thus result in changes at other levels.

The causes, recognition, impact, and treatment of disease can also be conceptualized from a systems viewpoint, as shown sequentially in Figures 1-1 to 1-3. In Figure 1-1, an individual suffers a heart attack as a result of insufficient blood supply to the heart. This results in physiological changes at the cellular, molecular, and organ system levels. As a result of the pain and other symptoms, the person becomes alarmed and tries to determine the problem. The victim seeks help from others. In Figure 1-2, the individual goes into cardiac arrest, which damages the heart and other organs. The person loses consciousness and others become alarmed. In Figure 1-3, successful medical intervention restores heart functioning, and enhances functioning, and at the cellular and organ levels. The person regains consciousness and can again relate to others. Those in the individual's social environment are relieved.

In a systems approach, a person is embedded in an environment having physical, social, and cultural dimensions. This individual must adapt to external environmental changes as well as to alterations in his internal environment. There is a constant, dynamic interplay in which the person is faced with an array of biological, psychological, and social demands that require a complex set of biological, psychological, and social responses. Clear boundaries between person and environment or between other levels cannot be defined. The person cannot be fragmented as in the biomedical paradigm but rather must be understood as a dynamic, multilevel system.

Health and disease reflect a person's ability to adapt. Adaptation takes place at many levels, from cultural to molecular. Illness is failure in adaptation; health is a successful adaptation. Persons are healthy when they can respond successfully to changes in their external and internal environment (Fabrega, 1974).

Systems theory thus emphasizes the psychological, social, and cul-

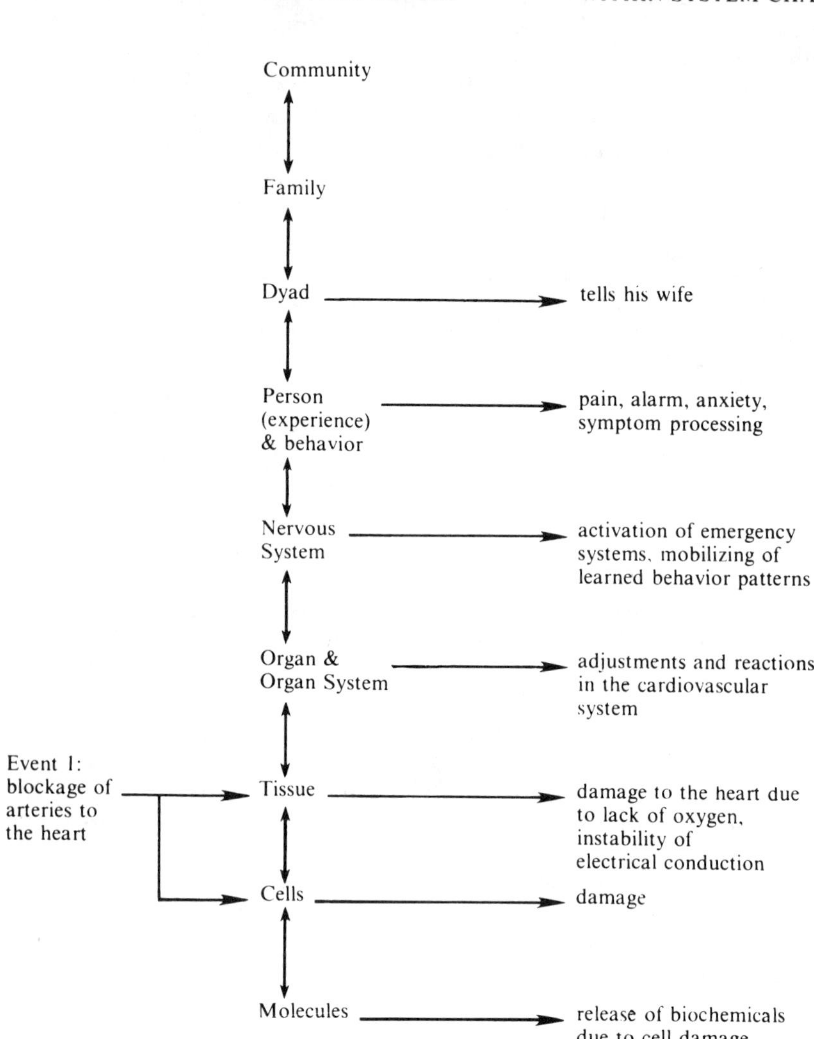

FIGURE 1-1 A Systems View of a Heart Attack—Event 1: The First Symptoms

tural as well as biological nature of persons. These various parts of the whole are closely interrelated. The focus on multiple elements and their dynamic interplay facilitates a clearer understanding of factors that influence health and provides a broader set of procedures to promote health.

In subsequent chapters, various topics related to health, illness, and medical intervention will be discussed using this systems perspec-

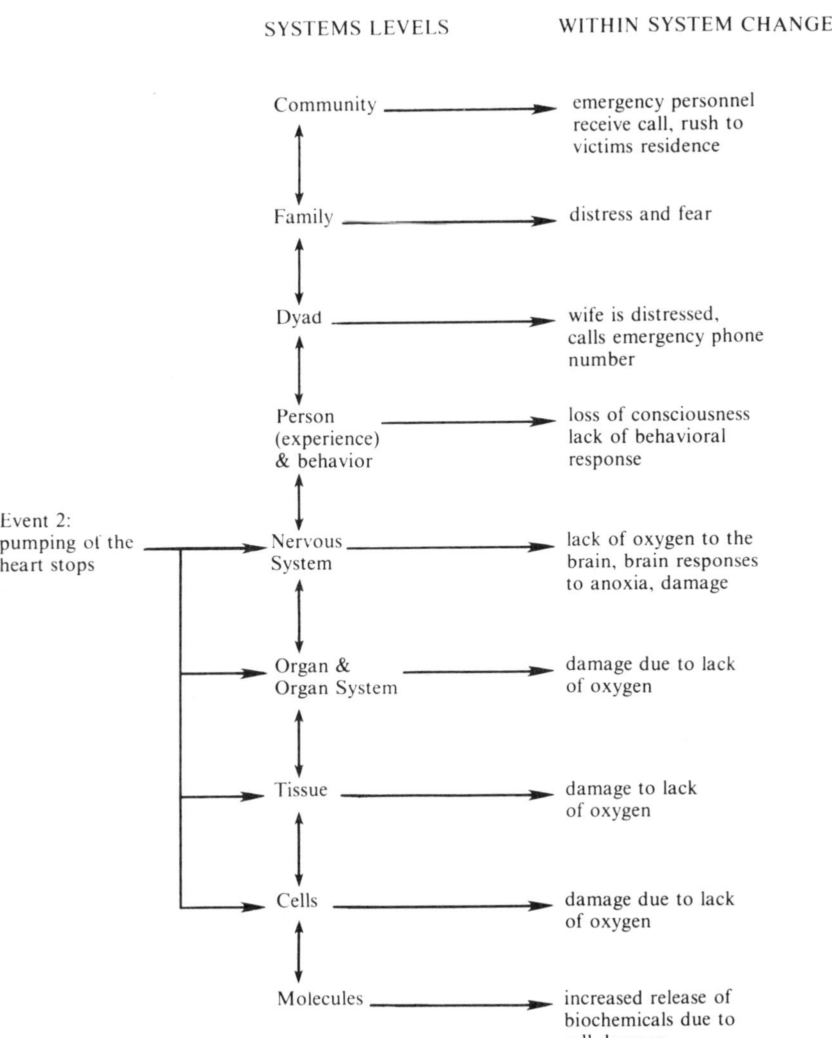

FIGURE 1-2 A Systems View of a Heart Attack—Event 2: Cardiac Arrest

tive. Particular attention will be paid to the interface between the person and the environment.

The Compensatory Paradigm of Helping: An Alternative to the Medical Paradigm of Helping

As described, the medical paradigm of helping does not hold persons responsible for the cause of their medical problem (or their health) or for the solution of the problem. Persons are assigned the role of pas-

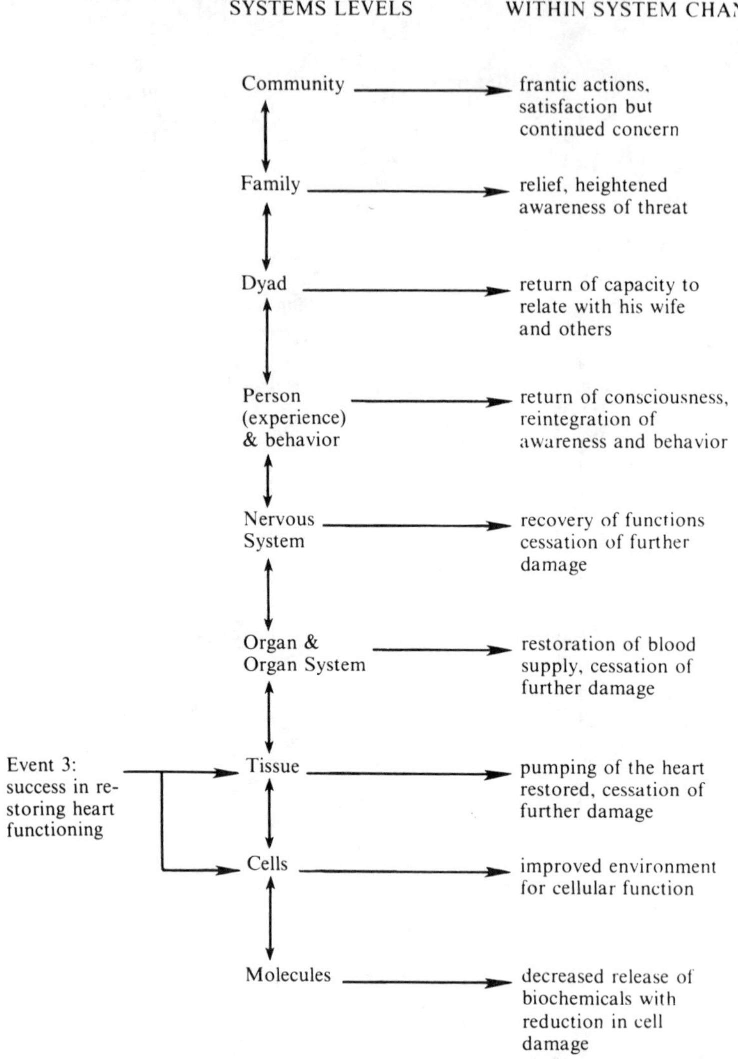

FIGURE 1-3 A Systems View of a Heart Attack—Event 3: Successful Intervention

sive, cooperative recipients of the health provider's treatment. The advantage to this approach is that people can seek medical services without being blamed for getting ill. However, the person's lack of active participation in the treatment of a problem or the maintenance of health often interferes with accomplishing either goal.

One of the dilemmas of helping is the notion that the attribution of responsibility for the cause of a problem and for its solution need to be consistent: People are responsible either for both the inception of a problem and its solution or for neither (Brickman et al., 1983). When a person is responsible for both the problem and its solution, it is hard to justify giving help. Yet if a person is not held responsible for the problem and its solution, it is difficult to enhance the individual's competence and to involve the individual in treatment. However, the attribution of responsibility for the problem and its solution do not need to be consistent. As Table 1-2 shows, Brickman et al. (1983) suggest four paradigms of helping relationships based on the attribution of responsibility.

Each model ascribes different roles to the client and has different implications. To recapitulate briefly the medical paradigm of helping, persons seeking help view themselves as ill, seek the help of an expert, are expected to accept the sick role, and are to cooperate with the helper. Clients are assigned a passive role and are seen as uninformed and subject to forces beyond their control. The relationship tends to depersonalize the client, foster dependency on the helper, and minimize the development of client competency, confidence, and control. This model is comparable to what Szaz and Hollender (1956) describe as the active-passive model of helping. In medicine, the clearest example of this relationship is typified by an emergency situation such as a coma in which the health care provider literally works on a person who cannot contribute or respond.

The moral paradigm of helping holds a person responsible for both the problem and its solution. Others are minimally involved or capable of helping. The person is seen as lazy, stupid, or lacking willpower. Helping entails reminding people that they are responsible and exhorting them to change. Within medicine, an example of the moral paradigm is the antismoking campaign. Smokers are portrayed as stupid or lacking willpower to quit. They are "helped" by reminders about the dangers of smoking and exhortations to stop before it is too late. The value of the moral paradigm is that it is unequivocable. People are responsible for their actions and for changing, but no one can really help them. However, this approach has two problems. First, exhortations and information provided by helpers are most likely to benefit those who have the resources and skills to use them; they are not sufficient unless persons have the means to engage in corrective practices. Thus, Farquhar et al. (1977) were successful in a media campaign to prevent vascular disorders because they offered people concrete suggestions on how to alter their risk-producing behavior rather than simply providing exhortations and information. The second problem with the moral model is that it takes personal responsibility to extremes: Victims are blamed for their problems.

In the enlightenment paradigm, persons are responsible for the cause of the problem but not its solution. The inception of the problem

TABLE 1-2 Consequences of Attribution of Responsibility in Four Models of Helping

ATTRIBUTION TO SELF OF RESPONSIBILITY FOR CAUSE OF THE PROBLEM	ATTRIBUTION TO SELF OF RESPONSIBILITY FOR PROBLEM SOLUTION	
	HIGH	LOW
High	Moral Model	Enlightenment Model
Perception of self	Lazy	Guilty
Actions expected of self	Striving	Submission
Actions expected of others	Exhortation	Discipline
Others besides self who must act	Peers	Authorities
Implicit view of persons	Strong	Bad
Potential problems	Loneliness	Fanaticism
Low	Compensatory Model	Medical Model
Perception of self	Deprived	Ill
Actions expected of self	Assertion	Acceptance
Actions expected of others	Mobilization	Treatment
Others besides self who must act	Consultants	Experts
Implicit view of persons	Good	Weak
Potential problems	Alienation	Dependency

Note: From "Models of helping and coping" by P. Brickman, V. C. Rabinowitz, J. Karusa, D. Coates, E. Cohn, and L. Kidder, 1982, *American Psychologist, 37*, p. 370. Copyright 1982 by the American Psychological Association, Inc. Reprinted by permission.

is directly related to the person's behavior or characteristics and could be avoided if the person were different. Because the person is weak, naïve, or uninformed, others need to intervene. The person must submit to experts, who use their moral, physical, or legal power to solve the problem. The person thus needs to be monitored and "disciplined." This thinking is typified by proposed regulations for air bags in cars. People can prevent severe injuries resulting from car accidents by using seat belts. Because they do not, car manufacturers may be legally required to provide another protective device. The deficiency of this paradigm lies in the reconstruction of the person's life around the method used to deal with the problem. There is potential for infringement of personal rights because great power is given to those in authority.

The last of the four paradigms is the compensatory paradigm of helping, which places responsibility for the solution but not the problem on the person. The problem is seen as the result of unfortunate circumstances over which the person—because of past learning, a lack of resources or knowledge, or social-environmental conditions—had minimal influence. The helper provides the information, resources, and interventions needed to remediate the problem. However, the client is expected to be actively involved in and has responsibility for using these resources as fully as possible. The idea is to do something not to the person but with the person such that the person's competence increases. The relationship between the helper and the client is a colleagial one, or comparable to what Szaz and Hollender (1956) call a mutual participatory relationship. In medicine, a good example of the compensatory model is prepared childbirth. The expectant parents are educated and given skills in order to participate actively in the birth of their child rather than having the physician deliver the child while the mother is anesthetized and the father is absent. Even in medical procedures like surgery, it is possible and therapeutically useful to involve the patient to the extent possible. This may be done by providing the person with information about what will happen, skills to cope with fear and post-operative discomfort, and instructions on how to facilitate recovery (Melamed & Seigel, 1980).

The compensatory paradigm is advantageous because it fosters the competencies of the clients to promote health. It provides them with a sense of control, utilizes their personal coping strategies, and fosters self-responsibility and independence. It recognizes the value of persons' activity on their own part. People are seen as clients, not patients, who are taken into an active, responsible partnership with the health provider to maintain, promote, or restore their health. It does not mean that the health provider is not responsible but rather responsible in a different way (Haan, 1979).

Each of the four paradigms has strengths and weaknesses. While the compensatory paradigm is not universally the most effective, it represents a method of helping that acknowledges the expertise and skills of the health care provider while involving the client. Studies suggest that attribution of responsibility for change to the client results in more persistent treatment effects, fewer deleterious effects when stressed, and less resistance to the assistance provided by the helper (Brickman et al., 1983). In fact, a compensatory paradigm may enhance the cooperation and manageability of the client (Wills, 1978). People have a tendency to resist one-sided influence. Although such resistance is often attributed to the personality of the client, it is also strongly influenced by situational and relational factors. By accepting a client as a partner in treatment, cooperation may be enhanced rather than diminished.

The previous evaluation of the biomedical paradigm suggested that people's behavior is intimately involved in health and health care. It was suggested that the promotion or restoration of health often necessitates changing people's behavior. The compensatory paradigm fosters client cooperation, motivation, and participation which are integral to such behavior change.

The utility of any paradigm of helping depends upon the specific client, helper, situation and problem. As noted by Szaz and Hollender (1956), the roles and responsibilities of the health provider and the client differ according to these characteristics. By definition, persons brought into an emergency room in a coma require immediate attention without participation on their part. However, in the majority of medical transactions, the client is conscious, aware, and capable of participating in the health intervention. In these cases, the compensatory paradigm may be more effective than the medical paradigm.

Another problem in using one paradigm of helping to the exclusion of others is that help is most effective when the client and helper use the same paradigm. The roles they assume must be congruent or complementary. When this does not occur, the efficacy of the helping is reduced. This can be seen in the dissatisfaction and noncooperation of a client who wants to be informed and involved (compensatory paradigm) but is interacting with a health provider who wants the patient to be passive and gives little information (medical paradigm). However, it is equally problematic to have a patient who does not want to be involved (figuratively unconscious) or informed (medical paradigm) interacting with a health provider who is trying to involve the client (compensatory paradigm). This does not mean that the health providers should alter their behavior to fit the client. The health provider needs to be aware of the client's paradigm and to alter that paradigm if such action would ultimately enhance the competency of the individual or the efficacy of treatment. There are data to suggest that, even though a client may not wish to actively participate in an intervention, actions by the health provider to involve that person may increase the efficacy of the intervention (Karusa, Zevan, Rabinowitz, & Brickman, 1983). The alteration of the client's expectations and role involves a presentation of alternate views and an indication of how those views may improve the effectiveness of intervention (Goldfried & Davidson, 1976).

In sum, the compensatory paradigm of helping provides solutions for health-related problems that are ineffectively addressed by the medical paradigm of helping. This is especially true for those problems that involve the person's environment and behavior. It may also serve to further personalize and humanize health care interventions.

In subsequent chapters, the usefulness of the compensatory paradigm of helping will be explored in relation to a number of health problems and interventions. While this model is not universally applicable, the goal of the book will be to promote a movement from a medical to a compensatory paradigm in which the client is viewed as an active, coping, information-seeking participant rather than a passive recipient of intervention.

SUMMARY

Paradigms are a set of assumptions about how to understand and solve a problem. Medicine entails the use of paradigms to understand health and disease and to promote health. In recent Western history, the prevailing paradigm of health and disease is called the biomedical paradigm. It emphasizes the biological characteristics of humans and attempts to understand individuals by viewing them as a complex collection of cells, tissues, and organs. The prevailing historical paradigm of helping is called the medical paradigm. In this model, clients are not held responsible for their health problems and solutions. They are instead expected to cooperate passively and comply with the health provider, who has the knowledge and expertise to solve the problem.

The tenets of the biomedical paradigm of disease and of the medical paradigm of helping are not truths but rather assumptions that developed in response to discernible historical events. These paradigms have proved to be very effective tools in dealing with acute diseases. In part, however, their success has also exposed their limitations, for they do not adequately recognize the importance of psychosocial variables in disease, health, prevention, and treatment.

As a consequence of these limitations, a paradigm shift is occurring in medicine. New models that incorporate the strengths of the older paradigms yet expand their scope and power are being developed. The systems paradigm views humans as complex organisms that can be analyzed at levels from molecular to environmental. Interaction can occur between all of these levels. In a sense, the systems paradigm attempts to glue the body-mind parts of dualism together again. As thinking, emotions, and behavior are again incorporated with biology, the importance of the active participation of the client in health care is apparent. The compensatory paradigm of helping considers the client and health providers as colleagues who actively work together to promote health.

This chapter provides the theoretical structure for the rest of the book. The problems and solutions discussed in the following chapters implicitly or explicitly examine how systems and compensatory paradigms enable us to provide humane, efficient, and effective health care.

REFERENCES

Belloc, N. B., & Breslow, L. (1972). Relationship of physical health status and health practices. *Preventative Medicine, 1,* 414–421.

Blair, L. (1961). *Essential works of Descartes*. New York: Bantam Books.
Brickman, P., Rabinowitz, V. C., Karusa, J., Coates, D., Cohn, E., & Kidder, L. (1982). Models of helping and coping. *American Psychologist, 37*, 368–384.
Dingle, J., Badger, G., & Jordan, W. (1964). *Illness in the home*. Cleveland: Case Western University.
Engel, G. (1968). A life setting conductive to illness: The giving up—given up complex. *Bulletin of the Menninger Clinic, 32*, 355–365.
Engel, G. (1977). The need for a new medical model: A challenge for biomedicine. *Science, 196*, 129–136.
Fabrega, H. (1974). *Disease and social behavior: An interdisciplinary perspective*. Boston: MIT Press.
Farquhar, J., Maccoby, N., Wood, P., Alexander, J., Breitrose, H., Brown, B., Haskle, W., McAlister, A., Meyer, L., Nash, J., & Stern, M. (1977). Community education for cardiovascular health. *Lancet, 1*, 1192–1195.
Feldman, J. (1966). *The dissemination of health information*. Chicago: Aldine.
Goldfried, M., & Davidson, G. (1976). *Clinical behavior therapy*. New York: Holt, Rinehart and Winston.
Haan, N. (1979). Psychosocial meanings of unfavorable medical forecasts. In G. Stone, F. Cohen, & N. Adler (Eds.), *Health Psychology*, 113–140. San Francisco: Jossey-Bass.
Johnson, J. (1975). Stress reduction through sensation information. In I. G. Sarason & C. D. Speilberger (Eds.), *Stress and anxiety* (Vol. 2. 278–291). New York: Wiley.
Karusa, J., Zevan, M., Rabinowitz, V., & Brickman, P. (1983). Attribution of responsibility by helpers and recipients. In T. A. Wills (Ed.), *Basic processes in helping relationships*, 107–130. New York: Academic Press.
Knowles, J. (1977). The responsibility of the individual, In J. Knowles (Ed.), *Doing better and feeling worse*, 57–80. New York: W. W. Norton.
Kübler-Ross, E. (1969). *Death and dying*. New York: Macmillan.
Kuhn, T. (1970). *The structure of scientific revolutions* (2nd ed.). Chicago: University of Chicago Press.
Ley, P. (1976). Toward better doctor-patient communication. In A. Bennett (Ed.), *Communications between doctors and patients*, 133–149. New York: Oxford University Press.
Melamed, B., & Seigel, L. (1980). *Behavioral medicine: Practical application in health care*. New York: Springer.
Miller, J. (1978). *The body in question*. New York: Random House.
Miller, J. G. (1975). The nature of living systems: An overview. In T. Murray (Ed.), *Interdisciplinary aspects of general systems theory. Proceedings of the Third Annual Meeting of the Middle Atlantic Regional Division, Society for General Systems Research*. College Park, MD: University of Maryland Press.
Rachman, S., & Phillips, C. (1980). *Psychology and behavioral medicine*. Cambridge: Cambridge University Press.
Reiser, D. E., & Rosen, D. H. (1984). *Medicine as a human experience*. Baltimore: University Park Press.
Sackett, D. (1976). The magnitude of compliance and noncompliance. In D. Sackett & R. Haynes (Eds.), *Compliance with therapeutic regimens*, 7–33. Baltimore: Johns Hopkins Press
Sklar, L., & Anisman, H. (1981). Stress and cancer. *Psychological Bulletin, 89*, 369–406.
Somers, H., & Somers, M. (1977). *Health and health care: Policies in perspective*. Germantown, MD: Aspen Systems.
Szaz, T., & Hollender, M. (1956). A contribution to the philosophy of medicine: The basic models of the doctor-patient relationship. *Archives of Internal Medicine, 97*, 585–592.
Walker, K. (1955). *The story of medicine*. New York: Oxford University Press.
Wills, T. (1978). Perception of clients by professional helpers. *Psychological Bulletin, 85*, 968–1000.
Zola, I. (1966). Culture and symptoms: An analysis of patients presenting complaints. *American Sociological Review, 31*, 615–630.

2

Health, Illness, and Behavior

INTRODUCTION

In the first chapter, it was suggested that health and illness are strongly influenced by psychosocial and behavioral as well as biological variables. Effective health actions by individuals and effective preventative and clinical interventions by health providers require recognition of all of these factors.

The link between psychosocial and behavioral variables and health takes three forms: (1) indirect psychophysiological effects of the environment and behavior on health; (2) direct effects of health-promoting and health-impairing behaviors on health; and (3) direct effects of health decisions and actions when ill (Krantz, Glass, Contrada, & Miller, 1981).

Indirect psychophysiological effects are changes in body structure and function mediated by neural, endocrine, and immune responses to psychosocial stimuli. These changes occur without the direct introduction of some agent into the body. Rather, physiology is indirectly influenced by our evaluation and behavioral response to stimuli impinging on our sense receptors. The usual term used to describe these indirect effects is stress. This link will be considered further in Chapter 4.

The first direct link between behavior and health consists of health-promoting and health-impairing behaviors. As a result of our behavior, we introduce into our bodies substances that may be detrimental (e.g., cigarette smoke, alcohol, and dietary fats) or conducive (e.g., vitamins, and serums to prevent disease) to our health. Our behavior may also be health promoting because it involves proper use of our body (e.g., exercise and sufficient sleep) or health impairing because it enhances the likelihood of injury or disease (e.g., not using seat belts and being sexually active with multiple partners). In short, our behavior directly influences our health state.

The second direct link between behavior and health consists of those decisions and actions we take when ill, including transactions with health providers. The speed and degree to which we recover from illness depend on our awareness and sensitivity to symptoms, the manner in which we interpret symptoms, and the actions we take to remediate symptoms. If we seek treatment, recovery is influenced by how we communicate and cooperate with health providers.

DIRECT LINKS BETWEEN BEHAVIOR AND HEALTH: BIOMEDICAL AND SYSTEMS PARADIGMS

The Biomedical Paradigm

Professionals who use the biomedical paradigm acknowledge the influence of behavior on health. From this perspective, persons' behavior is influenced primarily by biological variables. Persons should therefore engage in behaviors that have positive biological consequences and avoid those that have negative biological consequences. In other words, people should behave rationally.

When experiencing a symptom, for example, persons are expected to attend to the symptom, accurately evaluate its significance, and take appropriate action. As indicated in Chapter 1, persons with serious illnesses often do not seek treatment in a timely fashion, and those with minor, often self-limiting symptoms frequently seek treatment. When persons seek treatment, they are expected to cooperate with health providers and to comply with medical recommendations. Because providers are skilled and knowledgeable, these behaviors will lead to a positive biological outcome. However, clients do not reliably follow treatment recommendations.

Following a similar logic, persons should not engage in health-impairing behaviors like smoking and drinking alcohol because of their negative biological consequences. Conversely, they should engage in health-promoting behaviors like exercising and wearing seat belts. Again as indicated in Chapter 1, however, persons do engage in health-impairing behaviors and fail to engage in health-promoting behaviors, even when they know the consequences.

Before considering the direct behavior-health links in detail, let us consider which paradigms maximize our understanding and provide the most powerful means of altering behavior.

The Systems Paradigm

Behaviors related to health cannot be completely understood or effectively altered by focusing solely on biological variables. Health-related behaviors are a function of stimuli that either evoke and reinforce or punish the behavior. These cues and consequences occur at biological, cognitive, affective, social, and environmental levels of organization (Rodin, 1982). An overview of these multilevel cues and consequences is shown in Figure 2-1.

Let us consider this model in more detail. Cues and consequences can be internal or external to the person. Internal physiological stimuli like pain or hunger serve as strong cues for behavior, and actions that reduce these states are strongly reinforced. Cognitive and affective stimuli also function as internal cues and consequences for health behavior. We plan and evaluate our actions (e.g., going on a diet), and work to regulate our emotions (e.g., drinking when feeling tense).

Two broad categories of external stimuli influence health behavior: (1) immediate social and physical events, and (2) sociocultural norms and sanctions. The buzzer in your car is an immediate physical cue to buckle your seat belt, and doing so is reinforced by terminating the noise. Observation that others are exercising serves as a social cue to engage in exercise, which then may be reinforced by social approval.

FIGURE 2-1 Antecedent Cues and Consequences Controlling Health-Related Behavior

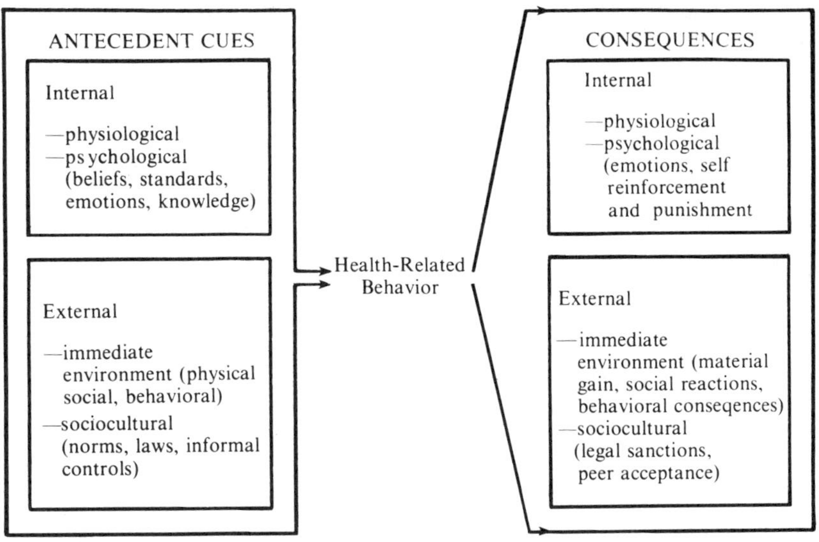

Sociocultural norms include explicit laws and sanctions and informal social controls. Laws and sanctions, like those concerning the legal age for drinking and mandatory immunization of schoolchildren, are imposed and enforced by recognized sociopolitical agents like police and legislatures. Failure to comply results in legal or administrative punishment. Informal social controls refer to rules and guides for behavior created by the ethnic, religious or other groups with which persons identify. Examples include religious proscription of alcohol and culturally based dietary preferences. There may be no formal codes or enforcement; but certain behaviors are unacceptable and lead to rejection by the group, whereas others are expected and lead to group acceptance and approval.

The performance of health-related behaviors (like quitting smoking, getting immunized, brushing teeth, and seeing a doctor) are determined by temporally proximate and salient stimuli from biological, psychosocial, environmental, and cultural sources. Which stimuli influence a specific health behavior as well as their strength and functional properties vary according to the developmental history of the individual. Health-related behaviors, whether adaptive or destructive, are acquired and shaped by past experience and observation (Bibace & Wallace, 1979; Jordan & O'Grady, 1982).

Those stimuli that are important determinants of a specific health-related behavior vary from one person to the next. Factors critical to alcohol use in one person are not necessarily critical to alcohol use in another. Variables that cue and maintain a health-related behavior during one period of a person's development may be less influential during a later period. For example, peer pressure may importantly contribute to smoking during adolescence, but exert little influence after the same person has smoked for ten years.

The determinants of adaptive and maladaptive health behaviors can be identified. Maladaptive behaviors that appear to be "irrational" from the narrow focus of the biomedical paradigm can be understood using the systems perspective. If we can identify the determinants of health-related behaviors, we can develop effective strategies to alter those behaviors to promote health. As discussed in the next section, the promotion of adaptive health behaviors frequently requires the active involvement of the client.

DIRECT HEALTH-BEHAVIOR LINK: HELPING PERSPECTIVES

The Medical Paradigm of Helping

In preventative and clinical interventions, health care providers who ascribe to the medical paradigm of helping rely on expert, informational, and legitimate sources of social influence to effect change in clients' health-related behaviors (Rodin & Janis, 1982). These sources of power are inherent in the roles assigned to health providers and clients in this paradigm of helping. Clients should adhere to the recommendations of health providers because those providers have the knowledge (informational power), the skills and status (expert power), and the responsibility (legitimate power) for solving problems.

There are two problems with using the medical paradigm of helping to alter clients' health-related behaviors. First, many clients do not ascribe to this paradigm. They want to have information and to play an active part in their own health care. Consequently, these clients "turn off" or rebel against the health provider. They do not automatically accept the premise that the health care provider is in charge, or behave as recommended because "the doctor says so." Second, the behaviors targeted for change must compete with habitual behaviors for which there are salient, routine-generated cues and immediate, powerful payoffs. The health provider's instructions provide temporally distant and functionally weak cues and consequences for behavior change in the natural environment. Barring powerful biological stimuli that evoke (e.g., pain) or reinforce (e.g., relief) the behavior, change is not likely to occur or to be sustained (Stone, 1979).

The Enlightenment and Moral Paradigms of Helping

The enlightenment paradigm can be used to influence clients' health-related behaviors. The fluoridation of public water supplies, mandatory seat belt laws, the minimum drinking age, and laws prohibiting the use of marijuana and cocaine are examples of this approach. Even more than the medical paradigm of helping, the enlightenment paradigm emphasizes the expert and legitimate power of the health provider and the irresponsibility and incompetence of the public. The basic premise of this model is; "If you aren't responsible enough to behave appropriately, we'll make you do it." This coercive approach is often ineffective.

Coercive control by those in power leads to countercontrol by clients. Frequently, persons do the exact opposite of what is desired. In the 1920s and 1930s, for example, Prohibition led to an increase rather than a decrease in the use of alcohol (Bringham, 1982). Persons may only engage in the prescribed behavior when being monitored by the authorities; people often obey the speed limit only when they see a police car. Persons find a substitute for proscribed behaviors. Historically, as recreational drugs were made illegal, persons simply switched to others that had not yet been proclaimed illicit (Goode, 1972). Even if coercive means are effective, once the controls are loosened, persons return to their old ways of behaving. Alcoholics who are forcibly "dried out" frequently resume drinking when released from the treatment program (Marlatt & Parkes, 1982). Human beings intrinsically desire control

(Bandura, 1977; White, 1959) and will try to maintain that control even in the face of aversive outcomes (Davidson, 1973). The loss of control is associated with negative psychological and physiological symptoms (Langer & Rodin, 1976).

The moral paradigm of helping suggests that clients are responsible for their own health behavior and that there is little health providers can do to effect change. Behavior is seen as a function of willpower, which is a personal trait only minimally subject to external influence. All the health provider can do is to remind clients of the need for change and hope that they develop the willpower to do so. Reminders and exhortations to change without providing the specific, concrete means to effect that change are not effective. Although there are helping strategies that are effective in overcoming client resistance to change (Haley, 1963, 1973; Janis, 1984), they require the development of a warm, trusting relationship between the health provider and the client.

The Compensatory Paradigm of Helping

The compensatory paradigm of helping holds promise as a means to effectively alter health-related behaviors, for it acknowledges an equity, a shared responsibility, and an active, collaborative role for clients and health providers. In this approach, health providers use referent as well as expert, informational, and legitimate sources of influence to foster adaptive health behaviors. Referent power (often called "a good bedside manner") is developed by establishing a caring, understanding and friendly relationship with clients. Clients in turn feel understood and appreciated as persons. Once this positive relationship is established, the social and emotional bonds can be used to motivate change and to overcome resistance. The development and use of referent power in helping relationships has been found to enhance the likelihood of positive change in clients' health-related behaviors (Rodin & Janis, 1982).

Because clients are seen as collaborators in the compensatory paradigm, this approach fosters a recognition of the importance of self-generated and environmental cues and consequences in encouraging health-related behaviors. The addition of these multilevel stimuli as focal points to effect change provides the potential for achieving greater, more consistent, and longer lasting changes in clients' health-related behavior than the other paradigms of helping (Kristeller & Rodin, 1984; Mahoney & Arnkoff, 1978).

The systems and compensatory paradigms provide effective means for understanding and altering health-impairing and health-promoting behaviors, and illness-generated health decisions and actions. In this chapter, a detailed analysis will be made of various health-impairing and health-promoting behaviors. Illness-related decisions and actions will be discussed in Chapter 3.

HEALTH-IMPAIRING AND HEALTH-PROMOTING BEHAVIORS

How much impact does routine behavior have on health? Let us begin to answer this question by examining the contribution of health habits to the causes of death in the United States. Table 2-1 presents a rank-order list of the most frequent causes of death for various age groups and the percentage of total deaths accounted for by each cause. As indicated in the table, the major cause of death from ages twenty to twenty-four is motor vehicle accidents; these accidents account for 31% of all deaths for this age group. The next most common cause of death for this group is other types of accidents, which account for 16.5% of all deaths.

TABLE 2-1 Leading Causes of Death in the United States by Age Group

CAUSE	TOTAL DEATHS (%)	CAUSE	TOTAL DEATHS (%)
Ages 20–24		*Ages 40–44*	
Motor vehicle accidents	31.0	Heart disease	23.2
Other accidents	16.5	Cancer	22.0
Homicide	12.6	Cirrhosis	7.1
Suicide	12.5	Other accidents	6.3
Cancer	5.6	Motor vehicle accidents	5.8
Heart disease	2.5	Suicide	5.3
Flu and pneumonia	1.3	Cerebrovascular disease	4.8
Cerebrovascular disease	1.1	Homicide	4.3
Congenital abnormality	1.0	Flu and pneumonia	2.0
All other causes	15.9	Diabetes	1.5
		All other causes	17.7
Ages 30–34		*Ages 50–54*	
Motor vehicle accidents	12.9	Heart disease	32.7
Suicide	11.1	Cancer	15.8
Heart disease	9.2	Cirrhosis	5.0
Cirrhosis	7.4	Cerebrovascular disease	4.5
Cancer	7.1	Bronchitis and emphysema	2.6
Homicide	6.3	Suicide	2.4
Other accidents	5.3	Motor vehicle accidents	1.8
Diabetes	1.6	Rheumatic heart disease	1.2
Cerebrovascular disease	1.3	Pneumonia	1.2
All other causes	37.8	All other causes	31.5

Note: Adapted from *Leading causes of death and probabilities of dying, United States: 1975 and 1976*, Centers for Disease Control, Public Health Service, 1979.

The rest of the table can be understood in a similar fashion. It is useful to study this data to get some notion of the changes in causes of death that occur with age.

The major causes of death listed in Table 2-1 are strongly associated with persons' daily health habits and lifestyle. Our behavior plays a major role in the likelihood of developing coronary heart disease, getting cancer, or being killed in a car accident (Robbins & Blankenship, 1982). In fact, our health habits and lifestyle have been estimated to play a stronger causative role in the major causes of death than either environmental or biological variables (CDC, 1979). The relative contributions of health habits and lifestyle, environment, and biology to major causes of death are shown in Table 2-2.

A nonexhaustive list of the risk factors for the major causes of death is given in Table 2-3. As the table indicates, health habits play an important role in nearly every leading cause of death. These include personal habits (e.g., smoking, drinking alcohol, and using seat belts), self-care behaviors (e.g., breast self-exams), and use of preventative health services (e.g., pap smears, rectal exams, and blood pressure checks). While we cannot totally avoid disease and death, we can promote our health and increase our longevity by behaving in a reasonable manner.

Space prohibits us from looking at the determinants of all of the health-promoting and health-impairing habits listed in Table 2-3. However, the biological, psychological, social, and cultural determinants (or a systems analysis) of several important health habits will now be discussed.

TABLE 2-2 Estimated Percentage of the Contribution of the Leading Causes of Death

CAUSE OF DEATH	HEALTH HABITS AND LIFESTYLE	ENVIRONMENT	HUMAN BIOLOGY
Heart disease	54	9	28
Cancer	37	24	29
Cerebrovascular disease	50	22	21
Motor vehicle accidents	69	18	0.6
Other accidents	51	31	4
Flu and pneumonia	23	20	39
Diabetes	26	0	68
Suicide	60	35	2
Average	48.9	18.7	23.3

Note: Adopted from *Leading causes of death and probabilities of dying, United States: 1975 and 1976*, Centers for Disease Control, Public Health Service, 1979.

TABLE 2-3 Influence of Health Habits on Risk Factors for Leading Causes of Death

Heart Attack
High blood pressure[+]
High cholesterol diet*
Diabetes[+]
Lack of exercise*
Family history
Smoking*
Overweight*
Type A behavior*

Lung Cancer
Smoking*

Breast Cancer
Family history
Breast self-exams*

Cervical Cancer
Family history
Obtaining pap smears
Age at first intercourse*
Number of sexual partners*

Colon / Rectal Cancer
Dietary habits*
Polyps
Obtaining rectal exams
Ulcerative colitis[+]

Cirrhosis of the Liver
Alcohol use*

Stroke
High blood pressure[+]
High cholesterol diet*
Diabetes[+]
Smoking*

High Blood Pressure
Lack of exercise*
Dietary habits*
Overweight*
Smoking*

Diabetes Mellitus
Family history
Overweight*
Dietary habits*

Suicide
Depression*
Family history

Homicide
Arrest record*
Use of weapons*

Pneumonia
Smoking*
Emphysema[+]
Alcohol use*
Bacterial contact

Motor Vehicle Accidents
Alcohol use*
Drug and medication use*
Miles driven per year*
Use of seat belts*

[+] Diseases that in turn are influenced by behavioral risk factors
* Behaviors that increase risk for the disease

EATING AND OBESITY

Obesity is a major health problem in the United States. Depending on the definition of obesity, it has been estimated that between 15 and 50% of American adults are overweight. Obesity is associated with high blood pressure, diabetes, heart disease, kidney problems, and stroke.

Why are people obese? Simply put, it is the result of consuming more calories than are expended by exercise or metabolism (Mayer, 1968; Stuart, 1971). The balance between consumption and expenditure of calories is a delicate one. The average, nonobese adult male consumes about 1 million calories of food per year. If he increases his caloric intake by 10% without simultaneously increasing exercise by a comparable amount, he will gain 30 pounds in that year (Stunkard & Mahoney, 1976). Two behaviors are thus critically involved in weight control: eating and exercise. We are overweight because we eat too much, exercise too little, or both.

There is no one simple cause for overeating. Cues and consequences at all organizational levels influence eating behavior. An overview of these multilevel factors are shown in Table 2-4. We will consider each level in detail, but as we do, note how the variables at each level interact.

Physiological Cues and Consequences

Body weight is relatively stable. When persons are put on forced diets that increase or decrease caloric intake and are then allowed to self-select their intake, they eat amounts that return them to their prediet weight. This has been demonstrated experimentally (Stunkard & Mahoney, 1976) and has been observed in the dieting actions of people in the natural environment (Polivy & Herman, 1985). Many of us have had this experience. We may lose weight when we diet, but we seem to

TABLE 2-4 Antecedent Cues and Consequences for Overeating and Obesity

VARIABLE	ANTECEDENT CUES	CONSEQUENCES
Physiological	Weight set point Number of fat cells	High food palatability Inefficient metabolism
Psychological	Poor discrimination of internal cues Hypersensitivity to external cues Excuses and rationalizations	Reduced tension and anxiety Self-punishment of attempts at dieting Any dietary failure is absolute
Environmental and sociocultural	Situations that evoke eating Availability and salience of food Invitations to eat Seeing others eat	Group approval and acceptance Praise and attention for "plate cleaning"
Behavioral	Cultural eating and dietary patterns Exercise Eating style	

quickly return to our prediet weight once we cease dieting. The body seems to have a "set point" for weight that functions much like a thermostat. Once weight differs from that set point, we adjust our food intake (and perhaps our metabolism) to return to the set point. The body seems to defend its weight when it is lowered by dieting or raised by eating more than usual (Keesey, 1980).

The number of fat cells in our bodies have an important influence on weight. Obese persons may have five times as many fat cells as those of normal weight (Hirsch & Knittle, 1971). The number of fat cells is influenced by genetics. Eighty percent of the children born to two obese parents are also obese, compared to 40% of the children born to one obese and one normal-weight parent and to 10% of the children born to two nonobese parents (Mayer, 1957). However, it is likely that this parent-child similarity is also influenced by learned dietary and eating habits (LeBow, 1984). The number of fat cells is influenced by nutritional patterns during childhood and adolescence when fat cell proliferation occurs (LeBow, 1984). Generally, the greater the number of fat cells, the more easily food is stored in the body. The bodies of obese persons are expert at storing fat. Obesity that begins during childhood or adolescence is very persistent and difficult to change (Abraham, Collins, & Nordsieck, 1971).

Overweight persons may also be particularly sensitive to the taste of food. They report greater food palatability than normal-weight persons, and thus good-tasting food may serve as a more powerful reinforcer. While food tastes particularly good to all of us when we are hungry (the first piece of pizza is better than the last), obese persons report a slower decline in palatability as they get full. Food is highly reinforcing even when they have just finished a big meal (Hagen, 1976). Palatability of food is also greater when persons are under their weight set point (Woody & Costanzo, 1981). In this way, the body defends its set point and seeks to restore the equilibrium upset by a negative energy imbalance.

Overweight persons may also have an inefficient metabolism. Basal metabolism (the number of calories burned while at rest) is similar in obese and nonobese persons. Caloric restriction results in a reduced basal metabolism; the body reacts to a diet by becoming more efficient so that some weight loss inhibits further weight loss. Repeated dieting may actually foster an increasingly efficient metabolism. Persons who repeatedly diet may "teach" their bodies to burn up fewer calories (Brownell, 1980). Overweight persons may have less efficient thermal metabolism than normal-weight persons. Thermal metabolism is the increase in metabolic rate after eating. It is like a furnace burning excess fuel. The thermal metabolism of obese persons is about 3 to 9% greater than their basal metabolism, whereas the thermal metabolism of slim persons is 20 to 25% greater (Hodgson & Miller, 1982).

Cognitive and Affective Cues and Consequences

Obese persons are reported to be less sensitive to internal, physiological cues of hunger (Stunkard & Koch, 1964). Their feelings of hunger are not strongly correlated with gastric contractions, for example. Obese persons may confuse nonhunger-related physiological cues with hunger. They may eat in response to anxiety, fatigue, tension, or any strong physiological arousal (Hodgson & Miller, 1982). Obese persons may also be particularly sensitive to external cues to eat (Schacter, 1968), eating in response to time of day, availability of food, and physical setting rather than physiological hunger. When overweight persons are exposed to appetizing foods either after eating or fasting, they experience a strong physiological as well as psychological reaction. At the sight of the appealing food, insulin is released from the pancreas, resulting in lowered blood sugar levels and physiological cues of hunger (Rodin, 1977). Years of overeating in response to multiple external cues results in either reduced sensitivity to physiological cues of hunger or a conditioned elicitation of physiological hunger cues to environmental stimuli.

There are also many cognitive cues and consequences that influence eating. Overweight persons frequently use excuses for eating (Janis, 1984; LeBow, 1984). "No use starting a diet until after the holidays," or "One more cookie won't make a difference" are common examples. Obese persons' thinking about their eating tends to be dichotomous: Changing eating habits is an all or nothing proposition. If they attempt to eat more reasonably, any violation of their dietary plan is seen as a total failure and serves as a cue to revert to their old eating pattern: "Now that I've had one cookie, my diet is broken and I might just as well have some more" (Marlatt & Parkes, 1982). The consequences applied to altering eating patterns focus on failures rather than successes: "It's no use, I'll always be fat," or "Because I ate that piece of cake, I don't have any willpower and may as well stop trying." These types of cognitive cues and consequences provide little incentive for change (LeBow, 1984). In fact, an eating binge frequently follows unsuccessful dieting attempts (Polivy & Herman, 1985). Eating may also reduce anxiety or tension, which consequently reinforces the eating (McKenna, 1972).

Setting Cues and Consequences

As indicated earlier, overweight persons may be particularly influenced by external cues to eat. Because they have eaten in so many settings (e.g., kitchen, bedroom, living room, car, and desk at the office), at so many different times of the day, and in conjunction with so many activities (e.g., watching TV, driving, talking to friends, and working), they are constantly bombarded with cues to eat.

Social Cues and Consequences

There are many social cues to (over)eat. As children, many of us were urged to eat everything on our plate and not to waste food. Well-meaning friends, relatives, and family members urge us to have another helping or to eat a specially prepared dessert. The amount and type of food eaten and when and where to eat are also affected by sociocultural norms.

While there is a strong social stigma attached to being overweight, many social messages are mixed and seem simultaneously to encourage excessive eating: "Clean your plate if you want dessert, but you're getting too fat from eating so much," "Food is splendid but fat is ugly," and "Eat to be friendly, but our friends are not fat" (Brownell, 1980; LeBow, 1984). In many cases, there is strong social pressure for eating; refusing food or eating small amounts may even be seen as an insult.

Behavioral Cues and Consequences

Noneating behaviors can also influence food intake. Food intake tends to covary with exercise. However, this relationship breaks down when physical activity falls below a certain level. A very sedentary lifestyle is often associated with a greater caloric intake than a less sedentary lifestyle. When these very sedentary persons begin to exercise, they often decrease their food intake (Mayer & Thomas, 1967).

Eating style may also influence intake. Overweight persons tend to eat rapidly, chew their food minimally, and add food to their mouths before swallowing the previous bite (LeBow, Goldberg, & Collins, 1977). These behaviors may interfere with satiety cues. Eating may also cue additional eating; once you start eating peanuts, you cannot stop.

FOOD PREFERENCES AND NUTRITION

What we eat is as important as *how* much we eat. Health-promoting diets require, along with water and fiber, five substances: the three basic components of food—proteins, carbohydrates, and fats— as well as vitamins and minerals.

Proteins, which are complex amino acids, are the constituents of living tissue. When we ingest foods containing protein (e.g., meat, fish, eggs, milk products, beans, and nuts), their amino acids supply the needed construction materials for our bodies. Not all important proteins can be made from simpler materials by our bodies. Therefore, the quantity of dietary sources of protein is important. The average adult, under average environmental conditions, should ingest between 40 and 60 grams of protein daily (The Food and Nutrition Board, 1974).

Carbohydrates, which are "fuel" foods, furnish the cheapest supply of energy in our diet. Carbohydrates include both sugars and starches. Most foods, especially grains, fruits, and vegetables, contain large quantities of carbohydrates. As these natural foods are processed or refined into such products as table sugar, white flour, and polished rice, they become almost pure sources of carbohydrates and contain fewer fibers and nutrients than unrefined foods. Both carbohydrates and proteins contain about four calories per gram. About 50% of our diet should come in the form of carbohydrates. The absolute recommended amount of daily carbohydrate intake depends on body weight, age, gender, and activity level. For the average woman weighing 120 pounds, about 1,400 calories are needed daily to meet basic metabolic requirements. The comparable figure for a 145-pound male is 1,600 calories. The consumption of additional calories must be offset by physical activity to maintain a constant weight.

Fats or lipids contain nine calories per gram, nearly twice as many as proteins and carbohydrates. Fats are found in saturated and unsaturated forms. Saturated fats, which tend to be solid at room temperature, include animal fat and shortening. Unsaturated fats, which remain liquid at room temperature, include corn, soybean, and peanut oil. A small amount of unsaturated fat is important in maintaining healthy tissues, especially the skin. However, the average American diet contains about 40% excess fat and includes more saturated than unsaturated fats.

In addition to proteins, carbohydrates, and fats, the body requires micronutrient vitamins and minerals. Vitamins are organic chemicals that work with body enzymes to carry out basic physiological processes. Some vitamins are fat soluble and easily stored in the body; they do not require daily replenishment. These are vitamins A, D, E, and K, which come from oils, milk, eggs, fish and meat. The water-soluble vitamins C and B complex must be replaced more frequently and are found in beans, nuts, grain, citrus fruits, vegetables, meat, and milk. A number of mineral elements are also needed for healthy body functioning. The major minerals required are calcium and phosphorous (for proper bone formation and maintenance), iron (for red blood cell transport of oxygen), iodine (for proper thyroid functioning), fluorine (for tooth and bone health), sodium and chlorine (for proper fluid balance), and potassium (for proper muscle functioning). Trace amounts of zinc, copper, magnesium, and manganese are also needed. All the necessary vitamins and minerals are found in a reasonably balanced diet. In the United States, over 100 million dollars are spent annually on vitamin and mineral supplements. Generally, however, it is much cheaper and better to get these substances from natural food sources. In fact, excess quantities of some vitamins and minerals may be toxic.

Disease may result from dietary insufficiency. This may occur because persons fail to ingest either enough calories to sustain their bodies (starvation) or the minimum requirements of proteins, carbohydrates, fats, vitamins, and minerals. A lack of protein, for example, may interfere with the manufacture of antibodies and thus lower resistance to infection. In the United States, the major nutritional problem is obesity. Compared to our counterparts at the turn of the century, we consume about the same number of calories but burn up fewer calories via exercise. We are eating more fats and getting more of those fats from meat sources (saturated rather than unsaturated). We consume about the same amount of carbohydrates as our grandparents, but obtain more of them from sugars and less from starches. We get more protein from meat and less from other sources. More of our foods are also highly processed, which removes vitamins, minerals, and fiber and concentrates calories (Hitt, 1982; Newman, 1981).

Standard recommendations for a healthy diet include: (1) eating a variety of foods (see Table 2-5); (2) maintaining ideal body weight; (3) avoiding excess fat, especially saturated fat; (4) eating foods with adequate starches and fiber; (5) avoiding excess sugar; (6) avoiding excess salt; (7) ingesting more potassium; and (8) using coffee and alcohol in moderation, if at all.

What variables influence the type of food we eat? Food preferences and selection have biological as well as cultural, familial, or learned determinants. Biologically, humans are omniverous; they can handle a wide variety of food substances. A few preferences appear to be innate, however. For example, there is an almost universal attraction toward sugar and a dislike of bitter foods. Yet these predispositions are readily modified, as is apparent in the acquired taste for coffee. There are also metabolic differences between individuals that are manifested in allergic reactions or intolerance for specific foods. Foods that are incidentally associated with nausea, vomiting, and stomach cramps (food poisoning) also result in strong and prolonged avoidance (Rozin, 1984).

The impact of cultural and familial socialization on food preferences is varied but powerful. Of the broad range of palatable foods, the types and quantity of food actually ingested are a product of learning. Food preferences depend on taste (like or dislike), anticipated consequences (value of various substances or satiation), and cognitive rules (some substances such as grass and sand, are inappropriate; feces and insects are disgusting). Taste, consequences, and rules are established by experience and modeling (Rozin, 1984). We are most likely to eat those foods to which we have been exposed and eaten in the past. We prefer foods that we observe others enjoying and valuing. Thus, preferred foods are established by the family dinner table, by peers and advertising, and by general socialization (e.g., telling a toddler not to eat sand or seeing someone become upset when there is a "fly in the soup"). Once developed, dietary preferences are remarkably resistant to change. Many cultural cuisines have retained their identities despite the great

TABLE 2-5 Daily Guide for a Well-Balanced Diet

FOOD GROUP	NUTRIENTS PROVIDED	ONE SERVING	RECOMMENDED SERVING		
			CHILD	TEEN	ADULT
Leafy green vegetables (lettuce, broccoli)	Folic acid, vitamins A and B, iron, riboflavin fiber	1 cup raw, 1/4 cup cooked	1	1	2
Vitamin C-rich fruits and vegetables (citrus, tomatoes, peppers)	Vitamins C and A, potassium, folic acid	1 orange, 2 tomatoes, 1 cup of fruit, 2 lemons	1	2	2
Other fruits and vegetables (beans, corn, potatoes, peas)	Carbohydrates, fiber, vitamin A, minerals	1 medium fruit, 1/2 cup of raw or cooked vegetable	2	3	4
Protein-rich foods (meat, seafood, eggs, nuts, beans)	Protein, iron, vitamins B and E, zinc, iodine	2 oz. of cooked lean meat, 2 eggs	1 1/2	3–4	2
Breads and cereals (rice, breads, rolls, pasta)	Carbohydrates, some protein, thiamin, niacin, iron, fiber, vitamins B and E	1 slice of bread, 1 cup of cereal, 1/2 cup of pasta or rice	4	5	4
Milk products (milk, yogurt, cheese)	Protein, calcium, vitamins A, B, and D	1 cup of milk or yogurt, 1 1/2 oz. of cheese, 1 1/2 cup of cottage cheese	2	3	2
Fats and oils (butter, margarine, vegetable oils, olives)	Energy, fatty acids, vitamin E (polyunsaturated)	1 tsp. of butter, oil, or margarine	3	4	4

Note: From *The Practice of Preventive Health Care* by L. J. Schneiderman (Ed.), 1981, Menlo Park, CA: Addison-Wesley Publishing Company. Copyright © 1981, the Williams & Wilkins Co., Baltimore. Reprinted by permission.

mobility and mass communications characteristic of our current world. "People eat food, not nutrients. Food is an aspect of culture and has implications beyond the act of eating" (Rozin, 1984, p. 482).

EXERCISE

Exercise has several beneficial effects. It burns calories, enhances weight loss, and increases the likelihood that weight loss will be maintained. It also increases metabolism, which counteracts the opposing effects of dieting, suppresses appetite, and minimizes the loss of lean tissue. Aerobic exercise in particular strengthens the heart; enhances general muscle tone, strength, and elasticity; and has a positive effect on serum lipids, coronary efficiency, and blood pressure (Brownell, 1980). At the same time aerobic exercise decreases the risk of coronary artery disease, diabetes, and high blood pressure. It is also associated with decreased anxiety and depression and an enhanced sense of well-being. However, exercise also carries some risks. If initiated by someone who is unfit or if carried to extremes, it may result in orthopedic discomfort and injury and, more rarely, may precipitate a heart attack (Haskell, 1984).

Most people think exercise is health promoting, but the majority of these individuals do not exercise regularly at a level that is genuinely health enhancing. Relatively little research has focused on the determinants of exercise.

General attitudes toward health are not good predictors of who decides to exercise. Perceptions that exercise is healthful and that one can exercise successfully are related to initiation of an exercise program. Persons who set realistic and attainable goals are more likely to continue to exercise once they have started (Dishman, 1982).

Along with these psychological variables, there are biological characteristics associated with exercise. Persons who are overweight are less likely to exercise, perhaps because exercise is simply harder for them, or perhaps because lean people are more active in the first place. Essentially those persons biologically less well equipped to exercise find it aversive, both behaviorally and biologically. Those who exercise regularly, on the other hand, frequently report it as pleasurable. There are several potential sources of such pleasure. Exercise may decrease negative affective states such as anxiety, depression, and tension, for it is associated with increased levels of endorphins and norepinepherine, which may mediate this enhanced sense of well-being. The pleasurable effects of such exercise may then become "addictive" (Dishman, 1982).

Exercise also depends on social and situational cues and consequences. The support of a spouse or significant other enhances the likelihood of exercise. Social participation and reinforcement from fellow exercisers or exercise leaders have similar effects. The convenience, in terms of time and location, of exercise is also important. Finally, the selection of an appropriate amount of exercise is important. This level appears to involve a balance between exercising vigorously and long enough to perceive benefits but not so much that the exercise is uncomfortable, unenjoyable, and excessive (Dishman, 1982).

Thus, biological, psychological, situational, and social cues and consequences appear to play a role in initiating and maintaining a health-promoting exercise program. A combination of personal and situational variables seems to be the best predictor of who will engage in physical exercise.

SMOKING

Smoking is a risk factor for coronary artery disease, cancer, and emphysema. It is estimated to cost 27 billion dollars in medical care, absenteeism, decreased productivity, and accidents each year (United States Department of Health, Education, and Welfare, 1979). In the United States, 54 million people smoke, and do so at a rate of 196 packs of cigarettes per year. A large number of children and adolescents are recruited into the ranks of smokers each year.

Smoking is a behavior that develops in a series of stages: preparation, initiation, and habitual smoking. If this developmental progression is followed further, persons may quit and remain abstinent, or they may quit unsuccessfully. Different variables are important at these various stages of smoking. An overview of the stages is shown in Table 2-6. Let us first look at the early stages.

Preparation for smoking begins early. Observation of smokers provides the young child with information about the nature of smoking, its functions, and its acceptability. Thus, a more or less appealing and positive image is engendered early. Social pressure from peers is one the prime initiators of experimentation. Smoking by family members and other important models may further promote experimentation. Initial experimentation is critical. Eighty-five to 90% of those who smoked four cigarettes when beginning to experiment became habitual smokers. Those children who are impulsive, less successful at school, rebellious, and "tough" are more likely to experiment early and to continue smoking.

After beginning smoking, it takes two to three years of continued use, or "practice," to fully establish the habit. There is a gradual increase in the number of cigarettes smoked. More situations, activities, and experiences cue smoking, and more reinforcers accrue to the behavior until the person becomes a habitual smoker (Leventhal & Cleary, 1980).

Once the habit is well established, smoking becomes a part of daily self-regulation. As shown in Table 2-7, smoking is evoked and reinforced by a wide range of stimuli. At a physiological level, nicotine is addictive. With continued use, the smoker's body "expects" a certain level of

TABLE 2-6 Developmental Stages of Smoking

Stage 1:	*Preparation* (psychological factors before smoking) Modeling by significant others Attitudes concerning the function and desirability of smoking
Stage 2:	*Initiation* (psychosocial factors leading to experimentation) Peer pressure and reinforcement Availability Curiosity, rebelliousness, and impulsivity Viewing smoking as a sign of adulthood and independence
State 3:	*Habitual* (psychosocial and physiological factors leading to continued smoking) Nicotine regulation Emotional regulation Cues in the environment Peer pressure and reinforcement Urges to smoke
Stage 4:	*Stopping* (psychosocial cues leading to attempts to stop) Health concerns Expense Aesthetic concerns Example to others (e.g., children) Availability of social support for stopping Notions of self-mastery
Stage 5:	*Resuming* (psychosocial and physiological factors leading to recidivism) Withdrawal symptoms Increased stress and other negative effects Social pressure Abstinence violation effects

nicotine and cues the person to smoke if actual levels are below those expected. Nicotine withdrawal symptoms are aversive, and smoking is negatively reinforced by a reduction in such symptoms. Smoking may be further reinforced by the stimulating and alerting effects of nicotine (Jarvik, 1979).

Smoking may also play a central role in emotional regulation. The experience of unpleasant emotions like anxiety, anger, boredom, and depression may cue smoking. A consequent relaxation or reduction in negative effect then reinforces the smoking response. Smokers also report cravings for cigarettes or other tobacco products. These cravings may be cognitive correlates of low nicotine levels, of affective arousal, or of the positive consequences associated with smoking, including taste, relaxation, or stimulation. Cravings may also be cued by external stimuli (e.g., seeing others smoke) or by other behaviors (e.g., a cup of coffee) (Leventhal & Cleary, 1980). Finally, a smoker may engage in self-

TABLE 2-7 Antecedent Cues and Consequences of Smoking

VARIABLE	ANTECEDENT CUES	CONSEQUENCES
Physiological	Nicotine dependence Withdrawal symptoms	Stimulation, relaxation Nicotine regulation Decreased withdrawal symptoms
Psychological	Anxiety, tension Craving Excuses and rationalizations	Relaxation Pleasure Positive self-image
Social and cultural	Peer and adult models Invitations and peer pressure Norms and laws	Peer approval Group affiliation Stress reduction
Environmental	Commercials Situations that evoke smoking Situational stressors Automatic behavior	Oral, manual and respiratory sensation
Behavioral	Multiple behavioral cues (e.g., with coffee, after meals)	

reinforcement (e.g., seeing oneself as mature, adult, or a "Marlboro man").

The social and physical environment along with the smoker's own behavior via past associative learning constantly bombard the habitual user with cues to smoke. Seeing others smoke, receiving invitations to smoke, seeing a pack of cigarettes, drinking coffee, finishing a meal, and watching TV are consequently all capable of evoking tobacco use. That use may in turn be reinforced by social approval, peer affiliation, and the oral, manual, and respiratory actions involved in smoking.

In summary, once established, smoking and other forms of tobacco use serve as regulating responses to physiological withdrawal, negative effect, cravings, and social interaction in a manner that achieves a powerful and immediate hedonic homeostasis. The cues and consequences for smoking combine and interact in a potentiating manner.

SUMMARY

Behavior plays a central role in health and illness. Health-impairing habits and lifestyles are important risk factors for chronic disease and death, whereas health-promoting habits and lifestyles enhance biological and psychosocial functioning. Maladaptive and adaptive health behaviors are acquired and maintained by the same processes. Their acquisition and shaping are a function of maturation and learning. Once established, their performance is evoked and maintained by the biological, cognitive-affective, social, environmental and behavioral cues and consequences that define an individual's daily experience.

The modification of health behaviors is a primary task in clinical and preventative medicine. Health behaviors are multiply determined and functionally involve the client and the natural environment. Consequently, effective intervention necessitates a collaborative, mutually active client-health provider relationship, and the utilization of cognitive, behavioral, and environmental as well as biological change strategies. Approaches to health habit modification will be detailed in Chapter 13.

REFERENCES

Abraham, S., Collins, G., & Nordsieck, M. (1971). Relationship of childhood weight status to morbidity in adults. *HSMA Health Reports*, 86, 273–284.

Bandura, A. (1977). *Social learning theory*. Englewood Cliffs, NJ: Prentice-Hall.

Bibace, R., & Wallace, M. E. (1979). Developmental stages in children's conceptions of illness. In G. C. Stone, F. Cohen, & N. E. Adler (Eds.), *Health psychology—A handbook*, 285–302. San Francisco: Jossey-Bass.

Bringham, T. (1982). Self management: A radical behavioral perspective. In P. Karoly & F. H. Kanfer (Eds.), *Self management and behavior change: From theory to practice*, 32–59. New York: Pergamon Press.

Brownell, K. D. (1980) Obesity: Understanding and treating a serious, prevalent, and refractory disorder. *Psychological Bulletin*, *88*, 370–405.

Centers for Disease Control, Public Health Service (1979). *Leading causes of death and probabilities of dying, United States: 1975 and 1976*. Atlanta: Author.

Davidson, G. C. (1973). Countercontrol in behavior modification. In L. A. Hamerlynck, L. C. Handy, & E. J. Mash (Eds.), *Behavior change: Theories, concepts and practice*, 153–168. Champaign, IL: Research Press.

Dishman, R. K. (1982). Compliance/adherence in health related exercise. *Health Psychology*, *1*, 237–267.

The Food and Nutrition Board (1974). *Recommended daily dietary allowances*. New York: National Academy of Sciences—National Research Council.

Goode, E. (1972). *Drugs in American society*. New York: Knopf.

Hagen, R. L. (1976). Theories of obesity: Is there any hope for order? In B. Williams, S. Martin, & J. P. Foreyt (Eds.), *Obesity: Behavioral approaches to dietary management*. New York: Brunner/Mazel.

Haley, J. (1963). *Strategies of psychotherapy*. New York: Grune & Stratton.

Haley, J. (1973). *Uncommon therapy: The psychiatric techniques of Milton H. Erickson, M.D.* New York: W. W. Norton.

Haskell, W. L. (1984). Overview: Health benefits of exercise. In J. D. Matarazzo, S. M. Weiss, J. A. Herd, N. E. Miller, & S. M. Weiss (Eds.), *Behavioral health: A handbook of health enhancement and disease prevention*, 409–423. New York: John Wiley & Sons.

Hirsch, J., & Knittle, J. L. (1971). Cellularity of obese and nonobese human adipose tissue. *Federation Proceedings*, *29*, 1516–1521.

Hitt, C. (1982). Nutrition and risk reduction. In M. Farber & A. Reinhardt (Eds.), *Promoting health through risk reduction*, 237–252. New York: Macmillan.

Hodgson, R., & Miller, P. (1982). *Self-watching addictions, habits and compulsions: What to do about them*. New York: Facts on File Publications.

Janis, I.L. (1984). Improving adherence to medical recommendations: Prescriptive hypotheses derived from recent research in social psychology. In A. Baum, S. E. Taylor, & J. E. Singer (Eds.), *Handbook of psychology and health* (Vol. 4), 260–278; Hillsdale, NJ: Lawrence Erlbaum.

Jarvick, M. E. (1979). Biological influences on cigarette smoking. In United States Department of Health, Education, and Welfare, *Smoking and health: A report of the surgeon general* (DHEW Publication [PHS] No. 79–50066), pp 135–139. Washington, DC: U.S. Government Printing Office.

Jordan, M. K., & O'Grady, D. J. (1982) Children's health beliefs and concepts: Implications for child health care. In P. Karoly, J. J. Steffen, & D. J. O'Grady (Eds.), *Child health psychology*, 58–76. New York: Pergamon Press.

Keesey, R. (1980). A set point analysis of the regulation of body weight. In A. J. Stunkard (Ed.), *Obesity*, 148–156. New York: Allen R. Liss.

Krantz, D. S., Glass, D. C., Contrada, R., & Miller, N. E. (1981). Behavior and health. In National Science Foundation, *The five year outlook on science and technology*. Boulder, CO: Westview Press.

Kristeller, J. L., & Rodin, J. (1984). A three stage model of treatment continuity: Compliance, adherence and maintenance. In A. Baum, S. E. Taylor, & J. E. Singer (Eds.), *Handbook of psychology and health* (Vol. 4), 279–294. Hillsdale, NJ: Lawrence Erlbaum.

Langer, E. J., & Rodin, J. (1976). The effects of choice and enhanced personal responsibility for the aged: A field experiment in an institutional setting. *Journal of Personality and Social Psychology*, *34*, 191–198.

LeBow, M. D. (1984). *Child obesity: A new frontier of behavior therapy*. New York: Springer.

LeBow, M. D., Goldberg, P. S., & Collins, A. (1977). Eating behaviors of overweight and nonoverweight persons in the natural environment. *Journal of Consulting and Clinical Psychology*, *45*, 1204–1205.

Leventhal, H., & Cleary, P. D. (1980). The smoking problem: A review of the research. *Psychological Bulletin*, *88*, 370–405.

Mahoney, M. J., & Arnkoff, D. B. (1978). Cognitive and self control therapies. In S. L. Garfield & A. E. Bergin (Eds.), *Handbook of psychotherapy and behavior change*, 689–722. New York: John Wiley & Sons.

Marlatt, G. A. & Parkes, G. A. (1982). Self management of addictive behaviors. In P. Karoly & F. H. Kanfer (Eds.), *Self management and behavior change: From theory to practice*, 443–488. New York: Pergamon Press.

Mayer, J. (1957). Correlation between metabolism and feeding behavior and multiple etiology of obesity. *Bulletin of the New York Academy of Medicine*, *22*, 744–761.

Mayer, J., & Thomas, D. W. (1967). Regulation of food intake and obesity. *Science*, *156*, 328–337.

McKenna, R. J. (1972). Some effects of anxiety level and food cues on the eating behavior of obese and normal subjects: A comparison of Schacterian and psychosomatic conceptions. *Journal of Personality and Social Psychology*, *22*, 320–325.

Newman, V. (1981). Nutrition in prevention. In L. J. Schneiderman (Ed.), *The practice of preventative health care*, 262–291. Menlo Park, CA: Addison-Wesley.

Polivy, J., & Herman, C. P. (1985). Dieting and binging: A causal analysis. *American Psychologist*, *40*, 193–201.

Robbins, L. C., & Blankenship, R. (1982). Prospective medicine and the health hazard appraisal. In R. B. Taylor, J. R. Ureda, & J. W. Denham (Eds.), *Health promotion: Principles and clinical applications*, 67–122. New York: Appleton-Century-Crofts.

Rodin, J. (1977). Bidirectional influences of emotionality, stimulus responsivity, and metabolic events in obesity. In J. D. Maser & M.E.P. Seligman (Eds.), *Psychopathlogy: Experimental models*, 217–241. San Francisco: W. H. Freeman.

Rodin, J. (1982). Biopsychosocial aspects of self management. In P. Karoly & F. H. Kanfer (Eds.), *Self management and behavior change: From theory to practice*, 60–92. New York: Pergamon Press.

Rodin, J., & Janis, I. L. (1982). The social influences of physicians and health care providers. In H. S. Friedman & M. R. DiMatteo (Eds.), *Interpersonal issues in health care*, 33–50. New York: Academic Press.

Rozin, P. (1984). The acquisition of food habits and preferences. In J. D. Matarazzo, S. M. Weiss, J. A. Herd, N. E. Miller, & S. M. Weiss (Eds.), *Behavioral health: A handbook of health enhancement and disease prevention*, 590–607. New York: John Wiley & Sons.

Schacter, S. (1968). Obesity and eating. *Science, 161*, 751–756.

Stone, G. C. (1979). Patient compliance and the role of the expert. *Journal of Social Issues, 35*, 34–59.

Stuart, R. B. (1971). A three-dimensional program for the treatment of obesity. *Behavior Research and Therapy, 9*, 177–186.

Stunkard, A. J., & Koch, C. (1964). The interpretation of gastric motility. Archives of General Psychiatry, *2*, 74–82.

Stunkard, A. J., & Mahoney, M. J. (1976). Behavioral treatment of eating disorders. In H. Leitenberg (Ed.), *Handbook of behavior modification and behavior therapy*, 45–73. Englewood Cliffs, NJ: Prentice-Hall.

United States Department of Health, Education, and Welfare. (1979). *Smoking and health: A report of the surgeon general* (DHEW Publication [PHS] No. 79–50066). Washington, DC: U.S. Government Printing Office.

White, R. W. (1959). Motivation reconsidered: The concept of competence. *Psychological Review, 66*, 297–333.

Woody, E., & Costanzo, P. (1981). The socialization of obesity-prone behavior. In S. Brehm, S. Kassem, & F. Gibbons (Eds.), *Developmental social psychology*, 211–234. New York: Oxford University Press.

3

Illness-Related Decisions and Actions

INTRODUCTION

As described at the beginning of Chapter 2, one of the two direct ways in which behavior influences health involves illness-related decisions and actions, which encompass a wide variety of behaviors: recognition and interpretation of symptoms, interactions with health providers, decisions concerning the nature of treatment, cooperation with diagnostic and treatment procedures, adherence to medical recommendations, and decisions and actions related to disease prevention.

In describing and understanding these behaviors, we will continue to use the multilevel framework of cues and consequences developed in Chapter 2. At the end of this chapter, we will consider another model of health-related behavior, which focuses on cognitive processing of these cues and consequences. This paradigm will help us understand how individuals utilize and process cues and consequences to decide on specific health actions.

SYMPTOM RECOGNITION

How do people determine if they are ill? What determines how they respond to symptoms once they are recognized? We frequently experience physical symptoms or illness episodes. To stay healthy, we need to make sense out of these symptoms and to take remedial action. This recurring process can be broken into several stages: becoming aware of a symptom, understanding and labeling the symptom, planning and taking action to remediate the symptom, and evaluating the outcome of these actions. In any one illness episode, we may cycle through these various stages more than once (Fabrega, 1974). Let us first consider symptom recognition.

It is adaptive to perceive potentially dangerous physical symptoms. Failure to recognize these symptoms may lead to health complications, unnecessary suffering, and increased health care costs. On the other hand, overattentiveness to minor symptoms may not be adaptive and may result in unnecessary emotional distress, overutilization of health care resources, and inflation of health care costs.

How do we become aware of physical symptoms? What factors influence awareness and attentiveness to our bodies? Perception of body sensations and symptoms involves the same processes as perception of stimuli in the external environment. Because we are constantly bombarded by stimuli from both sources, it is impossible to attend to all of them simultaneously. Rather, we selectively focus on certain stimuli and ignore others. We are most likely to attend to those stimuli, either external or internal, that are salient.

The salience of a physical symptom depends upon the strength and novelty of that symptom and of others competing for our attention. We are more likely to become aware of a symptom that is strong (Pennebaker, 1982, 1984). The nausea and dizziness of a hangover are attention riveting, whereas a mild sore throat may recede into the background as we go about our daily routine. The salience of a symptom also depends on its visibility to ourselves and others. Novel symptoms are also more likely to receive our attention. This novelty is related to the characteristics of the symptom; we attend to those that we have not previously experienced and tend to habituate to those that are common.

Novelty is also related to the persistence of the symptom and to the rate at which it appears. A pain that persists over time may become less salient because we habituate to its presence. Symptoms may likewise not be recognized because of their slow and subtle onset. This makes the early recognition of chronically developing diseases particularly problematic.

The salience of physical symptoms also depends on the number and salience of external stimuli with which they compete. We are more likely to notice symptoms when there is relatively little information coming in from the external environment. Thus, persons often notice symptoms when waking in the morning or lying in bed at night. Mild symptoms seem to recede during the day when we are actively engaged. Persons who hold boring jobs, are unemployed, or live alone report more symptoms, perhaps due to reduced environmental stimulation (Pennebaker, 1982).

Not all body symptoms are noticed. Awareness depends on the characteristics of the symptoms and the larger stimulus context in which they occur.

SYMPTOM INTERPRETATION

We are not passive recipients of stimuli. Once we attend to a symptom, we actively try to determine what it means. For example, if you wake some morning and have a sore throat, you may swallow a couple of times, feel the glands under your jaw, and look at your throat in the mirror to assess the nature and extent of the problem. You also label the sensation ("a sore throat"), think about its cause ("caught something going around"), and estimate its duration and consequences ("it'll last for a few days and then go away by itself").

Stated more formally, when we become aware of a symptom, we construct a representation or schema to explain it and to guide our action (Leventhal, 1983). Although the specific content of representations vary from symptom to symptom, they have four basic components: identity, cause, time line, and consequences. Identity refers to the question, "What do I have?" and involves naming the symptom. A sore throat, cough, and congestion may be represented as a cold. Cause refers to the question, "How did I get this?" The symptom may be seen as a result of our own behavior ("I didn't get enough sleep"), of external circumstances ("bad food in a restaurant"), or of both. Time line refers to the questions, "How long will this last?" and "Will it come back?" A symptom may be viewed as acute (e.g., a cold, the flu, or an infection) or chronic (e.g., allergies or high blood pressure). Consequences refer to the question, "What are the short- and long-term outcomes of the symptom?" These may be estimated to range from trivial to debilitating and life threatening. Short- and long-term consequences are not necessarily congruent. A hangover may be experienced as having extremely aversive short-term effects but only limited long-term consequences. Syphilis, on the other hand, may be seen as having only minor short-term implications but profound long-term consequences (Lau & Hartman, 1983; Leventhal, Meyer, & Nerenz, 1980).

The way in which a person represents symptoms can be construed as a kind of self-diagnosis. This self-generated schema is not necessarily congruent with the objective nature of the symptoms, however, since it depends on the symptoms being experienced, the information about illness available to the person is based on past experience and observation, and social communication and environmental cues (Leventhal, Nerenz, & Steele, 1984). A self-diagnosis may be quite different from the diagnosis of a skilled health provider.

Some symptoms are relatively unambiguous, observable, and commonplace; the construction of a schema for such symptoms may require little inference and is relatively accurate. Severe leg pain after a fall is likely to be labeled as a fracture. Its cause, time line, and consequences are relatively easily established. Many symptoms are more ambiguous and diffuse, and thus a schema for them requires more inference and is subject to greater error. Psychosocial variables play a stronger role in the development of a schema for ambiguous symptoms. "Medical student's disease" is a good example. The stress and fatigue engendered by medical school commonly results in vague symptoms like a racing heart, headaches, indigestion, and dizziness. The simultaneous study of the symptoms of diseases in pathology courses makes available a number of illnesses that could overlap with those being experienced by the student. As a result, over 70% of first-year medical students come to the conclusion that they have one of the diseases being studied (Woods, Natterson, & Silverman, 1966).

The representation of symptoms as serious often leads to emotional arousal. This arousal produces a concomitant physiological arousal that may in turn enhance or confuse the physical sensations on which the schema is based. Symptom reporting thus increases under stress and emotional arousal (Costa & McCrae, 1985; Kanner, Coyne, Schaefer, & Lazarus, 1981).

While illness representation is partially based on the symptoms we are experiencing, once constructed that representation influences the symptoms to which we attend. If we think we have a certain disease (a cold), we will attend to symptoms that fit the disease (cough and sore throat) and ignore those that do not (itchy eyes). The influence between symptoms and representation is therefore reciprocal (Leventhal et al., 1984).

Defining oneself as ill is a complex process that consists of perceiving symptoms and determining their meaning. The end product of this process is influenced by environmental, social, affective, cultural, and learning history variables in addition to the symptoms themselves. Self-evaluation of health and illness is thus subject to distortion and is not necessarily biologically objective. However, such representations do provide the person with a sense of control and serve as a guide for actions needed to remediate the symptoms.

ACTIONS IN RESPONSE TO ILLNESS

A wide range of actions may be taken in response to illness. Persons may: (1) ignore the symptoms, wait, and do nothing; (2) engage in self-medication or self-care (e.g., take aspirin, get more sleep, or use a heating pad); (3) seek information and care from family and friends, which is called popular care (e.g., ask others about what symptoms mean or what you should do, or have your mother make chicken soup); (4) seek information and aid from quasilegal or illegal helpers like herbalists or faith healers, which is called folk medicine; or (5) seek care from sanctioned professionals like physicians, dentists, nurse clinicians, and chiropractors (Chrisman & Kleinman, 1983). For any one illness episode, several of these responses may be used sequentially or simultaneously.

Symptoms are frequently experienced by most people; the average college student reports two to three discrete symptom episodes in a two-week period (Snyder, Rickson, & Parker, 1984). Most of these symptoms are minor and self-limiting, and thus require only that the person wait for them to recede. The majority of illnesses do not lead to seeking professional health care. Multiple factors influence the strategy selected to deal with an illness: the representation of the illness, the nature of the symptoms, social and cultural cues and consequences, and the cost of and access to the various response options. Within and between illness episodes, these factors shift. Thus actions taken in response to illness are highly situational. This is also an iterative process; if one response option is not successful, the person will select another. Let us look more closely at factors that influence the actions selected by persons who see themselves as ill.

Illness Representation

A person's representation of symptoms serves as an important guide to actions taken in response to an illness. Symptoms that are perceived as having serious short- and long-term consequences and that are not seen as self-limiting in terms of time line are likely to result in seeking professional health care (Andersen, 1968). Symptom seriousness also generates an emotional arousal (Leventhal et al., 1984) that affects the type of action taken. Moderate emotional arousal motivates people to seek care. Extreme arousal disrupts good problem solving and may cause a delay or avoidance in seeking health care. An illness schema that represents symptoms as less serious is more likely to result in a "wait and see" attitude and self- or popular care strategies.

On the basis of past experience, observation, and information from other people in the social environment, persons develop ideas about the types of action available for a given illness episode and the effectiveness and discomforts of those actions (Lau & Hartman, 1983; Safer, Tharps, Jackson, & Leventhal, 1979). Actions that are seen as potentially effective and as minimally aversive will be selected (Safer et al., 1979).

Social Influences

When ill, persons frequently seek information from family and friends to define the problem and to select appropriate action. They describe their symptoms and ask what they should do. This is called the lay referral process. As well as seeking information, the ill person may be testing the legitimacy of illness actions such as staying in bed, skipping work, and going to a doctor (Chrisman & Kleinman, 1983). There are strong positive and negative social consequences for various illness-generated behaviors. Exemptions from normal work and social roles and the attention of others strongly reinforce such behaviors (Fordyce & Steger, 1979). Illness behaviors may also lead to punishment in the form of social disapproval, stigmatization, and loss of income. The expected and actual consequences for illness actions thus influence an ill person's choices (Janis & Rodin, 1979).

The selection of illness actions is also influenced by values acquired during socialization that specify when it is legitimate to seek help and what illness actions will be approved by others. If a person strongly identifies with a group that has a negative view of professional health providers (like the Christian Scientists), that person is unlikely to seek help from such sources (Becker & Maiman, 1975).

Availability and Cost

Illness-generated actions are also affected by the availability of needed resources. Persons with adequate financial resources, like health insurance and sufficient income, are more likely to use health care services (Safer et al., 1979). The accessibility of health care in terms of travel time, ease in getting an appointment, and the existence of a regular physician also influence health care utilization (Andersen, 1968).

There are also personal costs to various illness actions. Social and vocational responsibilities may influence these behaviors. Statements like, "I don't have time to be sick," "Who would take care of my children while I was in the hospital?" and "I'll take care of it after I complete this project," all indicate that daily responsibilities influence the probability and timing of illness actions. For example, mothers who are dealing with personal problems are less likely to seek pediatric care for ill children than are mothers who are not distressed (Kirscht, Becker, & Eveland, 1976). Pressing work demands and social responsibilities are similarly associated with delayed use of health care services (Safer et al., 1979).

Summary: Response to Symptoms

In sum, actions in response to illness are influenced by many variables: the nature of the symptoms, our understanding of the symptoms, social suggestions and recommendations, and anticipated benefits and costs of the action. If a given behavior is implemented but is either ineffective or too costly, the person will shift to another action that appears to be potentially more successful. Illness behaviors are not necessarily consistent with what would be best biologically; cognitive, affective, social, cultural, and environmental variables all play a role in affecting those actions. Like health-promoting and health-impairing behaviors, actions in response to illness are determined by multiple, interacting cues and consequences that occur at many organizational levels.

CLIENT-HEALTH PROVIDER INTERACTION AND COMMUNICATION

Seeking treatment from a health professional initiates what appears, at first glance, to be a relatively straightforward process. The client describes the symptoms, responds to queries from the health provider, and cooperates with diagnostic tests and procedures. Using the information obtained from these sources, the provider uses technical knowledge, expertise, and clinical experience to determine the problem and to formulate an effective treatment. The health provider then communicates treatment information to the client, and the client follows these recommendations. The client and the health provider appear to share common goals and perspectives.

In reality, however, client-health provider interaction consists of a complex interpersonal exchange of information and social influence. It does not run as smoothly as suggested above. Each party has information not directly accessible to the other. This information can only be made available via communication. Each party also brings expectations, perspectives, and goals that may not be congruent with those held by the other person (Leventhal, 1975). These private perspectives are shown in Figure 3-1. Let us look at each party's perspective in more detail. Then we will analyze the clinical interchange in which these perspectives are shared and in which efforts are made to influence the other person.

The Client's Perspective

The client brings to the exchange his own subjective experience of the symptoms. Because symptoms are often ambiguous, the client may have difficulty in accurately describing the symptom experience. The symptom description may be further distorted by anxiety and by the schema used to represent the symptoms. The client's report may thus lack clarity and be far removed from the initial symptom experience. Based on past experience, the client has expectations about how the clinician ought to behave (the client's model of helping). Based on the schema developed to understand the current symptoms, the client also has expectations about the types of questions, tests, and treatment that will be utilized by the provider (Clymer, Baum, & Krantz, 1984). These private experiences, representations, and expectations guide the client's behavior during the interaction with the health provider, and are used to filter and understand what the provider is saying and doing.

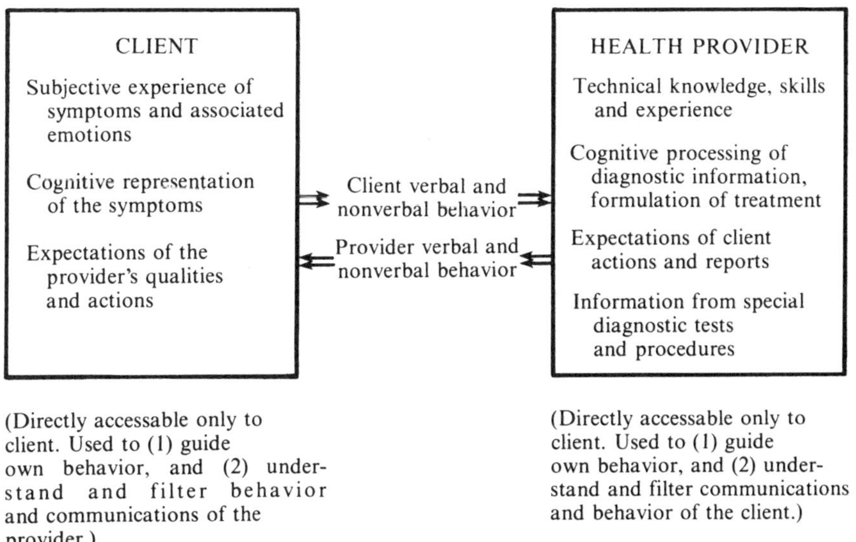

FIGURE 3-1 Client and Health Provider's Perspectives on Clinical Interaction

The Health Provider's Perspective

The clinician cannot directly access the client's symptom experience, but must depend on the client's verbal and nonverbal behavior to obtain that information. Consequently, the health professional expects the client to be as honest and accurate as possible in reporting symptoms, to be responsive to questions, and to be cooperative in diagnostic procedures. The clinician is interested in the "facts." Data obtained from the client, from the observation of overt signs of the illness, and from diagnostic tests and procedures are cognitively processed by the clinician to arrive at a diagnosis and treatment plan. The clinician's behavior is guided by her expectations of the client (the provider's model of helping), by her technical knowledge and clinical experience, and by data concerning the client's problem. These same expectations, knowledge, experience, and data are used by the health provider to filter and understand the client's behavior. The client does not have direct access to the health care provider's perspective, but must infer it from the provider's verbal and nonverbal behavior.

Clinical Interaction and Communication

In the clinical interaction, the health provider and the client attempt to make public their own experiences, expectations, and perspectives and to understand those of the other person. This verbal and nonverbal interchange is extremely important in that it serves as the basis for diagnosis and treatment. Both parties are attempting to influence the other, and both are active and responsible. The influence is reciprocal.

The importance of the interpersonal component in medical treatment is frequently minimized. It is considered an "art" and not a "science." This view of the interpersonal component is incorrect on two counts. First, the interpersonal component is subject to scientific scrutiny in the same manner as physiology and pharmacology: It can be observed, analyzed, and altered. It is a skill that can be taught to health professionals. Second, this component has a strong impact on the biological and psychosocial effects of treatment (DiMatteo & DiNicola, 1982). The quality of the interchange influences the data available to make a diagnosis, the client's responsiveness to the clinician's questions and cooperation with diagnostic procedures, and the client's willingness and care in carrying out treatment recommendations (DiNicola & DiMatteo, 1984; Kristeller & Rodin, 1984). Effective use of medical technology depends on good communication.

Good communication has additional benefits. It increases the information available to the client and enhances the client's perception of predictability and control. This sense of involvement improves the client's psychological well-being and physiological prognosis by reducing the stress inherent in many diagnostic and treatment procedures (see Chapter 4 for a further discussion). The quality of the interaction also affects the client's satisfaction with treatment (Ley, 1977), which in turn is correlated with "doctor shopping" and the probability of malpractice suits. Finally, health professionals who emphasize and foster good communication with clients report higher job satisfaction and less job "burnout" (Friedman & DiMatteo, 1979).

Medical and Compensatory Paradigms of Helping and the Clinical Interchange

The medical paradigm of helping minimizes the client's involvement in solving health problems. Its focus is on a goal-directed appraisal and solution of the problem that uses a line of inquiry to obtain as much information as possible in the shortest time possible. "Facts" about the symptoms are emphasized. The client's experience and understanding of the problem are peripheral to diagnosis and treatment. The body of the client is the primary concern, with an attendant objectification and depersonalization of the client. What the client thinks and feels is less important than the objective meaning of the symptoms. Most of the information flow is from the client to the health provider. The health provider is minimally communicative; all the client needs to know is what to do to get better. Being empathic and providing more complete information are more matters of courtesy and ethics than central facets of treatment. In the medical paradigm of helping, the provider relies primarily on expert and legitimate sources of power to obtain information and to solve the problem. The client should thus comply with the health provider's requests because the provider is responsible for treatment.

In the compensatory paradigm of helping, the client is viewed as an active participant in treatment. The client's subjective experience, worries, schemata, and expectations are important and thoroughly explored during the clinical interaction. The client is seen as a person who has a disease rather than as a disease. The client's perspective is met with interest and empathy. The clinician's expectations, the data available from diagnostic tests and procedures, and the meaning of those data are explicitly communicated to the client. In other words, an effort is made to access and clarify each party's perspective in order to develop a shared conceptualization of the problem and of treatment (Turk, Meichenbaum, & Genest, 1983). Based on this type of interchange, the health provider develops referent as well as expert, legitimate, and informational sources of influence to effect change in the client's behavior. This involvement communicates to clients that they are responsible, and provides clients with the means to take remedial and preventative actions. Client cooperation and adherence are thereby enhanced, and clients experience more control and predictability. They leave the interchange with increased knowledge and skills, which is compatible with the original meaning of the word *doctor*: "to teach."

In sum, the compensatory paradigm of helping emphasizes the importance of client-health provider communication in addition to the medical and technical aspects of intervention. A number of negative outcomes may result from a failure to foster good communication. Let us look at one example in some detail: adherence to treatment recommendations.

ADHERENCE TO TREATMENT RECOMMENDATIONS

Once a diagnosis has been made and a treatment plan has been developed, the clinician communicates the actions to be taken by the client to correct the problem or to prevent its recurrence. The actions requested of clients are quite diverse. They may entail taking medication at specified times for some specified interval. They may involve returning for an office visit or seeking treatment from a specialist. They may also consist of preventative actions like getting an immunization or changing a personal health habit. The clinician is attempting to influence the client's behavior outside the immediate clinical setting. The degree to which the client's behavior coincides with recommendations of the health provider is referred to as adherence (Haynes, 1979b).

If clients are experiencing discomfort and spend the time and money to seek treatment, it would make sense that they accurately follow the health providers' instructions. Although adherence is difficult to measure accurately (Kirscht & Rosenstock, 1979), 15 to 90% (an average of 30%) of medical recommendations are not accurately followed by clients (Davis, 1966; Sackett & Haynes, 1976). Nonadherence occurs across settings, across health problems, and across recommendations. It has been observed in clients in both hospital and outpatient settings and in clients with both symptomatic and nonsymptomatic disorders.

Nonadherence is a major health care delivery problem. No treatment is effective if it is not applied or is applied incorrectly. It is like bringing fire trucks to a fire and then not using them. Like other health-related behaviors, adherence can be understood in terms of the multiple cues that elicit and the multiple consequences that motivate the behaviors recommended by the health care provider. Let us look at factors that influence adherence behavior (see Table 3-1 for an overview).

Social Cues and Consequences in Client-Health Provider Interaction

Adherence is influenced by the nature of the interaction between the client and the health professional. To adhere to recommended actions, the client must be able to understand and remember the recommendations (DiNicola & DiMatteo, 1984). Clients have been found to forget 30 to 50% of the information provided by providers within an hour after leaving the clinical interchange (Ley & Spellman, 1967). Understanding and recall are influenced by how clearly the information is communicated and by the clients' attention and receptiveness to that information. Clients who are emotionally aroused because of the quality of the interaction or the nature of the information (a serious diagnosis) may not attend to what a health professional is saying. If the recommendations do not fit the client's representation of the problem (e.g., many clients with high blood pressure see it as an acute disorder rather than a chronic disorder) and if that difference is not clarified in the clinical interaction, the recommendations are likely to be ignored or to be inaccurately followed (e.g., clients take blood pressure medication for a week and then stop) (Leventhal et al., 1984). A careful, complete, and reciprocal exchange of information is needed to ensure client understanding and recall of and agreement with treatment recommendations. The private experiences of both the client and the clinician need to be exchanged until a shared conceptualization and clear understanding of the problem are developed and a commitment to action by the client is obtained.

The quality and affective tone of the relationship is important. Encouraging clients to disclose personal feelings and worries and listening

TABLE 3-1 Antecedent Cues and Consequences of Adherence Behaviors

VARIABLE	ANTECEDENT CUES	CONSEQUENCES
Physiological	Symptom salience	Salience and latency of symptom relief
	Pain or discomfort	Latency and quality of side effects
Psychological	Affective arousal	Alteration in affective arousal
	Illness representation Understanding and recall of instructions	Self-generated consequences
Social	Instructional clarity and complexity of recommendations from the health provider Quality of interaction with the health provider	Consequences provided by the health provider
	General and specific support from family, friends, and coworkers	Consequences provided by family, friends, and coworkers
Environmental	Salience of cues for adherence vs. competing routine-generated cues	Alteration in capacity to engage in normative roles and actions
Behavioral	Symptom interference with normative roles and actions	

to those disclosures in an accepting and caring manner foster the shared conceptualization and commitment needed for adherence. This approach establishes the referent power of the provider, which can then be used to motivate the client to take appropriate adherence actions. Clients are more likely to cooperate with a health provider who is seen as kind, caring, and understanding (Rodin & Janis, 1982).

Adherence also depends on the complexity and number of behavior changes being requested. Adherence decreases with the number of actions recommended, when clients are asked to sustain a new behavior over a long period, and with the passage of time since contact with the health provider (Kirscht & Rosenstock, 1979).

Social Cues and Consequences: The Client's Natural Environment

While the clinical interaction plays an important role in adherence, most of the recommended actions are implemented after the client leaves that interaction. Thus, cues and consequences for adherence in the client's natural environment are also very important (Haynes, 1979a). The client's family and friends can foster adherence by providing emotional support and acceptance, which reduce anxiety about illness and its treatment. Family and friends provide concrete cues and consequences for adherence behavior. They may offer reminders, remove temptations to nonadherence, and provide tangible socioemotional rewards for adherence (Caplan, 1979). On the other hand, a lack of support can quickly undermine and negate medical recommendations. The refusal of a spouse to cook low sodium, low fat foods for a client with hypertension is a strong barrier to adherence. Health providers need to be aware of the client's social system and, if necessary, involve important persons in the client's environment when planning and implementing treatment.

Physiological Cues and Consequences

Symptoms, especially those that are painful or discomforting, serve as salient, immediate cues for adherence behavior. A headache, for example, is sufficiently painful to elicit taking aspirin. Generally, symptomatic health problems result in better adherence than nonsymptomatic problems. Because preventative health care recommendations involve asking someone to take action in the absence of symptoms (i.e., no salient cues), adherence to such recommendations is particularly problematic (Kirscht & Rosenstock, 1979).

The nature and timing of the physiological consequences of adherence are also important. Those behaviors that lead to prompt relief from unpleasant symptoms (e.g., reduction of a headache after taking aspirin) are more likely to be sustained because they are strongly reinforced. Those actions that have no noticeable effect or a very delayed effect (e.g., taking medication for high blood pressure) are less likely to be sustained because there is a lack of reinforcement. In some cases, however, even immediate relief that is contingent on adherence is counterproductive. If a person has an earache, for example, the decreased pain resulting from taking an antibiotic reinforces that behavior. However, the person may prematurely stop taking the antibiotic because the pain is removed. The infection may then return because it is not totally eradicated (Becker, Drachman, & Kirscht, 1972).

Adverse side effects from adherence may decrease the probability of adherence because they effectively punish the behavior. To some degree, this can be counteracted by medical management or by anticipation of the side effects during the clinical interaction (Dunbar & Stunkard, 1979). Physiological cues and consequences can be powerful determinants of adherence because of their natural occurrence in the client's experience.

Setting Cues and Consequences

Clients' day-to-day physical environment and routine likewise affect the probability of adherence. Behavior required by treatment recommendations is a departure from routine. It therefore lacks salient environmental cues and competes with behaviors that are a part of that routine. Adherence is more probable if the recommended behaviors are tied to salient environmental cues. Daily adherence for taking medication could be enhanced by attaching a client's medication bottle to his toothbrush by a rubber band. The likelihood of adherence is also improved if its timing does not compete with other routine, strongly reinforced behaviors (Zifferblatt, 1975).

Clinicians can maximize adherence by fashioning the treatment program so that it is relatively simple and compatible with the client's routine and by building in social and setting cues that are salient and explicitly related to the desired behavior.

Cognitive Representation and Adherence

We have already learned that persons actively develop a representation of their illness in terms of its cause, time line, meaning, and consequences. This representation serves as a guide in determining not only whether to seek health care but also which actions are taken after the person leaves the clinical setting. Adherence by persons with high blood pressure is notoriously poor; let us consider how clients' representation of this illness may play a role in poor adherence.

Despite the general notion that essential hypertension is an asymptomatic disorder, most persons with high blood pressure report that they can use discernible symptoms like headaches or a flushed face to tell when their pressure is up. Many clients also view high blood pressure as an acute, episodic rather than a chronic, constant disorder (Meyer, 1981; Pennebaker, 1982). Taking medication for hypertension is influenced by these representations. If the specific symptom (e.g., a headache) thought to indicate elevation in blood pressure is not being experienced, there is no need (from the client's point of view) for the medication. If the medication has no influence on the symptom used to monitor blood pressure, the client sees the medication as ineffective and discontinues it. Similar findings are available for persons suffering from diabetes, ulcers, and cancer (Leventhal et al., 1980, 1984; Ley, 1977). Adherence is poor if the behaviors being recommended by the health provider do not make sense to the client. Clear communication and active involvement of the client in the medical transaction are needed to develop a shared conceptualization of the problem. This in turn promotes adherence.

SUMMARY

In this chapter, we have examined the nature and determinants of symptom recognition, actions to restore health, disease-preventative actions, interaction with health providers, and adherence. Using a multiple cues and consequences framework, we have learned that these behaviors are complexly determined by stimuli occurring at multiple organizational levels. These behaviors are integral to the maintenance or restoration of good health.

Individuals actively process information from multiple levels, develop schemata and expectations, generate and evaluate possible courses of action, and make decisions about what actions to take. To influence clients' health-related behaviors effectively, health professionals must find ways to interface with the multiple determinants of these behaviors and with clients' active processing, planning, and decision making. Such an interface entails the involvement of clients as coparticipants in clinical and preventative health care and the use of interventions that address clients' thinking, emotions, behavior, and environment as well as their physiology.

REFERENCES

Andersen, R. (1968). *A behavioral model of families' use of health services*. Chicago: University of Chicago, Center for Health Administration Studies.

Becker, M. H., Drachman, R. H., & Kirscht, J. P. (1972). Predicting mothers' compliance with pediatric medical regimens. *Journal of Pediatrics, 81*, 843–854.

Becker, M. H., & Maiman, L. A. (1975). Sociobehavioral determinants of compliance with health and medical care recommendations. *Medical Care, 13*, 10–24.

Caplan, R. D. (1979). Patient, provider, and organization: Hypothesized determinants of adherence. In J. Cohen (Ed.), *New directions in patient compliance*, 209–223. Lexington, MA: D. C. Heath.

Chrisman, N. J., & Kleinman, A. (1983). Popular health care, social networks and cultural meanings: The orientation of medical anthropology. In D. Mechanic (Ed.), *Handbook of health, health care and the health professions*, 569–590. New York: The Free Press.

Clymer, R., Baum, A., & Krantz, D. S. (1984). Preferences for self care and involvement in health care. In A. Baum, S. E. Taylor & J. E. Singer (Eds.), *Handbook of psychology and health* (Vol. 4), 174–189. Hillsdale, NJ: Lawrence Erlbaum.

Costa, P. T., & McCrae, R. R. (1985). Hypochondriasis, neuroticism and aging: When are somatic complaints unfounded? *American Psychologist, 40*, 19–28.

Davis, M. S. (1966). Variations in patients' compliance with doctor's orders: Analysis of congruence between survey responses and results of empirical investigations. *Journal of Medical Education, 41*, 1037–1048.

DiMatteo, M. R., & DiNicola, D. D. (1982). Social science and the art of medicine: From Hippocrates to holism. In H. S. Friedman & M. R. DiMatteo (Eds.), *Interpersonal issues in health care*, 9–32. New York: Academic Press.

DiNicola, D. D., & DiMatteo, M. R. (1984). Practitioners, patients and compliance with medical regimens: A social psychological perspective. In A. Baum, S. E. Taylor & J. E. Singer (Eds.), *Handbook of psychology and health*, (Vol. 4), 295–316. Hillsdale, NJ: Lawrence Erlbaum.

Dunbar, J. M., & Stunkard, A. J. (1979). Adherence to diet and drug regimen. In R. Levy, B. Rifkind, B. Dennis & N. Ernst (Eds.), *Nutrition, lipids and coronary heart disease*, 391–424. New York: Raven Press.

Fabrega, H. (1974). *Disease and social behavior: An interdisciplinary perspective*. Cambridge, MA: MIT Press.

Fordyce, W. E., & Steger, J. C. (1979). Chronic pain. In O. F. Pomperleau & J. P. Brady (Eds.), *Behavioral medicine: Theory and practice*, 125–154. Baltimore: Williams & Wilkins.

Friedman, H. S., & DiMatteo, M. R. (1979). Interpersonal issues in health care: Healing as an interpersonal process. In H. S. Friedman & M. R. DiMatteo (Eds.), *Interpersonal issues in health care*, 3–8. New York: Academic Press.

Haynes, R. B. (1979a). A critical review of the determinants of patient compliance with therapeutic regimens. In D. L. Sackett & R. B. Haynes (Eds.), *Compliance with therapeutic regimen*, 26–39. Baltimore: Johns Hopkins University Press.

Haynes, R. B. (1979b). Introduction. In R. B. Haynes, D. W. Taylor & D. L. Sackett (Eds.), *Compliance in health care*, 1–10. Baltimore: Johns Hopkins University Press.

Janis, I. L., & Rodin, J. (1979). Attribution, control and decision making: Social psychology and health care. In G. C. Stone, F. Cohen & N. Adler (Eds.), *Health psychology: A handbook*, 487–522. San Francisco: Jossey-Bass.

Kanner, A. D., Coyne, J. C., Schaeffer, C., & Lazarus, R. S. (1981). Comparisons of two modes of stress measurement: Daily hassles and uplifts versus major life events. *Journal of Behavioral Medicine, 4*, 1–37.

Kirscht, J. P., Becker, M. H., & Eveland, J. P. (1976). Psychological and social factors as predictors of medical behavior. *Medical Care, 14*, 422–428.

Kirscht, J. P., & Rosenstock, I. M. (1979). Patients' problem in following recommendations of health care experts. In G. C. Stone, F. Cohen, & N. Adler (Eds.), *Health psychology: A handbook*, 189–216. San Francisco: Jossey-Bass.

Kristeller, J. L., & Rodin, J. (1984). A three-stage model of treatment continuity: Compliance, adherence and maintenance. In A. Baum, S. E. Taylor & J. E. Singer (Eds.), *Handbook of psychology and health*, (Vol. 4), 317–334. Hillsdale, NJ: Lawrence Erlbaum.

Lau, R. R., & Hartman, K. (1983). Commonsense representations of common illnesses. *Health Psychology, 2*, 167–186.

Leventhal, H. (1975). The consequences of depersonalization during illness and treatment: An information processing model. In J. Howard & A. Strauss (Eds.), *Humanizing health care*, 119–162. New York: John Wiley.

Leventhal, H. (1983). Behavioral medicine: Psychology in health care. In D. Mechanic (Ed.), *Handbook of health, health care, and the health care professions*, 709–743. New York: The Free Press.

Leventhal, H., Meyer, D., & Nerenz, D. (1980). The common sense representation of illness danger. In S. Rachman (Ed.), *Medical psychology* (Vol. 2), 7–30. New York: Pergamon.

Leventhal, H., Nerenz, D. R., & Steele, D. J. (1984). Illness representations, and coping with health threats. In A. Baum, S. E. Taylor & J. E. Singer (Eds.), *Handbook of psychology and health* (Vol. 4), 132–149. Hillsdale, NJ: Lawrence Erlbaum.

Ley, P. (1977). Psychological studies of doctor-patient communication. In S. Rachman (Ed.), *Contributions to medical psychology* (Vol. 1), 9–42. New York: Pergamon Press.

Ley, P., & Spellman, M. S. (1967). *Communicating with the patient*. London: Staples Press.

Meyer, D. (1981). *The effects of patients' representation of high blood pressure on behavior in treatment*. Unpublished doctoral dissertation, University of Wisconsin, Madison.

Pennebaker, J. W. (1982). *The psychology of physical symptoms*. New York: Springer-Verlag.

Pennebaker, J. W. (1984). Accuracy of symptom perception. In A. Baum, S. E. Taylor & J.

E. Singer (Eds.), *Handbook of psychology and health* (Vol. 4), 150–173. Hillsdale, NJ: Lawrence Erlbaum.

Rodin, J., & Janis, I. L. (1982). The social influences of physicians and health care providers. In H. S. Friedman & M. R. DiMatteo (Eds.), *Interpersonal issues in health care*, 33–50. New York: Academic Press.

Sackett, D. L., & Haynes, R. B. (Eds.). (1976). *Compliance with therapeutic regimens*. Baltimore: Johns Hopkins University Press.

Safer, M. A., Tharps, O. J., Jackson, T. C., & Leventhal, H. (1979). Determinants of three stages of delay in seeking care at a medical clinic. *Medical Care, 17*, 11–29.

Snyder, J., Rickson, D., & Parker, R. (1984). *Health beliefs questionnaire: Measurement of cognitive schema used in processing health-relevant information and in selecting health action*. Unpublished manuscript, Wichita State University.

Turk, D. C., Meichenbaum, D., & Genest, M. (1983). *Pain and behavioral medicine: A cognitive-behavioral perspective*. New York: Guilford Press.

Woods, S., Natterson, J., & Silverman, J. (1966). Medical students' disease: Hypochondriasis in medical education. *Journal of Medical Education, 41*, 785–790.

Zifferblatt, S. M. (1975). Increasing patient compliance through applied analysis of behavior. *Preventative Medicine, 4*, 173–182.

4

Stress

INTRODUCTION

In Chapter 2, the term stress was used to refer to the third, indirect influence of the environment and behavior on health. Unlike health habits that directly introduce health-altering agents into the body, stress refers to psychophysiological changes occurring in response to stimuli perceived as threatening or harmful. What we think and how we feel affects our health; the mind and the body are intimately connected. In this chapter we will review the notion of stress and its impact on health and disease.

DEFINITIONS OF STRESS

Stress is an elusive concept. It has been variously defined as an environmental event, a physiological response, and a cognitive-behavioral process. These definitions focus on one organizational level to the relative exclusion of others, which results in much confusion. Each of these single-level definitions will be briefly reviewed to place theory and research concerning stress into a historical context. Each of these perspectives is inadequate. The notion of stress is inherently a multilevel one; it consists of cognitive, emotional, behavioral, and physiological responses to transactions with the environment. After reviewing single-level theories, an integrated systems perspective of stress will be presented.

Stress as a Biological Response

The concept of stress in relation to physical health originated in the biological sciences. From the biological perspective, stress is defined as "a specific syndrome which consists of all the nonspecifically induced changes within the biologic system" (Selye, 1956, p. 11). Stress is a physiological response that is nonspecific in terms of both cause and effect. Any event that requires adaptation can trigger the physiological responses that characterize stress. These responses are also nonspecific; the changes observed are similar across various types of stress-inducing events. Let us take a brief look at the physiological responses used to define the stress response.

While Selye (1956) first popularized the notion of stress, Cannon (1927) was the first researcher to describe thoroughly a physiological reaction to threat, which he called the "fight or flight" response. Cannon noted that when an organism is faced with a threat to its survival, a stereotyped pattern of physiological changes occurs. There is an increase in heart rate, blood pressure, and respiration. Blood is distributed to large muscles and gastrointestinal processes are shut down. These changes prepare the organism to take vigorous physical action in response to the threat: either to fight or to flee. The arousal is a built-in activation that enhances the chance of survival under threatening conditions. We have all experienced this activation. Immediately after a "near miss" automobile accident, your heart pounds, there are "butterflies" in your stomach, and your palms sweat.

Selye (1956) observed a related set of generalized physiological responses when organisms were exposed to noxious stimuli like overcrowding, cold temperatures, or toxins. He called these responses the general adaptation syndrome (GAS). The GAS refers to neural and endocrine activities that permit organisms to withstand noxious stimuli physiologically. The GAS is divided into three phases: alarm, resistance, and exhaustion. During alarm, there is an initial activation very much like the "fight or flight" response. During resistance, there is a sustained secretion of hormones from the adrenal gland, which is thought to protect the organism from the noxious stimuli. If the stimuli continue unabated, these adrenal hormones begin to have deleterious effects on the circulatory, digestive, and immune systems. If the stressor continues long enough, the organism may die as its adaptive resources are exhausted.

While Selye and Cannon nicely demonstrated the physiological aspects of stress, they failed to recognize the importance of psychological and behavioral variables in determining these physiological responses. The occurrence of the "fight or flight" and GAS responses depends on a person's awareness of the noxious stimuli and interpretation of them as threatening or harmful. When noxious stimuli occur without the person's awareness, the biological responses are not observed (Mason, 1975b). For example, dying patients who are in a coma show no physiological evidence of stress whereas those who remain conscious demonstrate the response (Symington, Currie, Curran, & Davidson, 1955).

Selye and Cannon used noxious physical stimuli as stressors. The "fight or flight" and GAS responses are also elicited by noxious *psychological* events like boredom, an exam, and a gruesome film (Frankenhaeuser, 1972, 1978). Physiological arousal occurs in response to psychosocial as well as physical threats. In the experimental settings studied by Selye and Cannon, organisms were not given the opportunity to respond behaviorally to the stressors. In the natural environment, persons can typically respond to stressful events. The occurrence of the "fight or flight" and GAS responses depends on the ability to predict and control the noxious events. A series of studies by Weiss (1968, 1971a, 1971b) demonstrate the importance of this predictability and control. In one study, two groups of rats were exposed to a series of electric shocks. Subjects in one group could press a lever to escape the shock. Subjects in the second group had no control over the shock but received the same shock as the first group. Those rats that had control showed less gastric ulceration than those that had no control. In a similar experiment, rats given a visual signal indicating when the shock would occur showed fewer ulcers, even with no behavioral control, than rats receiving the same shock but no signal and no control. Being able to predict when a noxious event will occur is thus better than having no information. In the last experiment, Weiss demonstrated that rats that received a signal that their behavioral response was effective in terminating the shock had fewer ulcers than rats that had the same control over the shock but received no informational signal. To summarize Weiss's findings, a threatening event has fewer deleterious effects if we know when it is going to happen, if we can do something about it, and if we get feedback about the effectiveness of our action. The importance of predictability and control has also been demonstrated in humans' response to stressors (Rodin, 1980).

The notion that the physiological response to stress is nonspecific (i.e., the same under all noxious conditions) has also been challenged. The exact physiological changes observed depend on how the person responds behaviorally and emotionally. Different physiological patterns have been found when persons respond to stressors with fear rather than anger (Mason, 1975a), with vigilance rather than action (Obrist, 1976), and with a competitive, hostile rather than a calm approach (Dembroski, 1981). How we interpret and deal with a threatening situation influences the pattern of physiological arousal associated with that situation. The biological response perspective on stress is not incorrect, but it is incomplete.

Stress as an Environmental Event

The notion of stress as an environmental event resulted from repeated observations of physiological and behavioral breakdown in persons exposed to extreme conditions like military combat (Grinker & Spiegal, 1945) and bereavement (Lindemann, 1944). If extreme environments resulted in negative effects, it was reasoned that the accumulation of less extreme events may also have deleterious effects. From this perspective, stress is defined as any enviromental event that places a demand on the individual, taxing available resources and requiring an unusual response (Holroyd, 1979). Stress resides in the "demandingness" of the event rather than in the person.

Research generated by the environmental perspective is epidemiological in nature; the number and severity of stressful events experienced by a person are predictive of that person's health status (Dohrenwend & Dohrenwend, 1981). Methodologically, individuals are asked to indicate which of a list of stressful events they experienced in a given period (e.g., the last six months). An example of such a list is the Schedule of Recent Events or SRE (Holmes & Rahe, 1967). The SRE includes such items as divorce, marriage, birth of a child, incarceration, taking out a mortgage, and Christmas. Each item is weighted based on the assumption that some experiences are uniformly more demanding (marriage) for people than are others (Christmas). The weighting of events explicitly assumes that a given event is uniformly stressful for all persons. Both positive and negative events are seen as stressors since both require adaptation.

Numerous studies have used the SRE to assess the relationship between stress and health. Studies attempting to predict future disease and to account for existing disease have found a relationship between the number and severity of stressors and the likelihood of diseases such as sudden cardiac death, heart attacks, tuberculosis (Rabkin & Struening, 1976), and a number of infectious ailments (Jemmott & Locke, 1984).

There are several problems with the environmental approach to stress. The strength of the relationship between stress and disease is modest; the average correlation is about .12 with a maximum of .30 (Tanig, 1982). Environmental measures of stress have limited predictive power. Contrary to the environmental perspective, not all change is necessarily stressful. Developmental changes like menopause and retirement are not experienced as stressful if they occur "on time" and are expected. In some cases, the lack of change may be stressful. For example, experiencing chronic boredom or not getting a promotion are often experienced as stressful (Lazarus & Folkman, 1984).

Nor are events uniformly stressful for all individuals. The degree of stress depends on the meaning of the event and the resources available to the individual. For example, Larazus, Opton, Nomikos, and Rankin (1965) had subjects view a film of gruesome woodmill accidents in which one worker saws off a finger and another is killed by a plank driven through his chest. Prior to observing the film, some subjects were told the film was staged and other subjects were given no explanation. Those who were told the film was staged experienced less arousal and distress, presumably because they appraised the events as "not real." Appraisal plays a central role in determining the degree to which an event is stressful.

The degree of stress also depends on the skills and resources available to the person for coping with an event. Nucholls, Cassel, and Kaplan (1972) assessed the effects of stress and coping during pregnancy on birth complications. They found that neither a life-events measure of stress nor an index of coping resources was related to medical complications during delivery. However, when life events and coping were considered jointly, a strong relationship was found. Ninety percent of the women with high life-change scores and low coping ability evidenced at least one complication, whereas only 33% of women with high change scores and high coping ability evidenced any complications.

The notion of stress as a demanding environmental event is inadequate. Recent revisions of stressful event inventories have remedied some of these weaknesses by asking individuals to rate the degree to which experienced events had a positive or negative impact (Sarason, Johnson, & Siegel, 1978). Via such ratings, these new measures attempt to account for persons' appraisal and coping abilities. Contrary to the notion that any kind of change is stressful, data from revised measures have shown that positive events may be health promoting rather than health destructive (DeLongis, Coyne, Dakof, Folkman, & Lazarus, 1982; Sarason et al., 1978).

The environmental and biological perspectives on stress are basically S-R (stimulus-response) models. They provide little insight into the variables and processes that mediate the relationship between noxious events and biological responses. If stressful events lead to negative health outcomes, just how does this occur?

Stress as a Cognitive-Behavioral Phenomenon

The cognitive-behavioral approach defines stress as a transaction between the person and the environment in which the person evaluates the environmental event as harmful or threatening and in which the person's adaptive resources are taxed or strained (Lazarus, 1966; Lazarus & Folkman, 1984). Stress does not reside in either the event or the person's response alone, but in both factors as well as the cognitive-behavioral responses mediating them. Because it explicitly emphasizes cognitive and behavioral (psychological) levels in understanding stress, this approach remedies many of the deficiencies of the biological and environmental models of stress.

Two processes are central to the psychological-behavioral perspective: cognitive appraisal and coping. Cognitive appraisal refers to an evaluative process by which a person determines whether and to what extent an event is threatening or harmful. An event is stressful only if it is appraised as noxious. Coping refers to a person's behavioral, cognitive, and emotional responses to an event. An event is stressful only in so far as a person lacks the means to cope. By integrating cognitive, affective, behavioral, and environmental aspects of stress, this perspective thus serves as a useful starting point in building a systems approach to stress. The cognitive-behavioral approach largely ignores biological aspects of stress and the mechanisms that connect the cognitive, affective, and behavioral levels with the biological level.

STRESS: A SYSTEMS VIEW

Stress is an organizing concept referring to many variables and processes occurring at many levels of analysis: physiological, cognitive-affective, behavioral, and environmental. Stress is therefore an integrated biopsychosocial response to events that are perceived as harmful and that strain a person's coping skills. We will explore each of these levels in detail and demonstrate their reciprocal influence.

Cognitive Appraisal

Aversive environmental, physiological, and mental stimuli do not reflexively elicit a stress response. Persons do not passively receive but rather actively appraise stimuli. Appraisal is the process by which we make sense of events that occur within and around us (Levine, Weinberg, & Ursin, 1978). We constantly evaluate the personal relevance and hedonic connotations of stimuli to which we attend. Based on past experience and the current situation, stimuli are evaluated as: (1) irrelevant (a state of no particular significance); (2) benign (a positive state of affairs that enhances personal well-being); or (3) negative (a potential or actual negative state threatens personal well-being) (Lazarus & Launier, 1978). Stress involves the appraisal of stimuli as threatening, harmful, or challenging.

Suppose you are driving to the mountains for a skiing vacation and encounter a blizzard. The roads are passable but very icy. Several cars and trucks can be seen in the ditches by the side of the road. It is difficult for you to control your car. You would probably feel both anxious and angry. You are in physical danger and may miss a long-planned and expensive vacation. As suggested by this vignette, a given situation can elicit several types of negative appraisal.

Once an event has been evaluated negatively, another evaluation is made that focuses on what can be done to deal with the event and the effectiveness of those actions. This is called coping appraisal (Lazarus & Folkman, 1984). While the major question addressed by stimulus appraisal is, "What does this event mean for me?," coping appraisal addresses the questions, "What can I do to respond to this problem?" and "How effective are those responses?" This step consists of generating strategies to cope with the stressor and estimating the effectiveness of those strategies.

To continue with the driving example, your concern about road conditions and your desire to go skiing would lead to an examination of your options. You could pull off the road and wait for a snowplow. You could drive slowly until the next exit and wait out the storm. You could also buy chains at that exit and continue your trip. You could look for an alternate route that may be less hazardous. You could implement any of these options, but would they help? None except stopping where you are would terminate the immediate physical danger. But that may result in a more serious long-term threat: having no food and limited gas to stay warm. The other options are better in the long run. However, if you stop at the exit and wait until the storm is over, your lodge reservations will be canceled. The other routes, according to the radio, are no better.

Both a negative evaluation of the stimulus event and an evaluation of insufficient or ineffective coping resources are needed for stress to occur. While these two types of cognitive appraisal have been discussed separately to clarify the process, they may occur simultaneously and relatively automatically. The degree to which an event is appraised as negative and to which coping resources are appraised as inadequate varies in intensity. Stimulus and coping appraisals interact in shaping the intensity of the stress experienced. The greatest stress occurs (as in the driving example) when the stimulus is very negative and no strategies are available to effectively mitigate the event. As the event is less negative or as coping efforts become available, the intensity of stress decreases. However, some stress will be experienced when the stimulus event is appraised as highly negative even if effective coping strategies are available (e.g., exams like the GRE, LSAT, and MCAT even when you are prepared) because of the importance of the event. Similarly, when the event is only slightly negative but no effective coping strategies are at hand (e.g., being in a dental chair or driving in an unpopulated area), some stress will be experienced because of the potential loss of control.

As described, the appraisal process seems quite detached and analytical, which does not fit with our subjective experience of threat or harm. An emotional reaction occurs simultaneously with the appraisal process (Leventhal & Nerenz, 1983). When an event is appraised as benign, positive emotions such as joy, love, happiness, exhilaration or peacefulness are experienced. When an event is appraised as negative, emotions such as fear, anxiety, anger, guilt, frustration, or depression are experienced. The appraisal process is affectively toned. Cognitive and affective processes influence each other (Schacter, 1964). In fact, a person may need to manage emotional arousal in addition to the negative stimulus event itself. In the driving example, driving on a slick road generated fear, and the delay or loss of a vacation evoked anger.

The appraisal process is subjective but not adventitious. It is influenced by the nature of the stimulus event and by characteristics of the person making the appraisal. This is the real meaning of the transactional notion of stress (Lazarus, 1966). Personality, past experience, and other person variables shape appraisal, especially when the stimulus event is ambiguous. But a person's appraisal is constrained by the nature of the stimulus event. When an event is relatively unambiguous, appraisal is usually congruent with the objective nature of that event. Let us look at person and stimulus factors that contribute to appraisal.

Person Factors in Appraisal. The appraisal of stimuli and the coping responses available to respond to those stimuli are strongly influenced by person variables (Wrubel, Brenner, & Lazarus, 1981). A large number of person variables have been studied in relation to stress (see Cohen, 1979, for a review). Following Lazarus and Folkman (1984), we will examine only two person variables: commitments and beliefs.

Commitments are what an individual values and considers important. This includes goals and activities into which energy is invested and groups and organizations with whom an individual identifies. Think about your commitments. What persons, activities and goals are very important to you? Any threat, harm, or challenge to your commitments potentially poses intense stress. If you love a person, threats to that person or to that relationship are particularly upsetting.

Commitments affect appraisal by influencing our sensitivity to certain stimuli. The more we have invested in a particular person, goal, or activity, the greater is the stress generated when that person, goal, or activity is threatened. Commitments increase our vulnerability. Think of a person with whom you are deeply in love. A rejection by that person would cause extreme hurt because of your strong attachment. On the other hand, your love for that person can also generate moments of great excitement, fulfillment, and pleasure. Commitment is a two-edged sword.

A more health-relevant example is the "will to live." The loss of a spouse (who represents a major interpersonal commitment) often results in illness and is associated with excess mortality of the surviving partner (Jacobs & Ostfeld, 1977; Parks, 1970). Conversely, finding meaning and having strong commitments can enhance the chances of survival, even in the worst circumstances. Almost all survivors of Nazi concentration camps reported finding some reason to survive: to bear witness, for the sake of relatives, or for revenge (Frankl, 1959). Commitments motivate us to persist in the face of adversity. When confronted with a threat to something we value, we will work particularly hard to eliminate that threat.

A second person variable affecting appraisal is our sense of control over events. A sense of control decreases stress, whereas a lack of control exacerbates stress. For example, Ferrare (1962) found that aging persons who were relocated to a nursing home by their own choice (i.e., had control) lived longer than those who were relocated without their choice (i.e., had low control). Similarly, Langer & Rodin (1976) examined the effects of enhancing the control of elderly nursing home residents. Residents in a group given responsibility and choice over daily activities and living arrangements, were more alert, active, and happy compared to a group encouraged to feel the staff would take care of them. The residents with enhanced control also demonstrated better physical health. Within eighteen months, 15% of those with enhanced control had died versus 30% of the residents in the other group.

The lack of control, perceived or real, is often called helplessness (Seligman, 1975). Helplessness occurs when individuals feel that their behavior has no effect on consequences or that events are uncontrollable. It is characterized by behavioral passivity, depressive affect, and thoughts centering on hopelessness. Helpless persons stop trying, even in a new set of circumstances (Miller & Seligman, 1975). They have negative expectations about themselves, the future, and the world (Beck, 1976); believing "I'm no good, the world's no good, and it's not going to get any better."

Perceived control influences the impact of stress on a person. Stress is exacerbated when persons feel behavior and outcome are unrelated. The lack of control has negative effects behaviorally, emotionally, and physiologically.

Situational Factors in Appraisal. Properties of the stimulus event also affect appraisal. We will focus on two such stimulus properties: predictability and timing. Predictability refers to knowledge about when an event will occur. Generally, predictable events are less stressful than unpredictable events. It is advantageous to know whether and when an aversive event will occur. Predictability reduces threat, harm, or challenge by allowing us to prepare for the event and to know when we are safe (Weinberg & Levine, 1980).

The importance of predictability was demonstrated in a study by Hunter (1979) of wives whose husbands were killed in action, missing in action, prisoners of war, or returned home from the Vietnam conflict. Predictability decreased for the wives in the following order: returned, killed in action, prisoner of war, and missing in action. Hunter found that the wives of men missing in action evidenced the worst emotional and physical health. They were faced with the greatest uncertainty concerning their marital status, roles, and responsibilities. They were in limbo.

The imminence, duration, and frequency of stress also affect appraisal. As an event becomes more imminent, it is appraised as increasingly threatening or challenging. Mechanic (1962) found that students preparing for doctoral exams experienced more anxiety and physical symptoms as the exams got nearer. Once the exams actually began, there was considerable emotional relief and the symptoms diminished. One student said, "Taking it was not as bad as anticipating it. . . .You don't have to worry while you are doing it" (p. 153).

The duration of stressors ranges from time-limited events, such as exams and dental work, to ongoing events, such as marital conflict, combat, and cancer. The duration and frequency of stressors are assumed to play a central role in determining the negative effects of stress on health. The assumption is that chronic stress wears a person down (Selye, 1956), but remarkably little research is available on the impact of stressors that vary according to frequency or duration.

The systems model of stress, as developed to this point, is shown in Figure 4-1. Stress consists of the appraisal of a stimulus as harmful, threatening, or challenging and of coping resources as inadequate or ineffective. These appraisals result from the interaction of the characteristics of the person (commitments, beliefs, memories, and experiences) and the event being appraised (predictability, timing, and ambiguity).

FIGURE 4-1 The Systems Model of Stress: Appraisal and Affect

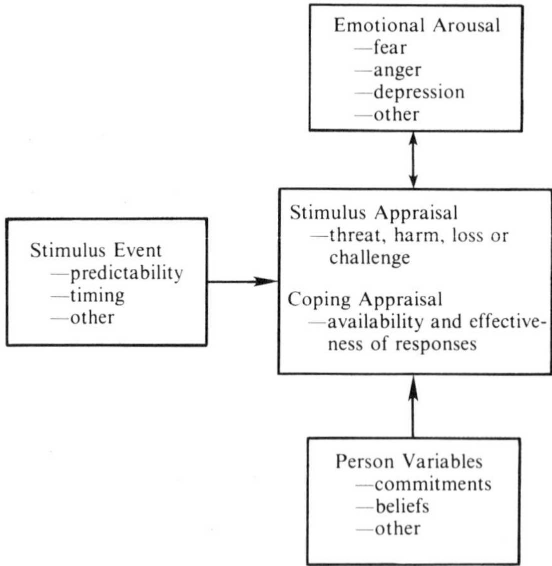

The appraisal of a stimulus as stressful also results in an emotional arousal that in turn interacts with the appraisal.

Coping

Coping refers to cognitive and behavioral actions taken to manage the demands of an event appraised as stressful. When faced with a stressor, individuals try to remediate the harm or prevent the threat. Limited data are available to identify how persons cope with stressors in the natural environment. The variety of possible coping strategies is immense. Table 4-1 outlines the major categories of coping strategies. Let us take a moment to understand this table.

There are two major targets of coping: changing ourselves or changing our environment. Persons can either make adjustments to fit better with the environment ("go with the flow") or change the environment to suit their own needs ("divide and conquer"). Imagine, for example, that your neighbors are having a noisy party that interrupts your sleep. You could join the party (change yourself) or call the police (change the environment). The self versus environment distinction is shown in Table 4-1.

Coping efforts can be either emotion oriented or problem oriented. Emotion-oriented coping focuses on reducing the emotional arousal caused by the stress. Problem-oriented coping focuses on altering the event appraised as threatening or harmful. Problem- and emotion-oriented coping may be implemented simultaneously or separately and may be incompatible. In most stressful situations, coping efforts focus on both (Folkman & Lazarus, 1980). Imagine you are very anxious about the midterm exams scheduled for next week. Problem-oriented coping would consist of intensive studying. Emotion-focused coping could involve taking tranquilizers to reduce your anxiety. It may appear that problem-oriented coping is preferable because it "gets at the root of the problem," but coping with emotional responses to stress is also important. Emotions are often painful and distressing and may consequently be a source of stress. Emotional arousal can also interfere with skilled cognitive and behavioral efforts to deal with the problem. We have to

TABLE 4-1 A Conceptual Scheme of Coping Strategies

	GOAL OF CHANGE	
Target of Change	Emotional Regulation	Problem Solution
Self	Cognitive Behavioral	Cognitive Behavioral
Environment	Cognitive Behavioral	Cognitive Behavioral

get ourselves under control before we can tackle the problem. In some cases (e.g., natural disasters or enduring disabilities), there may be little we can do to deal with the problem. The primary task is to cope with the emotional arousal elicited by those events. Our coping strategies take three major forms: cognitive, behavioral, and social.

Cognitive Coping Strategies. We can cope with a stressor or our emotions by problem solving, self-talk, and reappraisal. Problem solving involves analyzing the situation to generate possible courses of action, to evaluate the efficacy of those actions, and to select an effective plan of action (Janis & Mann, 1977). To continue with the midterm exams example, problem solving could focus on how to reduce our anxiety (emotion oriented, self as target), on how to study to get good grades (problem oriented, self as target), on which classes to drop to reduce worry (emotion oriented, environment as target), or on how to enlist the aid of fellow students to study (problem oriented, environment as target).

Self-talk refers to covert statements or thoughts that are used to direct our efforts at coping with the stressful event and its associated emotional arousal. This internal talk directs attention to relevant stimuli, facilitates the formulation and implementation of coping strategies, and provides corrective feedback (Meichenbaum, 1977). Imagine reclining in a dental chair, awaiting a root canal procedure. You might use the following self-statements: "The dentist is a caring person: he'll take care not to hurt me" (emotion oriented, environment as target); "I'm really tense, need to take a couple of deep breaths to relax" (emotion oriented, self as target); "Maybe I can make this easier by distracting myself with pictures on the ceiling" (problem oriented, environment as target); or "I need to develop a plan to deal with this" (problem oriented, self as target).

Reappraisal involves reducing the impact of a stressful event by altering how that event is interpreted. In other words, the event is given a different meaning. A student could deal with an F on an exam by thinking, "The test was unfair" (problem oriented, environment as target), or "I just had a bad day" (problem oriented, self as target). The anger engendered by the F could be reappraised by thinking, "The teacher is a real creep, I have a right to be angry" (emotion oriented, environment as target), or "No big deal, this course isn't important anyway" (emotion oriented, self as target).

Behavioral Coping Strategies. Persons also respond to stress behaviorally. There are four general classes of behavioral responses to stress: seeking information, direct action, inhibiting action, and turning to others. Seeking information refers to gathering data on the nature of the stressor and on possible coping strategies. An individual faced with a diagnosis of cancer, for example, may seek information about prognosis from a health care provider (Haan, 1977). That individual may use changes in the size of a palpable tumor to assess the effectiveness of chemotherapy (Nerenz, Leventhal, & Love, 1982). Information thus provides useful, instrumental coping strategies and enhances feelings of control and predictability.

Direct action refers to overt verbal and motor responses that alter the stressor or stress-related emotional arousal. An individual with a sprained ankle may rest, take pain pills, or see a physician to find relief. An individual who has recently experienced the death of a loved one may bury himself in his work or look at old pictures to deal with his grief.

Inhibiting action involves not doing something in order to reduce stress and emotional arousal. A person with a persistent cough may stop smoking. Avoidance of anxiety provoking situations would also fit in this category. For example, persons frequently "miss" their appointments with health providers because of the pain and embarrassment associated with those visits. The last class of behavioral coping, turning to others, has been traditionally labeled social support.

Social Support. The phrase "turning to others" is used here because it emphasizes the active, interactional nature of this coping strategy. Our relationships with other persons provide an important resource in dealing with stress. We can gain material, emotional, and informational support from others. Material support includes the money, goods, and services available from significant others (Cohen & McKay, 1984). Emotional support is the feeling of being loved and valued by others and the opportunity to reciprocate those feelings (Cobb, 1976). Informational support is available when others make suggestions about the meaning of stressful events or recommendations concerning coping strategies, and provide feedback about the appropriateness of coping efforts (Cohen & McKay, 1984).

Social support may modulate stress in two ways. First, such support may prevent stress. Knowing that others care and will help are stress protective because the events are then perceived as less threatening (Singer & Lord, 1984). The lack of social support is related to poor health. Berkman and Syme (1979), for example, found social support to be a modest but significant predictor of mortality, even when controlling for initial health status, health-impairing behaviors, and social status. Those persons with few social ties had higher mortality rates.

Social support may also mitigate the negative effects of stress that have already occurred. For example, social support is associated with longer survival time among those with cancer (Weisman & Worden, 1975). A large proportion of the problems most frequently reported by persons with the disease are interpersonal. These include difficulty communicating with significant others about the cancer, speaking with family members about the future, and gaining information from health providers (Wortman & Dunkel-Schetter, 1979). Health providers, family, and friends can provide cancer victims with clarification and reassurance about what is happening, show love and caring, and assist in developing strategies to deal with the physical and emotional demands of cancer and its treatment. Social support also promotes recovery by enhancing adherence to treatment regimens (Suls, 1982).

Caring relationships enhance physical and mental health. The timing and manner in which social support is offered significantly influence its impact. Well-meaning assistance that is not wanted is not helpful. Social support is not a reservoir from which a person passively borrows but rather an interpersonal exchange in which both parties are active (Cohen & McKay, 1984). Social support may also have negative effects. For example, significant others can interfere with adherence to treatment regimens, suggest ineffective coping strategies, or create a dependence by a person who is ill (Suls, 1982).

Determinants of Coping. A wide variety of coping strategies can be used to respond to stress. The selection of strategies is influenced by person and situational variables. Such person variables as values and beliefs that prescribe and proscribe certain types of action affect how a person copes with a stressor. A response must also be in a person's repertoire before it can be used to cope with a stressor. While divorce may seem to be the logical solution to marital conflict or abuse, this alternative may be unacceptable to persons who hold religious beliefs that divorce is sinful. An assertive response may seem the logical choice in dealing with persons who are unreasonable or abrasive, but some people have not learned to express their feelings and opinions in a direct, forceful manner. In sum, coping actions must be available and acceptable to the person.

The situation in which a stressor occurs may also affect the means by which a person copes. Obviously, the stressor itself can constrain the availability and effectiveness of coping strategies. The loss of a loved one through death requires largely an emotion-oriented form of coping; it is not possible to bring the person back. The context in which the stressor occurs may also constrain coping. Slugging the boss in response to an unreasonable job request is unlikely because of its consequences. Our coping efforts usually fit with our environmental demands and constraints.

THE PHYSIOLOGY OF STRESS

In Chapter 1, we learned that disturbances at one level in a system often result in changes at other levels in the system. While stress entails a cognitive appraisal of threat or harm, this appraisal evokes physiological as well as affective and behavioral responses. In this section, we will detail the physiology of stress.

Biological Pathways Activated During Stress

The physiological response to stress is mediated via the nervous, endocrine, and immune systems. An overview of these response systems is shown in Figure 4-2. Neural, endocrine, and immune responses to stress occur under differing temporal gradients. Immediate physiological responses are mediated by the autonomic nervous system (ANS). In-

FIGURE 4-2 Physiological Pathways in the Stress Response. (From *The Physiology of Stress* by M. F. Asterita, 1985, New York: Human Sciences Press. Copyright 1985 by the Human Sciences Press. Reprinted by permission.)

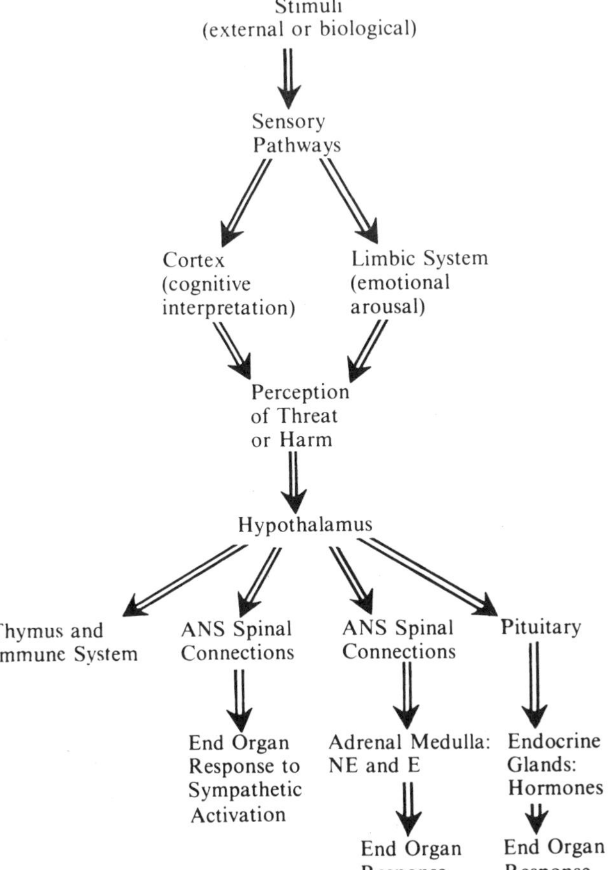

termediate responses are mediated by the adrenal medulla, an endocrine gland under the control of the ANS. The long-term responses are mediated by the endocrine and immune systems. Each of these systems has broad effects on target tissues in the body (Allen, 1983). These responses are in turn controlled by the hypothalamus, a group of neurons at the base of the brain. The hypothalamus along with the limbic system (that part of the brain mediating emotions) controls basic body functions such as eating, drinking, sexual activity, emotions, pleasure, and punishment. The limbic system and the hypothalamus are influenced by the cerebral cortex, the outer portion of the brain that mediates higher order functions such as thinking, reasoning, and memory. These structures are shown in Figure 4-3.

The Autonomic Nervous System

The autonomic nervous system controls basic body processes such as heart rate, respiration, blood pressure, and digestion. The ANS also controls visceral functions with minimal awareness on our part. There are two divisions of the ANS: sympathetic and parasympathetic. The sympathetic division prepares the organism to take action; its general effect on target tissues is arousal. The parasympathetic division is concerned with the maintenance of basic body requirements; its general effects could be described as housekeeping chores: getting rid of wastes, building up energy stores, and taking care of infections. These two divisions often have antagonistic effects on the body. For example, the sympathetic division increases heart rate while the parasympathetic slows it. They act respectively like an accelerator and brake pedal in a car. The net effect on a given organ is a function of the relative activation of the two divisions.

The effects of sympathetic and parasympathetic activation on various body organs are shown in Table 4-2. Understanding and recalling all of these effects appear to be formidable tasks. However, sympathetic activation most commonly occurs under stress and prepares the person to take vigorous action, either "fight or flight," to deal with the stressor. Increased heart contraction rate, force, and volume speed delivery of the oxygen and energy needed for the vigorous activity of large skeletal muscles (i.e., to fight or flee). Blood vessels to the skeletal muscles dilate, increasing the blood supply needed for large muscle activity. Blood vessels to the gut contract, slowing food absorption. Blood vessels to the skin also contract, minimizing blood loss in case of injury. Enhanced blood coagulation also minimizes blood loss in case of injury. Both systolic and diastolic blood pressure increase.

The increase in respiration rate and the dilation of the bronchi enhance the exchange of oxygen and carbon dioxide to meet metabolic demands of vigorous action. Perspiration increases to rid the body of excess heat. Body functions not immediately contributing to survival via

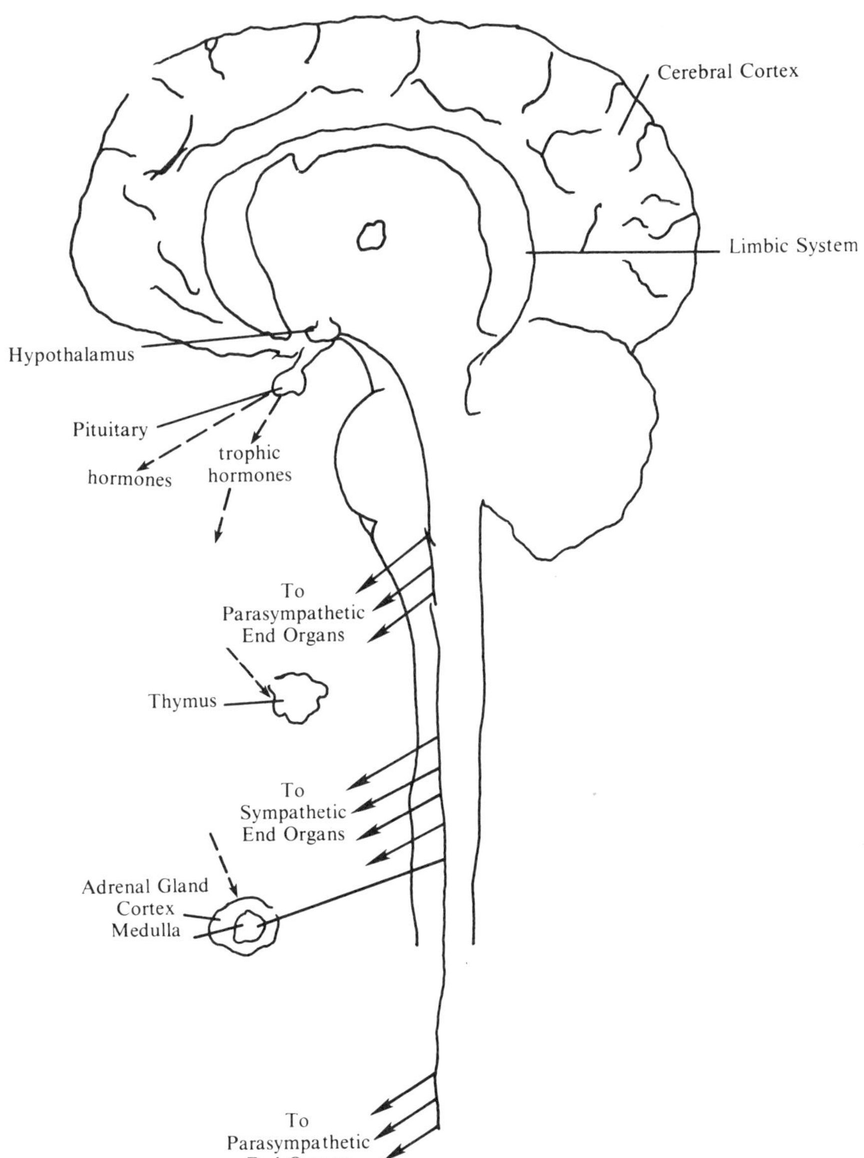

FIGURE 4-3 Anatomy of the Structures Involved in the Stress Response

TABLE 4-2 Functional Effects of the Sympathetic and Parasympathetic Activation

ORGAN	SYMPATHETIC EFFECT	PARASYMPATHETIC EFFECT
Eye	Dilates pupil Relaxes ciliary muscle	Contracts pupil Contracts ciliary muscle
Glands		
Lacrimal	——	Stimulates secretion
Salivary	Inhibits secretion	Stimulates secretion
Sweat	Stimulates secretion	Inhibits secretion
Heart	Increases contraction rate, force, and volume	Decreases contraction rate and force
Blood vessels	Vasodilates vessels to heart and large muscles Vasoconstricts vessels to skin and gut	—— ——
Lungs	Dilates bronchi	Constricts bronchi
Gut		
Lumen	Decreases peristalsis and tone	Increases peristalsis and tone
Sphincters	Increases tone	Decreases tone
Secretions	Decreases	Increases
Blood		
Coagulation	Increases	——
Glucose	Increases	——
Liver	Releases glucose	——
Basal metabolism	Increases	——
Piloerectors	Stimulated	——

fight or flight are shut down. There is decreased activity in the digestive system. Peristalsis is slowed, and sphincters in the gastrointestinal tract and in the urinary bladder constrict to minimize the elimination of body wastes.

The sympathetic, or "fight or flight," response is quickly elicited in response to stress because it is mediated by neural connections. It is a relatively automatic and biologically programmed response to physical and psychosocial stressors. We have all experienced these changes when physically threatened by someone, when suddenly coming upon a snake, or when nearly having an automobile accident. These changes also occur in response to threats to our psychosocial well-being: taking tests, feeling angry at someone, or speaking before a large crowd. But our body reacts the same under both conditions; it does not know the difference.

The Adrenal Medulla

The effects of sympathetic activation are short-lived. Arousal is maintained by an intermediate mechanism—the release of epinephrine (E) and norepinephrine (NE) from the adrenal medulla. The adrenal gland is located at the top of the kidneys and consists of two functionally distinct parts: the medulla and the cortex. As a result of sympathetic activation, E and NE are released by the adrenal medulla. Once in the bloodstream, E and NE circulate and influence target organs. Their effects are very similar to those of sympathetic activation. They reinforce and prolong the physiological arousal resulting from sympathetic activation and thus also foster the "fight or flight" response. The specific effects of E and NE are shown in Table 4-3. The net results of those effects are an increase in heart rate, blood pressure, respiration, and blood sugar levels and a decrease in gastrointestinal activity.

The adrenal response is slower to occur but lasts longer than the sympathetic response because it involves both neural and chemical pathways. Generally it takes 20 to 30 seconds for the physiological effects of E and NE to be observed. These effects last an hour or more, because E and NE are slowly removed from circulation. The duration of E and NE effects is about ten times that of sympathetic effects.

TABLE 4-3 Physiological Effects of Epinephrine and Norepinephrine

ORGAN	NOREPINEPHRINE	EPINEPHRINE
Heart	Increases contraction rate and force	Increases contraction rate and force
Blood vessels	Vasoconstricts blood vessels	Vasoconstricts blood vessels to skin and gut, vasodilates vessels to muscle
Lungs	Dilates bronchi, increases respiration rate	Dilates bronchi, increases respiration rate
Gut		
Lumen	Decreases peristalsis and tone	Decreases peristalsis and tone
Sphincters	Increases tone	Increases tone
Blood		
Coagulation	—	Increases
Glucose	—	Increases
Liver	—	Releases glucose
Basal metabolism	—	Increases
Pancreas	Inhibits insulin secretion	Inhibits insulin secretion

The Endocrine and Immune Systems

The endocrine and immune systems mediate the third set of physiological changes in response to stress. Four endocrine glands are primarily involved in the stress response: pituitary, thyroid, adrenal cortex, and pancreas. These glands secrete hormones into the circulatory system that affect target organs sensitive to those chemicals. In contrast to sympathetic activation and the effects of E and NE from the adrenal cortex, the latency of hormonal activation in response to stress is long, requiring minutes to hours before an end organ response is observed. The effects of these hormonal changes also last longer. Figure 4-4 presents an overview of the endocrine system. Let us consider each of the endocrine glands in more detail.

The pituitary gland is located at the base of the brain and is controlled by the hypothalamus. The pituitary is often called the master gland because of its controlling influence over other endocrine glands. The pituitary is divided into two parts: the anterior and posterior lobes. The anterior lobe secretes six hormones. Five of these hormones are called trophic hormones because they influence the secretions of other endocrine glands. In terms of the stress response, we will focus on two of these trophic hormones: adrenocorticotrophic hormone (ACTH) and thyroid-stimulating hormone (TSH). The sixth hormone released by the anterior pituitary is growth hormone (GH). GH has a direct effect on body tissue independent of other endocrine glands; it is not a trophic hormone. The release of hormones from the anterior pituitary is controlled by chemical messages from the hypothalamus. Hypothalamic release of these chemical messages is in turn controlled by circulating levels of hormones in the bloodstream (a negative feedback loop arrangement) and by neural input from the limbic system and the cerebral cortex.

FIGURE 4-4 Endocrine Responses to Stress

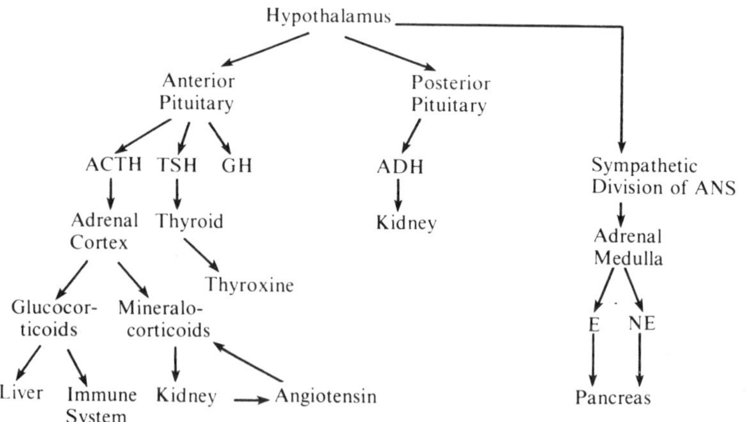

The posterior pituitary secretes two hormones: antidiuretic hormone (ADH) and oxytocin. Both of these hormones have a direct influence on body tissue; they are not trophic hormones. Only ADH is involved in the stress reponse. ADH is actually manufactured in the hypothalamus and then transported by small blood vessels to the posterior pituitary for storage. Its release is controlled by osmoreceptors in the hypothalamus, which are sensitive to body fluid levels. Because ADH influences body fluid levels, there is again a negative feedback loop.

Under stress, there is an increased release of growth hormone by the pituitary. GH enhances the cellular utilization of energy and effects an increase in blood sugar (Asterita, 1985). The resulting increase in available energy and efficient utilization of that energy prepare the person to take vigorous physical action in response to the stressor. Under stress, the pituitary also releases ADH, which acts on the kidney to increase fluid reabsorption to raise fluid levels in the body (Asterita, 1985), which protects against potential blood loss and shock due to injury. It also results in increased blood pressure because of an increase in blood volume.

The adrenal cortex is the outer portion of the adrenal gland. Two classes of hormones are released by the adrenal cortex: glucocorticoids and mineralocorticoids. The release of glucocorticoids is controlled by ACTH from the pituitary. The amount of circulating glucocorticoids affects hypothalamus-pituitary release of ACTH. Under stress, there is an increase in ACTH release and consequently in the secretion of glucocorticoids from the adrenal cortex. The glucocorticoids mobilize proteins and fats from body tissues and cause the liver to convert these proteins and fats to glucose. This results in an increase in sugar and fat levels in the blood, providing the person with the readily available supply of energy needed for a physical response to a stressor. The glucocorticoids also affect the body's response to injury and infection. They suppress inflammation in response to injury and infection by inhibiting the passage of plasma out of the bloodstream and the ability of white blood cells to reach the site of injury or infection. The glucocorticoids also inhibit the immune response by shrinking the thymus, spleen, and lymph nodes and by suppressing the development of lymphocytes and antibodies (Asterita, 1985). The increased release of glucocorticoids under stress thus not only keeps the "furnace stoked with fuel" but suppresses the body's built-in defenses against injury and infection. This makes sense if we keep in mind that the immediate goal of the physiological response to stress is to prepare the body for physical action. Reduced inflammation keeps blood plasma in the bloodstream, where it transports energy and promotes the physical mobility needed for "fight or flight." The manufacture of lymphocytes and antibodies requires protein; the glucocorticoids are mobilizing this available protein for conversion to glucose for energy. The housekeeping chores dealing with injury and infection are sacrificed to deal with the immediate threat. The second major class of hormones released by the adrenal cortex is the mineralocorticoids. The mineralocorticoids act on the kidney to enhance the retention of salt and fluid in the body. This increases blood volume and blood pressure, thus complementing the action of ADH (Asterita, 1985).

The thyroid gland is located in the neck just below the larynx. The release of thyroxine by the thyroid is controlled by thyroid-stimulating hormone (TSH) from the pituitary. Thyroxine enhances glucose metabolism and utilization. It also increases oxygen utilization by cells. Under stress, increased thyroxine is secreted. The mobilization of available energy and the enhanced utilization of that energy prepare the person to take action in response to stress (Asterita, 1985).

The pancreas is located next to the stomach. It functions as an endocrine gland and secretes two hormones, glucagon and insulin. Their secretion is under the control of blood glucose levels. Glucagon stimulates the release of stored sugars into the bloodstream. Under stress, the heavy utilization of blood sugars as a result of physical activity stimulates the release of glucagon to replenish blood sugar levels, keeping the person ready for physical action. Insulin has the opposite effect. When blood sugar levels are high, insulin secretion is stimulated, resulting in the storage of sugar in liver, muscle, and fat tissue. The lowered blood sugar levels resulting from vigorous activity under stress inhibits insulin release. While the increase in blood sugar levels resulting from the increased release of E, NE, thyroxine, and glucocorticoids under stress would normally stimulate insulin release, E from the adrenal medulla counteracts the release of insulin. The net result is an increased level of blood sugar, which supplies the person with ready energy to fuel "fight or flight" (Asterita, 1985).

We have learned that high levels of glucocorticoids tend to suppress the immune system. In fact, the proper functioning of the immune system is dependent on normal levels of other hormones. The endocrine changes associated with stress consequently alter immune functioning. The thymus and other tissues serving the immune response may also be altered by the autonomic nervous system. The effect of stress on immune functioning is very complex. Both enhanced and decreased immune functioning have been associated with stress, depending on the conditions under which the stress occurs and on which facet of immune functioning is observed. The effect of stress on immune functioning will be considered in more detail in Chapter 7.

Physiological Responses to Stress: A Summary

A complex set of physiological responses are observed under stress: short-term sympathetic activation, intermediate adrenal medulla secretion of E and NE, and long-term alteration in endocrine and immune functioning. These responses are complementary. They prepare the person physiologically for vigorous and sustained physical action in the face of physical and psychosocial stressors. The major physiological consequences of stress are increases in heart rate, blood pressure, blood glucose levels, blood coagulation, metabolism, and respiration and decreases in digestive, eliminative, and inflammatory processes. Under certain conditions, stress may also suppress the immune system. Thus stress has widespread and powerful biological effects.

Physiological Responses to Stress and Cognitive-Behavioral Coping Strategies

We have treated physiological responses to stress and cognitive-behavioral coping strategies as independent entities. Actually, they are interdependent. What is the nature of their relationship? There are two theories that address this question. One emphasizes the generality and the other the specificity of physiological responses to stress. Those holding the generalized viewpoint (Selye, 1956; Wolf, 1950) suggest that all stressors are equivalent in producing a generalized, biologically preprogrammed mobilization. Physiological changes are thus considered to be the same under all stress and coping conditions. Those holding the specificity viewpoint suggest that the intensity and pattern of physiological responses vary according to the person's appraisal, emotional arousal, and cognitive-behavioral response to a stressful event (Mason, 1975a).

There are insufficient data to support either position definitively. There does appear to be some variation in the pattern of physiological arousal depending on the strategy used to cope with the stressor. For example, different cardiovascular patterns are associated with active versus passive (Obrist, 1976) and avoidant versus vigilant (Lacey & Lacey, 1978) types of coping. Different patterns of hormone secretion are associated with feelings of denial versus worry (Mason, 1975a) and anger versus fear (Ax, 1953). Thus, the physiological response to stress is not uniform or general. Only a subset of the responses enumerated in previous sections may be observed in any one stressful transaction. In some cases, physiological responses are highly fractionalized; one response may change without another (e.g., blood pressure increases but heart rate is unchanged).

Cognitive-behavioral and physiological responses are usually complementary. The physiological responses correspond with the cognitive-behavioral coping strategy being used. Our thoughts, actions, and physiology are interrelated; one level affects another. Otherwise, we would be trying to do one thing while our body was preparing us to do something else. In defense of the generalized mobiliztion hypothesis, there is probably no one unique pattern of physiological arousal for each event appraised as stressful, for each coping strategy, and for each emotional response because there is limited plasticity in the physiological responses to stress (Holroyd, 1979).

STRESS AS A PROCESS

Figure 4-5 integrates the various facets of stress considered to this point. From a systems point of view, stress is a person's multilevel, integrated response to external and internal stimuli. The various response levels are interdependent.

There is a tendency to think of stress in a linear stimulus-organism-response manner. Some event occurs, the person processes the event as threatening, and then responds emotionally, behaviorally, and physiologically. The transaction is then completed. However, this is not an accurate representation of a stressful transaction as it occurs in the natural environment (Lazarus & Folkman, 1984). Stress is better conceptualized as an iterative, bidirectional, ongoing process (Leventhal & Nerenz, 1983). When faced with a stressor, our initial coping and physiological responses alter the event. We then reappraise the altered event and adjust our coping and physiological responses accordingly, which further changes the event and so on. Problem-oriented coping directly alters the original stimulus input. Emotion-oriented coping indirectly affects the input by altering appraisal or the emotional reaction to the event. Thus stress and coping are a circular process in which our coping efforts alter the event in a feedback loop. To add to the complexity, we often face multiple stressors that overlap and combine in complex ways.

FIGURE 4-5 The Systems Model of Stress: Appraisal, Affect, Coping, and Physiology

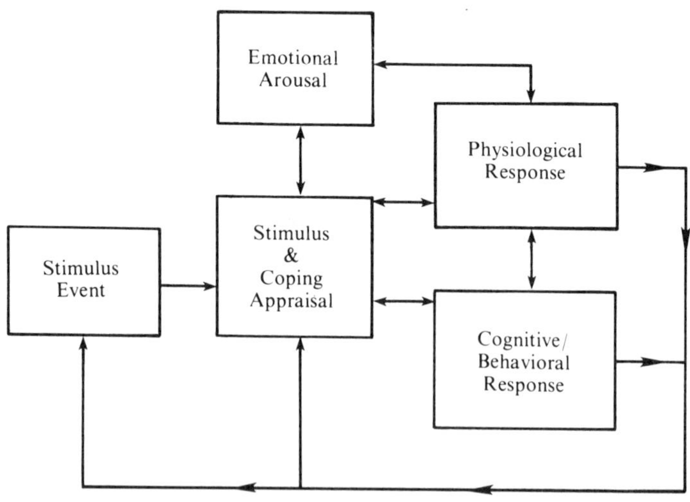

In summary, stress can be conceived as a person's multilevel response to stimuli that are appraised as threatening or harmful. This response may be more or less successful in ameliorating the stressful stimuli.

ADAPTATIONAL OUTCOMES

The notion of stress as an ongoing, recursive process leads to the consideration of adaptational outcomes, or the progressive, accumulating effects of our efforts to cope with stressors over time. Adaptational outcomes can be thought of as the biopsychosocial status of an individual at one point in time; they are like a freeze frame on a videotape. The action that is depicted on that frame can be understood on the basis of what occurred in a few previous frames (short-term adaptational outcomes) or in a very large number of previous frames (long-term adaptational outcomes). We can evaluate adaptational outcomes at physiological, cognitive, affective, behavioral, and social levels. Put another way, persons' physical health, affect, satisfaction, attitudes, behavioral competence, and social relationships are in part the net result of their ability to transact with their environment.

Before discussing adaptational outcomes more fully, it is important to keep two points in mind. First, stress does not necessarily have a negative impact. Stress can also be viewed as a motivating force that promotes growth and expands resilience and competencies. This is implicit in the notions of challenge, commitments, and social support. Persons who are overly protected from stress may be at risk because they have failed to develop coping skills needed in day-to-day living (Murphy & Moriority, 1979). The lack of stress can thus have a negative impact (Frankenhaeuser, 1978). Stress may result in positive outcomes. Successfully dealing with threats and challenges lead to positive affect, enhanced feelings of personal efficacy, and physical health.

Second, adaptational outcomes are the result of a number of factors in addition to stress. It would be a mistake to replace the biomedical germ theory of disease with the notion that stress is the only or the most important determinant of physical and psychosocial adjustment. To treat stress as such would only create a psychosocial germ theory that would be as incomplete as the biomedical theory. The multiple determinants of health and illness will be elaborated in the next chapter. Let us now consider the means by which stress can influence physiological adaptation.

Physiological Adaptation

From Stress to Disease. The physiological arousal associated with the stress response is an adaptive, short-term response to physical threat or harm. Physiological arousal mobilizes the individual to take vigorous physical action to avoid, escape, or overcome the physical threat. If you come upon a grizzly bear when backpacking in the Rocky Mountains, arousal assists in your escape. Because of sociocultural developments in the last one hundred years, we are faced with relatively few threats to our physical well-being. Today most stressors are psychosocial in nature and are thus not amenable to "fight or flight" solutions, yet the physiological mobilization still occurs. When facing a physical threat, the mobilization is relatively brief. Either we are successful in dealing with the threat or we are likely to be killed. But with psychosocial stressors, the mobilization occurs frequently and is of long duration. What is an adaptive biobehavioral mechanism for dealing with physical threats appears less adaptive when dealing with psychosocial threats.

When the frequency, intensity, or duration of the physiological mobilization associated with stress becomes excessive, it may have deleterious effects (Depue, Monroe, & Shachman, 1979). The frequency, intensity, and duration of mobilization depend on individuals' appraisal of the environment and on their coping skills. Excessive mobilization is more likely to occur when persons inaccurately appraise relatively innocuous events as substantively threatening or harmful and when they have inadequate skills and resources to effectively cope with stressors.

Correlational, epidemiological (Cohen, 1979), and experimental research (Miller, 1980) has found a significant although modest relationship between the frequency, intensity, and perhaps duration of stress and health. Stress is not the sole determinant of health status. It interacts with the health-related behaviors discussed in Chapters 2 and 3 and with other environmental and biological factors discussed in Chapter 5 in determining health.

From Disease to Stress. Not only does stress contribute to disease, but disease and its treatment are also often stressful. The relationship is bidirectional. Illness and its treatment present individuals with threats to their physical, psychological, and social well-being. Disease and treatment represent multilevel adaptational tasks. The stress induced by disease and treatment can affect the course and prognosis of the disease and complicate recovery. Table 4-4, adapted from Cohen and Lazarus (1979), outlines the multilevel threats that may result from illness and treatment.

The quality of health care technology available to the client plays an important role in physiological recovery. However, disease and treatment are often stressful and require problem- and emotion-oriented coping. If a client lacks coping skills, disease and treatment may result in frequent, intense, and chronic physiological mobilization that may interfere with recovery. The client-health provider relationship affects

TABLE 4-4 Threats Presented by Illness and Treatment

Threats to life and fear of dying

Threats to body integrity and comfort
- Body injury or disability
- Permanent physical changes
- Pain, discomfort, and other negative aspects

Threats to self-concept and future plans
- Alteration of self-image and sense of efficacy
- Uncertainty about the illness and the future
- Endangering life goals and personal values

Threats to emotional equilibrium
- Anxiety
- Anger
- Depression
- Embarrassment

Threats to fulfillment of usual roles and activities
- Separation from social support network
- Loss of central self-defining roles
- Dependence on others

Threats involving adjustment to new physical and social environments
- Adjustment to hospital and other treatment settings and routines
- Understanding diagnostic, prognostic, treatment, and other medical communications
- Decision making under threatening and unfamiliar conditions

Note: From "Coping with the Stresses of Illness" (p. 229), 1980, by F. Cohen and R. S. Lazarus in G. C. Stone, F. Cohen, & N. Adler (Eds.), *Health Psychology: A Handbook,* San Francisco: Jossey-Bass. Copyright 1980 by Jossey-Bass Publishers. Reprinted by permission.

recovery because it plays an important role in the client's ability to cope with the stress of disease and treatment.

Correlational and experimental research suggests that clients who are provided with accurate information and effective coping strategies adapt better emotionally, behaviorally, socially, and physiologically (Turk, Meichenbaum, & Genest, 1983). For example, studies assessing the effects of prepared childbirth have found that the information, control, predictability, and coping strategies offered to expectant parents lead to a reduction in perceived pain and in the use of analgesics and anesthetics, an increase in cooperation by the mother during labor, and a reduction in blood loss, extreme obstetric interventions, and length of labor. Such training also benefits the neonate by fostering increased oxygenation of fetal blood, higher apgar scores, and decreased illness and mortality (Genest, 1981).

Other Stress-Health Relationships. Responses used to cope with stress can also be assessed in terms of their health-impairing and health-promoting outcomes. Common forms of coping with stress, like smoking and drinking alcohol, introduce pathogenic substances into the body (see Chapter 2). Other forms of coping, like relaxation and exercise, may have beneficial effects.

If frequent, intense, chronic stress contributes to disease, can frequent, intense, recurring positive events and emotions have a health-enhancing or curative effect? While there is some anecdotal evidence to suggest that this may be the case (Cousins, 1979), there are insufficient data to draw even tentative conclusions.

SUMMARY

From a systems paradigm, disturbances at one level in the system have an impact at other levels. The relationship of stress to health represents just such an effect. Stress not only elicits emotional and behavioral coping but also profound physiological changes. When there is a continued imbalance between the perceived demands placed on a person and the person's ability to cope, negative physiological effects are likely to ensue.

Stress is not necessarily negative and is certainly not the sole (or perhaps even the most important) determinant of health. Stress cannot be avoided. It is the product of a person's transaction with the environment. It is an implicit part of an open system. Stress can even be motivating and growth producing. However, when it surpasses our coping abilities and resources, it may have deleterious effects.

A person's health is complexly determined. It is influenced via indirect psychophysiological mechanisms that we have termed stress. It is also affected by health-promoting and health-impairing behaviors, and by actions and decisions made in response to illness and treatment, as detailed in Chapters 2 and 3. Psychosocial variables thus play an important role in health.

REFERENCES

Allen, R. J. (1983). *Human stress: Its nature and control.* Minneapolis, Minnesota: Burgess Publishing.

Asterita, M. F. (1985). *The physiology of stress.* New York: Human Sciences Press.

Ax, A. F. (1953). The physiological differentiation between fear and anger in humans. *Psychosomatic Medicine, 15,* 433–442.

Beck, A. T. (1976). *Cognitive therapy and the emotional disorders.* New York: International Universities Press.

Berkman, L. F., & Syme, S. L. (1979). Social networks, host resistance and mortality: A nine-year follow-up study of Alameda County residents. *American Journal of Epidemiology, 109,* 186–204.

Cannon, W. (1927). The James-Lange theory of emotions: A critical examination and alternate theory. *American Journal of Psychology, 39,* 106–124.

Cobb, S. (1976). Social support as a moderator of life stress. *Psychosomatic Medicine, 38,* 300–314.

Cohen, F. (1979). Personality, stress, and the development of physical illness. In G. C. Stone, F. Cohen, & N. Adler (Eds.), *Health psychology: A handbook,* 77–112. San Francisco: Jossey-Bass.

Cohen, F., & Lazarus, R. S. (1979). Coping with the stresses of illness. In G. C. Stone, F. Cohen, & N. Adler (Eds.), *Health psychology: A handbook,* 217–254. San Francisco: Jossey-Bass.

Cohen, S., & McKay, G. (1984). Social support, stress, and the buffering hypothesis: A theoretical analysis. In A. Baum, S. E. Taylor & J. E. Singer (Eds.), *Handbook of psychology and health* (Vol. 4), 364–383. Hillsdale, NJ: Lawrence Erlbaum.

Cousins, N. (1979). *Anatomy of an illness as perceived by the patient.* New York: Bantam Books.

DeLongis, A., Coyne, J. C., Dakof, G., Folkman, S., & Lazarus, R. S. (1982). Relationship of daily hassles, uplifts and major life events to health status. *Health Psychology, 1,* 119–136.

Dembroski, T. M. (1981). Environmentally induced cardiovascular responses in Type A and B individuals. In S. M. Weiss, J. Herd, & B. H. Fox (Eds.), *Perspectives on behavioral medicine,* 321–328. New York: Academic Press.

Depue, R. A., Monroe, S. M., & Shachman, S. L. (1979). The psychology of human disease: Implications for conceptualizing depressive disorders. In R. A. Depue (Ed.), *The psychobiology of the depressive disorders: Implications for the effects of stress,* 3–22. New York: Academic.

Dohrenwend, B. S., & Dohrenwend, B. P. (1981). *Stressful life events and their contexts.* New York: Prodist.

Ferrare, N. A. (1962). *Institutionalization and attitude change in an aged population.* Unpublished doctoral dissertation, Western Reserve University.

Folkman, S., & Lazarus, R. S. (1980). An analysis of coping in a middle-aged community sample. *Journal of Health and Social Behavior, 21,* 219–239.

Frankenhaeuser, M. (1972). *Biochemical events, stress and adjustment.* (Rep.) Stockholm: University of Stockholm, Psychological Laboratories.

Frankenhaeuser, M. (1978). *Coping with job stress: A psychobiological approach.* (Rep.) Stockholm: University of Stockholm, Department of Psychology.

Frankl, V. (1959). *Man's search for meaning.* Boston: Beacon.

Genest, M. (1981). Preparation for childbirth: A selective review of evidence for efficacy. *Journal of Obstetric, Gynecologic and Neonatal Nursing, 10,* 82–85.

Grinker, R. R., & Spiegal, J. P. (1945). *Men under stress.* New York: McGraw-Hill.

Hann, N. (1977). *Coping and defending: Processes of self-environment organization.* New York: Academic Press.

Holmes, T. H., & Rahe, R. H. (1967). The social adjustment rating scale. *Journal of Psychosomatic Research, 11,* 213–216.

Holroyd, K. A. (1979). Stress, coping and the treatment of stress related illness. In J. R. McNamara (Ed.), *Behavioral approaches to medicine: Application and analysis,* 191–226. New York: Plenum Press.

Hunter, E. J. (1979). *Combat casualities who remain at home.* Monterey, CA: Naval Postgraduate School.

Jacobs, S., & Ostfeld, A. (1977). An epidemiological review of the mortality of bereavement. *Psychosomatic Medicine, 39,* 344–357.

Janis, I. L., & Mann, L. (1977). *Decision making.* New York: The Free Press.

Jemmott, J. B., & Locke, S. E. (1984). Psychosocial factors, immunologic mediation and human susceptibility to infectious diseases: How much do we know? *Psychological Bulletin, 95,* 78–108.

Lacey, B. C., & Lacey, J. I. (1978). Two way communication between the heart and the brain. *American Psychologist, 33,* 99–113.

Langer, E. J., & Rodin, J. (1976). The effects of choice and enhanced personal responsibility for the aged: A field experiment in an institution setting. *Journal of Personality and Social Psychology, 34,* 191–198.

Lazarus, R. S. (1966). *Psychological stress and the coping process.* New York: McGraw-Hill.

Lazarus, R. S., & Folkman, S. (1984). *Stress, appraisal and coping.* New York: Springer.

Lazarus, R. S., & Launier, R. (1978). Stress related transactions between person and environment. In L. Pervin & M. Lewis (Eds.), *Internal and external determinants of behavior,* 163–198. New York: Plenum Press.

Lazarus, R. S., Opton, E. M., Nomikos, M. S., & Rankin, N. O. (1965). The principle of short circuiting threat: Further evidence. *Journal of Personality, 33,* 622–625.

Leventhal, H., & Nerenz, D. R. (1983). A model for stress research with some implications for the control of stress disorders. In D. H. Meichenbaum & M. E. Jaremko (Eds.), *Stress reduction and prevention,* 140–167. New York: Plenum Press.

Levine, S., Weinberg, J., & Ursin, H. (1978). Definition of the coping process and statement of the problem. In H. Ursin, E. Baade, & S. Levine (Eds.), *Psychobiology of stress: A study of coping men,* 3–22. New York: Academic Press.

Lindemann, E. (1944). Symptomatology and management of acute grief. *American Journal of Psychiatry, 101,* 141–148.

Mason, J. W. (1975a). Emotions as reflected in patterns of andocrine integration. In L. Levi (Ed.), *Emotions: Their parameters and measurement,* 143–182. New York: Raven Press.

Mason, J. W. (1975b). A historical view of the stress field. *Journal of Human Stress, 1,* 22–36.

Mechanic, D. (1962). *Students under stress: A study in the social psychology of adaptation.* New York: The Free Press.

Meichenbaum, D. (1977). *Cognitive behavior modification.* New York: Plenum Press.

Miller, N. E. (1980). A perspective on the effects of stress and coping on disease and health. In S. Levine & H. Ursin (Eds.), *Coping and health,* 323–334. New York: Plenum Press.

Miller, W. R., & Seligman, M.E.P. (1975). Depression and learned helplessness in man. *Journal of Abnormal Psychology, 84,* 228–238.

Murphy, L. B., & Moriority, A. E. (1979). *Vulnerability, coping and growth: From infancy to adolescence.* New Haven: Yale University Press.

Nerenz, D. R., Leventhal, H., & Love. R. R. (1982). Factors contributing to emotional distress during cancer chemotherapy. *Cancer, 50,* 1020–1027.

Nucholls, C. B., Cassel, J., & Kaplan, B. H. (1978). Psychosocial assets, life crises and the prognosis of pregnancy. *American Journal of Epidemiology, 46,* 932–946.

Obrist, P. A. (1976). The cardiovascular-behavior interaction as it appears today. *Psychophysiology, 13,* 95–107.

Parks, C. M. (1970). The first year of bereavement. *Psychiatry, 33,* 444–467.

Rabkin, J. G., & Struening, E. L. (1976). Life events, stress and illness. *Science, 194,* 1013–1020.

Rodin, J. (1980). Managing the stress of aging: The role of control and coping. In S. Levine & H. Ursin (Eds.), *Coping and health,* 171–202. New York: Plenum Press.

Sarason, I. G., Johnson, J. H., & Siegal, J. M. (1978). Assessing the impact of life changes: Development of the Life Experiences Survey. *Journal of Consulting and Clinical Psychology, 46,* 932–946.

Schacter, S. (1964). The interaction of cognitive and physiological determinants of emotion. In L. Berkowitz (Ed.), *Advances in experimental social psychology* (Vol. 1), 49–81. New York: Academic Press.

Seligman, M.E.P. (1975). *Helplessness.* San Francisco: W. H. Freeman.

Selye, H. (1956). *The stress of life.* New York: McGraw-Hill.

Singer, J. E., & Lord, D. (1984). The role of social support in coping with life-threatening illness. In A. Baum, S. E. Taylor & J. E. Singer (Eds.), *Handbook of psychology and health* (Vol. 4), 383–398, Hillsdale, NJ: Lawrence Erlbaum.

Suls, J. (1982). Social support, interpersonal relations and health: Benefits and liabilities. In G. Sanders & J. Suls (Eds.), *Social psychology of health and illness,* 255–278. Hillsdale, NJ: Lawrence Erlbaum.

Symington, G., Currie, R. C., Curran, T. M., & Davidson, S. K. (1955). Nonspecific indications of physiological change: Comatose and non-comatose patients. *Journal of Psychiatry, 3,* 67–71.

Tanig, M. (1982). Measuring life events. *Journal of Health and Social Behavior, 23,* 78–108.

Turk, D., Meichenbaum, D., & Genest, M. (1983). *Pain and behavioral medicine.* New York: Guilford.

Weinberg, J., & Levine, S. (1980). Psychobiology of coping in animals: The effects of predictability. In S. Levine & H. Ursin (Eds.), *Coping and health,* 39–60. New York: Plenum Press.

Weisman. A. D., & Worden, J. W. (1975). Psychosocial analysis of cancer deaths. *Omega: Journal of Death and Dying, 6,* 61–75.

Weiss, J. M. (1968). Effects of coping response on stress. *Journal of Comparative and Physiological Psychology, 65,* 251–260.

Weiss, J. M. (1971a). Effects of coping behavior in different warning signal conditions on stress pathology in rats. *Journal of Comparative and Physiological Psychology, 77,* 1–13.

Weiss, J. M. (1971b). Effects of coping behavior with and without feedback signal on stress pathology in rats. *Journal of Comparative and Physiological Psychology, 77,* 22–30.

Wolf, H. G. (1950). Life stress and body disease—A formulation. In H. G. Wolf, S. Wolf, & C. C. Hare (Eds.), *Life stress and body disease,* 137–146. Baltimore: Williams & Wilkins.

Wortman, C. B., & Dunkel-Schetter, C. (1979). Interpersonal relationships and cancer: A theoretical analysis. *Journal of Social Issues. 35,* 120–155.

Wrubel, J., Brenner, P., & Lazarus, R. S. (1981). Social competence from the perspective of stress and coping. In J. Wine & M. Smye (Eds.), *Social Competence,* 61–99. New York: Guilford.

5

Health and Illness: A Systems View

INTRODUCTION

In the last three chapters, we have reviewed the role that psychosocial and behavioral variables play in determining health and illness. Stress, health-impairing and health-promoting behavior, and illness-related decisions and actions clearly make important contributions to health and illness. However, biological and genetic variables, as emphasized by the biomedical model, also play a significant role. This chapter has two goals. First, the role of biological and genetic variables in health and illness will be described. Second, a systems model of health and disease will be formulated in order to understand the relative contribution of biological, genetic, psychosocial, and behavioral variables. This second goal entails developing answers to several questions. Do biological-genetic and psychosocial-behavioral variables play separate or interactive roles? Is each variable always involved in all diseases? Does each variable contribute equally to health? How much contribution does each variable make? In answering these questions, we will summarize and integrate the material presented in Chapters 2 through 4 and in the early portion of this chapter to develop a complete and coherent model of health and disease.

BIOLOGICAL AND GENETIC FACTORS IN HEALTH AND ILLNESS

Fossils demonstrate that diseases such as infections, tooth decay, cancer, and arthritis have plagued persons since earliest evolution. According to current scientific theories, disease is the result of physical, chemical, or biological agents that cause biological injury or malfunction. These pathological agents are classified as hereditary, traumatic, physical, chemical, and infectious (Sheldon, 1984). Let us look at each of these causes in more detail.

Heredity

Each of us has inherited a general biological code from our parents. This code is carried by our chromosomes and accounts for similarities in the anatomy, physiology, and psychological capacities of human beings. The particular manner in which genes are organized on a chromosome varies from person to person. External characteristics like hair color, height, and facial features are readily ascribed to genetic variation between individuals. Less recognized is the fact that our internal anatomy and physiology also vary depending on genetic make-up. While we think of a normal heart rate as 72 beats per minute, some normal hearts are observed to beat twice as fast as others. Persons with no known stomach pathology have been found to exhibit variation in the gastric secretion of pepsin ranging from 0 to 4,300 units (Williams, 1967). This tremendous variation in biological structure and function plays an important role in susceptibility to disease.

We cannot consider genetic contributions to health and disease without recognizing the interaction of heredity and the environment. The entire collection of genes form a person's genotype. The environment plays an important role in determining how each gene will be expressed. The outward expression of the genotype is called the phenotype, which depends on the environment in which a gene is expressed. Because of this, we cannot speak of health or disease as either purely genetic or purely environmental in determination; health and disease are the result of both.

The conventional approach is to classify genetic disorders into three main groups: (1) chromosomal, (2) monogenetic, and (3) multifactorial. Chromosomal disorders refer to diseases shown to be due to abnormalities in the structure or number of chromosomes. The incidence of chromosomal disorders is about 6.5 per 1,000 live births; most embryos with chromosomal abnormalities are spontaneously aborted. A well-known chromosomal disorder is Down's syndrome, or Trisomy 21. A child with Down's syndrome is often characterized by slanted eyes, hyperextensibility of the joints, short stature, and mental retardation.

Monogenetic disorders are diseases that clearly follow a genetic pattern but for which there are no observable chromosomal abnormalities. These disorders are most frequently expressed as errors of metabolism. Some examples are Huntington's disease, phenylketonuria, sickle cell anemia, and hemophilia. Huntington's is a disease of the central nervous system that results in nervous system degeneration, involuntary muscular movements, and premature death. The folk singer Woody Guthrie died of this disease. Sickle cell anemia, most frequently found in blacks, consists of a biochemical deficit that alters red blood cells. These abnormal cells are destroyed by the spleen faster than the person can manufacture mature replacement cells, and these immature red blood cells lead to anemia. In hemophilia, a biochemical deficit results in the inadequate synthesis of proteins needed for normal blood clotting. Physical injury then leads to excessive bleeding. Many of the royal families in Europe carry genes for hemophilia.

Multifactorial disorders result from the interaction of several genes with multiple environmental factors. These disorders tend to run in families, but the inheritance pattern is complex. Rather than directly causing the disorder, the information carried by many genes influences a person's susceptibility for the disease. Whether that risk is expressed depends on other factors like stress, diet, and exercise. Most traits affecting health are polygenic. Coronary heart disease, cancer, ulcers, and hypertension are polygenic disorders. Insofar as life span is a measure of health, it also has a polygenic component.

Genetic factors, then, play an important role in health and illness. Not all genetic effects are apparent at birth. Huntington's disease, for example, does not occur until between ages thirty and forty. The impact of genetic make-up on health depends on its interaction with the environment. Phenylketonuria, a metabolic disorder that results in mental retardation, can be minimized with a corrective diet. The likelihood of coronary heart disease, given a genetic predisposition, depends on behavioral factors like diet, smoking, and exercise.

Trauma

Trauma is a mechanical injury that damages tissue. It is the result of a blow to the body, a wound, a fracture, or a sprain. Mechanical injury can predispose a person to other types of disease, such as infection. As noted in Chapter 2, traumatic injuries resulting from motor vehicle accidents, homicides, and suicides are a leading cause of death of young adults in the United States. The likelihood of traumatic injuries is closely related to day-to-day behavior (e.g., using drugs, driving recklessly, wearing seat belts, and carrying a weapon) and to sociopolitical factors (e.g., drinking and gun laws).

Physical Agents and Chemical Poisons

A number of physical agents are also health destructive. These include extremes in temperature (e.g., burns, heatstroke, and frostbite), electrical hazards, and radiation. We are also exposed on a daily basis to a large number of toxic chemicals in our homes and in the work place. These chemicals are found in our water, food, and air. They include such agents as asbestos, nitrates, carbon monoxide, coal dust, lead, PCBs, and herbicides and insecticides (Brandt-Rauf & Weinstein, 1983). Some of these agents occur naturally in the environment, but their concentration is often exacerbated by our industrial and personal economic actions. Still other agents exist only as a result of socioeconomic choice and cultural evolution.

Infectious Agents

Infectious diseases are those in which the body is invaded by a living organism. There are six types of infectious agents: bacteria, viruses, rickettsiae, fungi, protozoa, and worms. Some of the diseases associated with these organisms are listed in Table 5-1. We will focus on bacteria and viruses. Bacteria are single-celled organisms found in the soil, air, and water. After invading the host, bacteria cause illness by producing poisons that disrupt cellular functioning. Many regions of the body are normally inhabited by bacteria. Viruses are the most minute form of life. They consist of a bit of DNA or RNA in a protein coat. After invading a host, a virus enters cells, takes over their machinery, and produces hundreds of new virus particles that are spewed forth to capture new cells and to maintain the cycle.

Contact with infectious agents does not necessarily result in disease. Whether disease occurs depends on natural lines of defense. The effectiveness of these defenses is also influenced by our behavior. Infectious agents more successfully invade the body when natural defenses are suppressed or altered as a result of stress (see Chapter 7 and Jemmott & Locke, 1984). The likelihood of getting an infectious disease also depends on health-promoting behaviors like receiving immunizations and on social behavior that differentially exposes persons to various infectious organisms. If natural body defenses are insufficient, control of an infection may ultimately depend on the timely use of medical services to obtain antibiotics or other medications and on subsequent adherence to treatment recommendations. In sum, the likelihood of disease is determined by the presence of the infectious agent and the susceptibility of the person. These in turn are related to psychosocial factors such as stress, health-related behavior, and collective socioeconomic decisions and actions.

TABLE 5-1 Diseases Associated with Infectious Agents

AGENT	DISEASE
Bacteria	Pneumonia Food poisoning Cholera, malaria, tuberculosis, bubonic plague Syphilis, gonorrhea
Viruses	Cold, flu, mononucleosis Chicken pox, smallpox, polio, rubella, mumps Hepatitis Rabies AIDS
Rickettsiae	Typhus Rocky Mountain fever
Fungi	Ringworm Athlete's foot
Protozoa	Malaria Amoebic dysentery
Worms	Trichinosis Tapeworms, pinworms, flukes

Biological Factors in Health and Disease: A Summary

Biological and genetic variables play a significant role in health and disease. Genetic make-up influences individual variations in anatomy and physiology, which account in part for differences in persons' biobehavioral capacity, resistance, and resilience. In the environment, there is an array of physical, chemical, and biological agents that may have deleterious effects on health. These genetic factors and pathogenic environmental agents interact in a complex manner with psychosocial and behavioral variables to determine health. Let us now turn to how we may conceptualize the interactive contribution of biogenetic and psychosocial variables to health and disease.

HEALTH AND DISEASE: A SYSTEMS PERSPECTIVE

Let us consider what phenomena must be included and integrated to develop an adequate model of health and disease. First, the model must be applicable to manifestations of disease at behavioral as well as biological levels of organization. Pain and depression are as legitimate and important targets of explanation as heart disease, cancer, and infections. Second, the determinants of health and disease occur at multiple systems levels, ranging from physical, chemical, and biological to social, psychological, and behavioral. Some of these determinants are temporally close to (proximal) and others are temporally removed from (distal) the level of biobehavioral functioning to be explained. For example, the cause of pneumonia is not solely the successful invasion of bacteria (proximal physical and chemical cause) but also entails social and behavioral conditions that result in contact with the bacteria and that alter resistance to the bacteria (distal psychosocial causes). The cause of heart attacks is not solely clogged arteries (proximal physical and chemical cause) but also smoking, high fat diets, and stress (distal psychosocial causes) as well a genetic predisposition to heart disease (distal physical and chemical cause). Third, the model must adequately describe and account for successful functioning or health as well as disease. Such an inclusive and integrative model provides the basis for effective interventions for health promotion, disease prevention, and clinical treatment.

In Chapter 1, systems theory was offered as a useful paradigm for understanding health and disease. The essence of this paradigm is that persons' health status can be understood at many organizational levels and that these levels interact in a reciprocal manner. As a result of our discussion of specific physical, chemical, biological, and sociopsychological determinants of health and disease in this and previous chapters, we can now develop an inclusive and integrative systems theory of health and disease.

Self-Regulation

A basic principle in the systems paradigm of health and disease is that persons are self-regulating systems (Carver & Schreier, 1981, 1982). The origin of this notion is evident in the concept of homeostatic physiological mechanisms (Cannon, 1929, 1932). Self-regulation is also congruent with current medical physiology (Guyton, 1976), and has been used to describe overt behavior (Bandura, 1977), thinking and emotion (Leventhal, 1980), and social relationships (Cantor & Mischel, 1979). Thus this principle has been successfully applied to multiple organizational levels describing the human organism.

The basic unit of any self-regulatory system is a negative feedback loop (see Figure 5-1). The function of such a loop is to reduce deviations from some reference value. The components of a negative feedback loop unit include current system status (e.g., room temperature), a mechanism to perceive that status and to compare it to a reference value (e.g., thermostat), and a corrective output mechanism that alters the status of the system (e.g., furnace). If a discrepancy is perceived between the current state and the reference value (e.g., the room temperature is colder than the thermostat setting), corrective output is generated to reduce that discrepancy (e.g., the furnace turns on) until the perceived state and the reference value are the same. Negative feedback loops reduce discrepancies above or below the reference value. In our example,

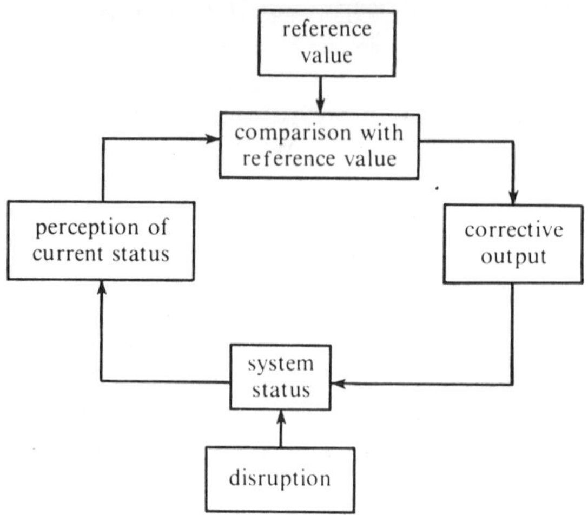

FIGURE 5-1 Essential Components of a Negative Feedback Loop

the thermostat would also need to be connected with an air conditioner to reduce room temperature when it is above the thermostat setting. The purpose of a negative feedback loop is to maintain homeostasis within the system.

Homeostatic feedback loops are evident at all organizational levels in human organisms. Cells, for example, have the digestive, excretory, communication, and transportation mechanisms needed to maintain their existence. Specialized cellular functions also depend on homeostatic mechanisms. A nerve cell, in order to transmit information, must generate a resting membrane potential via the active and passive transportation of molecules across its cell membrane. Information is transmitted by changes in the membrane potential. The integrity and functioning of tissues, organs, and organ systems are similarly dependent on homeostatic mechanisms. The maintenance of blood pressure, for example, requires an exquisite interaction of multiple feedback loops between and within the cardiovascular, nervous, endocrine, respiratory, skeletal-muscular, and excretory systems (see Figure 5-2).

Human functioning at the psychosocial and behavioral levels also involves self-regulatory, negative feedback loops. The concepts of stress, coping, and adaptation presented in Chapter 4 provide a good example. An event (current system status) is perceived and appraised (primary and secondary appraisal can be construed as comparison of the current status with a reference value) as threatening or harmful. A negative appraisal of the event results in emotional, physiological, and cognitive-behavioral responses (corrective output) in an attempt to cope with the stressor. The success of such strategies determines adaptation (homeostasis). Other cognitive and behavioral phenomena, such as thinking and reinforcement, can also be construed in self-regulatory terms (for example, see Carver & Schreier, 1981, 1982).

There are two components of the negative feedback loop that we have not considered: disturbance and reference value. Most systems, including human organisms, are open systems. They do not exist in a vacuum. Forces from outside the system impinge on the system and alter its status. In the thermostat-furnace example, room temperature (current status) is affected by the weather and the time of day. Disturbances can produce discrepancies (a blast of cold air when the door is open) that require corrective feedback (the furnace turns on to bring room temperature back up to the thermostat setting). However, disturbances can also reduce discrepancies (warm sunshine coming through the window raises the room temperature to the thermostat setting). In humans, disturbances can occur at biological, psychosocial, and behavioral levels of or-

FIGURE 5-2 Mechanisms Mediating Blood Pressure Regulation. (From "Learned control of Physiological Function and Disease" (p. 109), by D. Shapiro and R. S. Surwitt, 1976, in H. Leitenberg (Ed.), *Handbook of Behavior Modification and Behavior Therapy*, Englewood Cliffs, NJ: Prentice-Hall. Copyright © 1976 by Prentice-Hall, Inc. Reprinted by permission.)

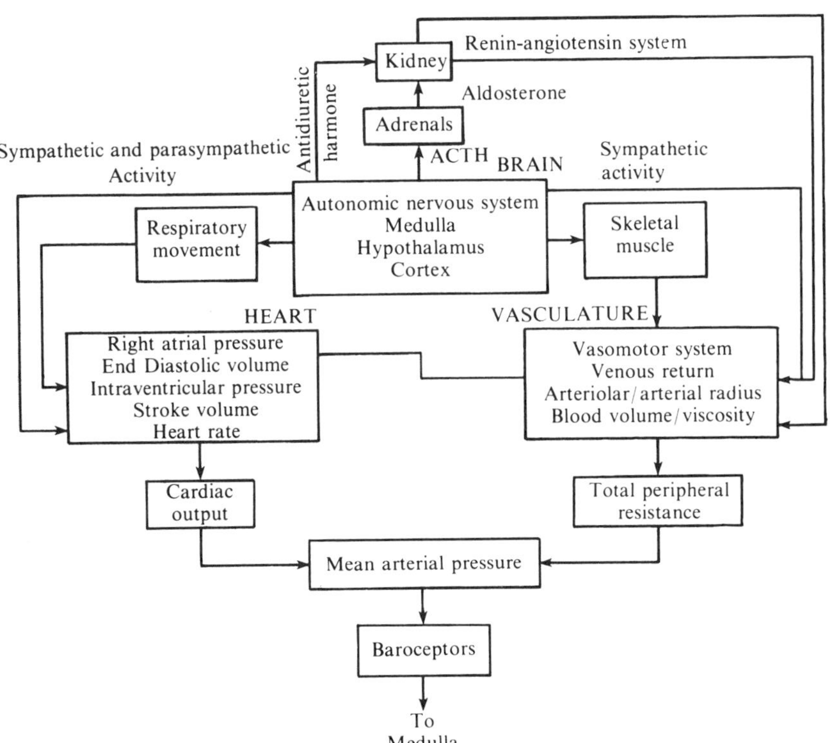

ganization. At the cellular level, for example, homeostasis can be influenced by the availability of nutrients in the extracellular space or by chemical messengers (like hormones) that impinge on the cell. In fact, the specialized function of cells often involves systematic disruptions by other cells; the membrane potential of one neuron is altered by neurotransmitters secreted by adjacent neurons. At the organ system level, the multiple feedback loops that regulate blood pressure have to adjust to disturbances like exercise, temperature, salt intake, stress, and medication. In each case, external disturbances can be discrepancy producing or discrepancy reducing. If blood pressure is too high, increased salt intake would be discrepancy enhancing but the ingestion of antihypertensive medication would be discrepancy reducing.

The last component in the negative feedback loop is the reference value. Where does this value come from? In the thermostat-furnace example, the reference value (thermostat setting) is determined by the person residing in the room, that is, from outside the feedback loop. This is also true in living organisms. The reference value for a feedback loop at one organizational level is set by the output of a loop at the next superordinate level. That level in turn receives its reference value from the feedback loop superordinate to it and so on.

Let us make the notion of downward causation (i.e., the reference value of a negative feedback loop comes from the output of the loop at the next higher level) more tangible with a couple of examples. At the biological level, organ systems should provide the reference value for organs. Using the interacting organ systems involved in the regulation of blood pressure (see Figure 5-2), let us focus on the relationship of these systems to the heart. Blood pressure is monitored by baroreceptors in the arteries. If blood pressure is low, the baroreceptors send information via the nervous system to the heart to increase its contraction rate to raise blood pressure. If blood pressure is high, the baroreceptors send information to the heart to decrease its contraction rate to thereby lower blood pressure. Thus the heart (lower level organ) receives its reference value from the circulatory and nervous systems (higher level organ systems).

In a similar manner, psychological processes provide reference values for physiological levels. Suppose you want to visit a friend. This goal is implemented by a series of complex physiological and biochemical processes. The brain sends signals to the muscles to carry out the motor processes involved in walking. These processes are effected by the contraction of the cells that compose the skeletal musculature. Their contraction in turn entails changes in cellular physiology and so forth. Heart rate and blood pressure will also be altered to meet the physical and metabolic demands of motor activity.

In a hierarchically arranged self-regulatory system, the attainment of subordinate goals is requisite to the attainment of superordinate goals. Although a person may set the thermostat at a certain temperature (reference value from a higher organizational level), the attainment of the desired room temperature depends on the correct functioning of the thermostat, furnace, gas supply, and electricity (subordinate levels). If a lower level feedback loop is not functioning properly, higher level self-regulatory demands cannot be carried out. Blood pressure cannot be adequately regulated if the heart is malfunctioning. You cannot walk to your friend's house if you have a broken leg.

When a lower level feedback loop is malfunctioning, higher level self-regulation is suspended, and attention is focused on solving the lower level problem (Carver & Schreier, 1982). For example, the pain of a heart attack will demand our attention despite the press of job and social responsibilities. While minor disruptions in the functioning of lower level negative feedback loops may be ignored for a time, major disruptions demand our attention. Along with environmental changes, lower level malfunctions serve, as a source of disruption for higher level self-regulatory feedback loops.

Thus, there are both upward (subordinate to superordinate) and downward (superordinate to subordinate) interactions between negative feedback loops at various levels of organization. The nature of these upward and downward interactions differs. Downward influences reflect goals descriptive of the constant adjustment required of organisms as open systems. Upward influences reflect disregulation in the system and serve notice that actions need to be taken to correct the malfunction.

A Systems View of Health

Health is an elusive concept. The word itself, comes from roots meaning whole or hale. This etymology is congruent with persons' subjective experiences of health. Persons describe health as a feeling of equilibrium or well-being. On an organic level, it is "not knowing your body is there." Health is described as a natural property, as an implicit characteristic of oneself. Health is not something accomplished by the person; it *is* the person. Illness, on the other hand, is experienced as an external intrusion, as something that is "not me." It is an imposition that renders the person powerless.

The subjective experiences of health are also congruent with theoretical definitions of health. Audy (1971, p. 33) defines health as the property of an individual that can "be measured in terms of one's ability to rally from challenges, to adapt" on physical, psychological, and social levels. Antonovsky (1979) defines health as a sense of control, predictability, and coherence that consists of the ability to adapt to physical and psychological demands and disruptions. Milsum (1984) similarly defines health as a person's resilience in the face of insults and stressors.

Let us develop a systems model of health. We have conceptualized humans as hierarchically organized systems composed of interacting self-regulatory mechanisms at cellular, tissue, organ, organ system, psychological, behavioral, and social levels of organization. Humans are living, open systems who engage in goal-directed behavior. Because they are living, they need to make constant adjustments to maintain internal homeostasis (e.g., adequate levels of nutrients, elimination of wastes, and regulation of heart rate). Because they are open systems, they must adapt to continuing changes in the external environment (e.g., temperature, availability of food and water, social stimuli, and cultural norms). Because they are sentient, intelligent, social beings, humans also perform the cognitive, motor, and verbal behaviors needed to effect goal-directed behavior (e.g., work, social relationships, education, and recreation).

Via evolutionary processes, humans have developed built-in biobehavioral mechanisms to carry out these tasks. Insofar as the self-regulatory mechanisms at various organizational levels work together to address internal physiological demands, to respond adaptively to external environmental changes, and to effect goal-directed behavior in a manner that fosters homeostasis across all organizational levels, individuals are healthy. Health is not a state. It is a continuing process by which persons adjust to internal and external demands and pursue goals in a manner that promotes equilibrium.

A few concrete examples may be helpful. As discussed earlier in this chapter, we live in an environment in which we are frequently exposed to various bacteria and viruses that are potential threats to our health. Contact with such pathogens can be limited by our personal and social behavior (e.g., food preparation and sexual habits). If we do come into contact, we have a built-in line of defense: the skin, mucous membranes, white blood cells, inflammation, and specific immunity. When this built-in health care system is functioning well, we can resist the pathogens. The integrity of the system (host resistance) may depend on how well we cope with stress. When these natural defenses fail and infection successfully invades the body, we can seek health care to regain our health.

If our blood sugar is low, stored energy is released into the bloodstream. We also experience hunger and seek food. The ingestion of food raises our blood sugar and replenishes our body's food stores. The availability of food depends on goal-oriented planning and work. Food selection can also influence future health depending on its nutritional constituents.

Vocational, interpersonal, and recreational goal-directed behaviors are integral to health and happiness. As we saw in the last chapter, the ability to develop close interpersonal relationships (social support) may be health protective. The sense of hopefulness, control, and efficacy associated with the successful pursuit of goals is central to the definitions of health cited above, and their absence is apparent in disorders like anxiety and depression. However, the pursuit of these goals must be reasonable. As we will see in the next chapter, individuals who pursue goals in a hostile, hard-driving manner increase their risk of heart disease.

Thus, adjustments to demands at any one organizational level require the actions of self-regulatory mechanisms at several levels. Successful adaptation, or health, requires an integrated, multilevel response. Frequently, we are faced with demands at several levels. Your bladder is full in the middle of an exciting movie. You are tired but you have two finals tomorrow. You have a headache but cannot miss an important meeting. To maintain health, these multiple demands have to be addressed in a coordinated manner, and each demand may require adjustments at several levels. Health refers to our biobehavioral ability to successfully deal with such multiple and seemingly contradictory demands and disruptions.

In summary, the systems view of health suggests that we have a built-in biobehavioral capacity that promotes the constant adaptation to the goals, stressors, and disruptions that are a natural part of life. This view of health is closely related to the old concept or *vis medicatrix naturae* (the healing force of nature), which asserts that we have within us a strong natural force that promotes our wholeness and integrity and that opposes forces that threaten our well-being.

A Systems Model of Disease

In contrast to health, disease is the result of converging and interacting disregulatory processes at one or more levels in the system. Up to this point, we have described such disregulatory forces separately. These forces include the behavioral and lifestyle factors considered in Chapters 2 to 4: health-impairing habits, nonadaptive illness-related decisions and actions, and excessive stress. They also include the biological, physical, and chemical factors considered earlier in this chapter: genetics, trauma, physical and chemical agents, and infectious organisms. Using the notion of hierarchically arranged negative feedback loops, there are four types of disregulation: (1) dysfunctioning system-perceptual mechanisms or corrective output devices at a given level; (2) inadequate coping with disruptions or demands from the external environment; (3) higher levels' setting of maladaptive reference values for lower levels; and (4) failure to respond adequately to lower level disruptions. Let us consider each of these in more detail.

Successful regulation at any one organizational level requires the accurate perception of the system status and some means to correct that status if it differs from the homeostatic reference value. Disregulation can result from a malfunction of either of these mechanisms. Diabetes, for example, may result from a lack of production of insulin (disordered corrective output) or from tissue insensitivity to circulating insulin (disordered perceptual mechanism). Depression may result from negatively biased perceptions of the environment or oneself (disordered perceptual mechanism) or from a failure to produce behaviors that lead to satisfaction and self-esteem (disordered corrective output) (Beck, 1967; Lewinsohn, 1974).

Successful self-regulation requires the availability of effective corrective responses to environmental demands and challenges. These demands may be psychosocial (e.g., interpersonal conflict and work demands) or physical-chemical (e.g., infectious agents, toxins, and temperature). Acquired immune deficiency syndrome (AIDS), for example, is a condition in which an individual's immune system is malfunctioning such that the person cannot resist infectious agents. Once established, infections run rampant and are life threatening. In the absence of sufficient coping resources and skills, psychosocial demands may result in psychophysiological responses that promote disease (see the discussion of adaptational outcomes in Chapter 4).

Disregulation may also occur when superordinate organizational levels set destructive, nonhomeostatic reference values for subordinate regulatory systems. Type A behavior, characterized by hostility and competitiveness, may be adaptive in terms of psychosocial success and achievement. But it also results in a physiological response pattern that promotes heart disease. Likewise, drinking alcohol and smoking tobacco may help regulate anxiety but also introduce pathogenic toxins into the body.

Finally, disregulation may occur when disruptions in the functioning at lower levels are ignored or improperly addressed at higher levels. The body has an innate "wisdom." If something is wrong, there is usually some kind of symptom. Recurrent abdominal pain and blood in the stools, for example, may indicate an ulcer. The body is signaling that something is wrong and that corrective action is required. Our recognition of and response to such symptoms influence whether lower level disregulation will continue, improve, or worsen (Schwartz, 1978). Individuals may attempt to ignore or cover up such symptoms, but this is like unplugging the oil light on your car when it comes on. Existing disease and disability may severely limit our ability and normal roles. Paralysis from stroke, disfigurement from burns, and kidney failure requiring dialysis provide challenges to a person's self-image, social and vocational pursuits, and self-esteem. The manner in which someone copes with these challenges is integral to physiological recovery and rehabilitation as well as meaning and quality of life. Genetically mediated disorders can be construed as the incorrect programming of the regulatory system.

Disease is the result of several types of disregulation, that occur and interact at several levels of organization over a period of time. Proximal physiological and anatomical causes of disease can usually be identified. But these proximal causes are in turn the result of converging sources of disregulation or distal causes of disease. Figure 5-3 provides a schematic summary of the multiple distal and proximal causes of disease.

Several additional notions are implied by this model. First, any one type of distal disregulation has the potential to contribute to several types of disease. Smoking increases the risk of cancer, heart disease, stroke, and emphysema. Hostile coping styles may enhance the risk of heart disease, ulcers, and hypertension. One type of disregulation often leads to others. Diabetes increases the risk of heart, retinal, kidney, and peripheral vascular diseases.

Second, the probability of developing a specific disease depends on the pattern of disregulatory forces that are operating and the interaction of those forces (Weiner, 1977; Zegans, 1983). For example, stress and smoking in the presence of exposure to asbestos and air pollution may lead to lung cancer. Stress and smoking, when combined with high blood pressure, high blood cholesterol, and Type A behavior may result in heart disease.

Third, the importance of various disregulatory forces that contribute to a specific disease may be differentially important in the etiology of the same disease in two persons. The primary distal causes of heart disease in one individual may be diabetes, high blood pressure, and Type A behavior, whereas the primary distal causes of the disease in a second individual may be obesity, genetic predisposition, smoking, and high serum cholesterol. Different combinations of distal disregulatory forces may thus lead to the same proximal pathogenic process and clinical disease.

FIGURE 5-3 A Systems Model of Disease: Converging and Interacting Disregulatory Processes

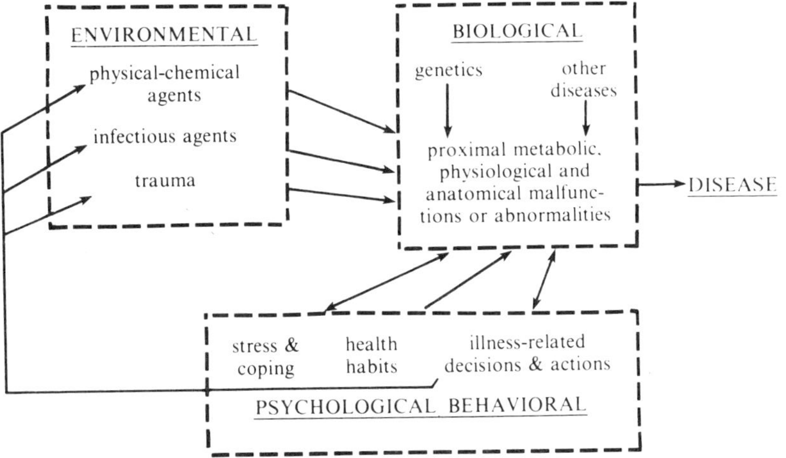

Fourth, symptoms of disease typically occur at multiple levels. This is reflective of the multiple, interacting nature of disregulatory forces. Depression, for example, is characterized by negative affect, altered patterns of sleep, decreased appetite, disrupted endocrine and neurotransmitter levels, and disturbances in behavior. Angina pectoris (a form of heart disease) is characterized by chest pain, occlusion of the coronary arteries, and limitations in activity level and physical exertion.

In the systems paradigm, the etiology of disease cannot be adequately understood, and the diagnosis of disease cannot be adequately accomplished by focusing solely on proximal causes or on one organizational level of the system to the exclusion of others. This is equally true of psychological and biological disorders. Disease involves the whole person.

THE SYSTEMS PARADIGM OF HEALTH AND DISEASE: IMPLICATIONS FOR INTERVENTION

Conceptualizing disease solely in terms of proximal physical causes and symptoms is inadequate. A focus on proximal causes emphasizes surgical and pharmacological interventions aimed at correcting the symptoms of disregulation. While useful and effective, it is "after the fact" intervention. It does not insure the correction of the disregulation that led to the disease. Consequently, it does not prevent the recurrence of the disease. Conceptualizing a person with coronary artery disease totally in terms of clogged arteries, and then treating those arteries by performing a coronary bypass operation is certainly useful as far as it goes. But it is also quite short-sighted. The arteries are clogged as a long-term result of disregulation at a number of levels: biological (multifactorial genetic predisposition, high blood cholesterol, and high blood pressure), behavioral (smoking, diet, and exercise), and psychosocial (stress and Type A behavior). Without a consideration of the whole person, disease and consequent suffering cannot be prevented, and relapse is likely. Performing the bypass without focusing attention on the distal disregulation that led to the symptoms fosters in the client the notion that the disease be "fixed" and that the client can thus continue to act in a disregulatory fashion. Medical intervention, to be maximally effective, needs to promote a return to self-regulation (Schwartz, 1978).

In some cases, a purely somatic, symptomatic focus may override or disrupt normal regulatory mechanisms and consequently exacerbate problems. For example, the prescription of sedatives (minor tranquilizers) like Librium and Valium may be effective in the short-term treatment of anxiety. These drugs may relieve distressing symptoms that interfere with effective coping. As the only intervention, however, such drug treatment may be inadequate. Drugs do not teach anything. Insofar as stress and the lack of adequate coping and instrumental skills are associated with the experience of anxiety, interventions aimed at addressing these deficits are also needed. The use of Librium and Valium may also inadvertently promote long-term disregulation. Functionally, these drugs are very similar to alcohol. Primary, long-term reliance on such chemical means of coping may result in psychological and physical dependence on the drugs.

The systems model also emphasizes the importance of health promotion and disease prevention in addition to clinical medicine. This requires genuine efforts in health education, risk appraisal, and early intervention. To be successful, such programs must address the distal social, psychological, and behavioral forces that lead to disease. The systems paradigm provides the theoretical model and methodology needed to design and implement effective health education and disease prevention programs.

The systems paradigm of health and illness also reinforces the importance of the compensatory model of helping. Because health and disease are dependent on behavioral, psychological, and social as well as biological variables, clients need to be actively involved in their health care. Enhancing a client's self-regulatory capacity implicitly necessitates responsibility and participation by the client. By endorsing clients' responsibility and participation, the compensatory model of helping enhances their sense of control and self-efficacy. This is consistent with the notion of health as persons' ability to self-regulate and adapt.

SUMMARY

From the systems perspective, persons are self-regulating organisms. They have built-in biobehavioral mechanisms and capacities to sustain life by maintaining internal homeostasis, adapting to shifting environmental demands, and engaging in planned, goal-directed behavior. Health and disease are reflections of persons' ability to self-regulate biologically and behaviorally. Health entails successfully addressing multiple, complex needs and demands in a manner that promotes ongoing regulation and homeostasis. Disease is the result of a number of converging and interacting disregulatory forces that can be observed at biological (e.g., genetics, trauma, and infections) and psychosocial (e.g., health-impairing behavior and stress) levels of organization. In the next section of the book, we will apply this systems paradigm to the etiology, manifestations, and course of a number of prevalent diseases.

REFERENCES

Antonovsky, A. (1979). *Health, stress, and coping*. San Francisco: Jossey-Bass.

Audy, J. R. (1971). Measurement and diagnosis of health. In P. Shepard & D. McKinley (Eds.), *Environment/Health*. Boston: Houghton Mifflin.

Bandura, A. (1977). *Social learning theory*. Englewood Cliffs, NJ: Prentice-Hall.

Beck, A. T. (1967). *Depression: Causes and treatment*. Philadelphia: University of Pennsylvania Press.

Brandt-Rauf, P. W., & Weinstein, I. B. (1983). Environment and disease. In D. Mechanic (Ed.), *Handbook of health, health care, and the health care professions*, 240–280. New York: The Free Press.

Cannon, W. B. (1929). Organization for physiological homeostasis. *Physiological Review, 9*, 399–431.

Cannon, W. B. (1932). *The wisdom of the body*. New York: Noeron.

Cantor, N., & Mischel, W. (1979). Prototypes in person perception. In L. Berkowitz (Ed.), *Advances in experimental social psychology* (Vol. 12), 4–52. New York: Academic Press.

Carver, C. S., & Schreier, M. F. (1981). *Attention and self-regulation: A control theory approach to human behavior*. New York: Springer-Verlag.

Carver, C. S., & Schreier, M. F. (1982). Control theory: A useful framework for personality-social, clinical, and health psychology. *Psychological Bulletin, 92*, 111–135.

Guyton, A. C. (1976). *Textbook of medical physiology*. Philadelphia: Saunders.

Jemmott, J. B., & Locke, S. E. (1984). Psychosocial factors, immunologic mediation and human susceptibility to infectious diseases: How much do we know? *Psychological Bulletin, 95*, 78–108.

Leventhal, H. (1980). Toward a comprehensive theory of emotion. In L. Berkowitz (Ed.), *Advances in experimental social psychology* (Vol. 13), 140–208. New York: Academic Press.

Lewinsohn, P. M. (1974). Clinical and theoretical aspects of depression. In K. S. Calhoun, H. E. Adams, & K. M. Mitchell (Eds.), *Innovative treatment methods in psychopathology*, 169–184. New York: Wiley.

Milsum, J. H. (1984). *Health, stress, and illness: A systems approach*. New York: Praeger.

Schwartz, G. E. (1978). Psychobiological foundations of psychotherapy and behavior change. In S. C. Garfield & A. E. Bergin (Eds.), *Handbook of psychotherapy and behavior change: An empirical analysis*. (2nd ed.), 63–100. New York: John Wiley & Sons.

Sheldon, H. (1984). *Boyd's introduction to the study of diseases*. Philadelphia: Lea & Febiger.

Weiner, H. (1977). *Psychobiology and human disease*. New York: Elsevier North-Holland.

Williams, R. J. (1967). *You are extraordinary*. New York: Random House.

Zegans, L. S. (1983). Emotions in health and illness: An attempt at integration. In L. Temoshok, C. Van Dyke, & L. S. Zegans (Eds.), *Emotions in health and illness: Theoretical and research foundations*, 117–139. New York: Grune & Stratton.

Part II
Prevalent Diseases: Etiology, Symptoms, Course, and Prognosis

6 Coronary Artery Disease

In Chapters 6 through 9 the research and theories reviewed in Part I are applied to understanding the etiology, symptoms, course, and prognosis of four specific health problems: coronary artery disease, infectious diseases, cancer, and pain. Proximal and distal biobehavioral variables that predispose and precipitate each of the disorders are described to include health habits, stress and coping, genetics, and physical, chemical, and biological pathogenic agents. Individuals' behavioral responses to symptom appearance and their psychobiological reaction to the symptoms and medical intervention are considered in terms of treatment outcome and prognosis.

INTRODUCTION

Coronary artery disease is the leading cause of death in the United States, accounting for about 50% more deaths than all forms of cancer. The annual economic cost of coronary artery disease in the United States is $50 billion (United States Department of Health, Education and Welfare, 1977). Based on the combined data of several prospective studies, an average group of 1,000 men, ages 40 to 49, will have the following incidence of coronary heart disease after ten years: 150 (15%) will develop symptomatic coronary heart disease; 75 (7.5%) will have a heart attack; 50 (5%) will have angina; 25 (2.5%) will die suddenly before treatment; and 25 (2.5%) will die despite treatment. Only 45 (4.5%) will die from other causes (Stokes, Froelicher, & Brown, 1981). If all cardiovascular disease could have been eliminated for infants born between 1969 and 1971, it would have increased their life expectancy by twelve years (Tsai, Lee, & Hardy, 1978).

Coronary artery disease is a major health problem. Its development is closely tied to individuals' behavior and lifestyle. In this chapter, the causes of the disease will be detailed. But first it is necessary to understand the anatomy and physiology of the cardiovascular system and to define coronary artery disease.

CARDIOVASCULAR ANATOMY AND PHYSIOLOGY

The heart and blood vessels make up a closed hydraulic system that works under pressure. The heart is a pump that pushes blood through the vessels to deliver oxygen and nutrients and to remove waste products from the body. Assuming an average heart beats 70 times per minute, the heart beats over 100,000 times per day, or more than two and a half billion times during a seventy-year life span. In this same day, the heart pumps 1,800 gallons of blood, or 46 million gallons during a lifetime. The heart is a four-chambered muscle whose contractions provide the pumping force. The two smaller chambers, the atria, receive blood. The two larger chambers, the ventricles, force the blood into circulation.

The heart beats rhythmically at a complexly determined rate. The average normal heart rate is about 72 beats per minute. While external neural and hormonal influences can alter the heart rate, the heart will continue to beat even if all nerves to it are cut. One part of the heart, the sinoatrial node, initiates the contraction of the heart muscle to provide the pumping action.

The heart is innervated by both the parasympathetic and sympathetic divisions of the autonomic nervous system. The parasympathetic input, which decreases the heart rate, has a constant influence and tends to slow the heart below the intrinsic rhythm generated by the sinoatrial node. Cutting the parasympathetic nerves to the heart causes the heart rate to increase to about 160 beats per minute. The sympathetic input increases the heart rate. It has a constant effect. Cutting the sympathetic nerves to the heart results in a reduction of the normal heart rate from 72 to around 60 beats per minute. The sympathetic division also has transient effects on the heart rate, raising it as high as 250 beats per minute. The heart rate is also raised by circulating epinephrine and norepinephrine from the adrenal medulla. As a muscle, the heart itself needs a supply of blood that is carried by the coronary arteries (see Figure 6-1).

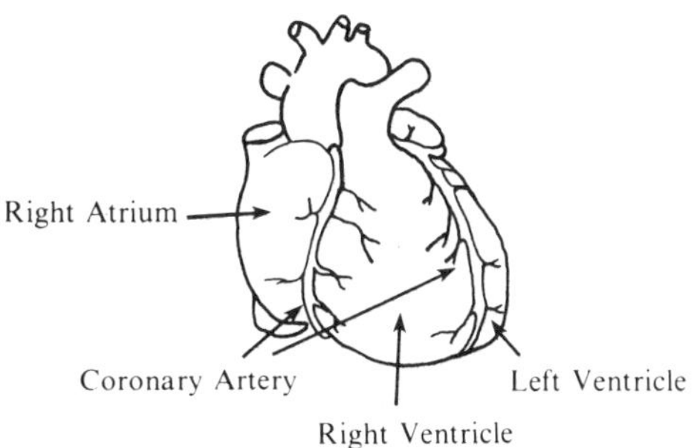

FIGURE 6-1 The Heart and Coronary Arteries

Cardiac output is the amount of blood pumped by the heart per minute. The output is complexly determined. It depends on the amount of blood returned to the heart from the veins. It depends on temperature; heat tends to increase the heart rate. It is influenced by psychosocial factors like stress, which, via the autonomic nervous system, alter the rate of the heart's pumping action. Cardiac output also depends on the conditioning of the heart. A heart that is well conditioned as a result of exercise is strong and efficient. It requires fewer beats per minute to achieve a given output than does a poorly conditioned heart. Diseased hearts are inefficient. They must beat rapidly to sustain needed cardiac output.

CORONARY ARTERY DISEASE: A DEFINITION

Coronary artery disease is a general term used to describe those illnesses that result from a narrowing or occlusion of the coronary arteries, which supply the heart muscle with blood. When these arteries narrow or close, the flow of oxygen and nourishment to the heart is partially or completely stopped. This results in two major manifestations of coronary artery disease: angina pectoris or myocardial infarction.

Angina is chest pain caused by anoxia (lack of oxygen) to the heart muscle following the narrowing of one or more of the coronary arteries. The pain is localized in the upper chest and often radiates to the left shoulder and arm. Angina is often precipitated by physical exertion or psychological stress, and is relieved by rest or the ingestion of drugs that dilate the coronary arteries and reduce the blood pressure. Anginal episodes usually do not involve permanent and substantial damage to the heart.

Myocardial infarction, or a heart attack, involves the death of heart tissue due to the sustained insufficiency of the blood supply to the heart. This is caused by a severe narrowing of the coronary arteries or by a clot or thrombosis that closes the arteries. The pain experienced is similar to that of angina but is more intense and lasting. It is often independent of physical exertion. Other symptoms of a heart attack are shortness of breath, weakness, blanching of the skin, and sometimes nausea. Myocardial infarction not only damages the heart's muscle but also may damage its conduction system, which causes cardiac arrhythmia (irregular heartbeat) or ventricular fibrillation that may result in sudden death.

The narrowing of the coronary arteries is due to a process called atherosclerosis. Atherosclerosis consists of the building up of a deposit on the inside lining of the arteries that is analogous to mineral deposits on the inside of a water pipe. This deposit is called plaque and consists of a mound of tissue composed of cholesterol (fats) capped with scar tissue. While the exact mechanism by which plaque develops has yet to be identified, it is hypothesized that mechanical injury to the lining of the arteries is involved. This mechanical injury is the result of blood being pumped through the arteries under pressure. Fats and scar tissue accumulate at these injury sites. This process begins during childhood and continues into adulthood. As the number and size of these plaque deposits increase over the years, they may impede or entirely cut off the blood supply to the heart. When the coronary arteries are unable to deliver sufficient blood, angina or myocardial infarction occurs (Surwitt, Williams, & Shapiro, 1982). This atherosclerotic process is shown in Figure 6-2.

CAUSES OF CORONARY ARTERY DISEASE

Coronary artery disease results from a combination of many disregulatory, predisposing factors that can be observed at the biological, behavioral, and environmental levels of organization. This section will review these factors.

Traditional Psychobiological Risk Factors

Based on prospective research such as the Framingham Study (Kannel, McGee, & Gordon, 1976), several factors have been shown to increase an individual's risk of coronary artery disease. These risk factors focus on psychobiological variables: past and existing disease states, genetic predisposition, and health habits. The exact mechanisms by which these factors contribute to the development of coronary artery disease are not always clear, but each factor has been found to be statistically related to the incidence of the disease.

Blood Cholesterol. Animal studies suggest that it is impossible to induce coronary heart disease without high levels of blood cholesterol or fat. In humans, coronary artery disease is especially associated with certain types of blood cholesterol called low density lipoproteins. Other

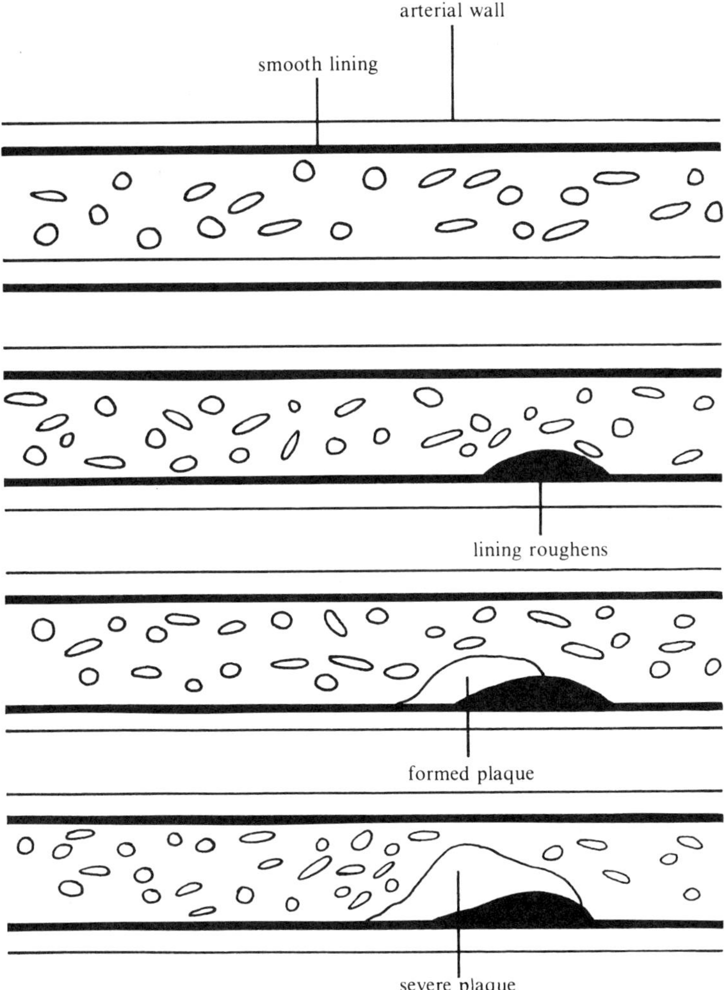

FIGURE 6-2 The Process of Atherosclerosis. (From *Essentials of Life and Health*, Second Edition. Copyright © 1972, 1974 by Ziff-Davis Publishing Co. Copyright © 1977 by Random House, Inc. Reprinted by permission of CRM Books, a Division of Random House, Inc.)

types of blood cholesterol, called high density lipoproteins, are associated with the *reduced* risk of coronary artery disease. High levels of low density lipoproteins increase the chances of coronary artery disease because they supply fats that accumulate as plaque (Stokes et al., 1981). Levels of blood cholesterol are determined by genetic factors, diet, and exercise.

High Blood Pressure. Coronary artery disease is more probable in those persons who have high blood pressure. Individuals with a resting systolic blood pressure of 180 or more are seven times as likely to develop coronary heart disease than those with a systolic blood pressure of 120. High blood pressure accelerates atherosclerosis by either damaging the lining of the arteries or "driving" fats into that lining or both (Stokes et al., 1981). High blood pressure is the result of genetic influences, other diseases, and health habits.

Tobacco. Smoking cigarettes and other forms of tobacco use are likewise associated with the occurrence of coronary artery disease. Persons who smoke one pack of cigarettes per day are twice as likely as nonsmokers to develop coronary heart disease. Although smoking is associated with atherosclerosis, the exact causative mechanism is unknown. Nicotine constricts the coronary arteries and thereby reduces the blood supply to the heart. It also increases blood platelet aggregation (the "stickiness" of the blood) and consequently enhances the development of plaque or a clot. Finally, nicotine increases the heart rate, thus putting a greater demand on the coronary blood supply (Stokes et al., 1981).

High Fat Diet. As indicated above, high blood cholesterol is associated with the development of atherosclerosis. The level of circulating cholesterol is influenced by the diet. No more than 25% of a person's caloric intake should come from fats, but the average American diet includes more than 40%. Unsaturated fats such as corn and peanut oil are preferable. Saturated fats such as butter, animal fat, and shortening are more strongly associated with atherosclerosis. The effects of a high fat diet are observable early in a person's life. Seventy-seven of one hundred American soldiers who were killed in Korea, with an average age of 22, were found to have observable atherosclerosis. More than fifteen had at least one coronary artery that was more than 50% blocked, and 3% had one coronary artery that was totally blocked. All of these men were in good health and had no signs of coronary artery disease prior to their death. A comparable sample of Japanese men were found to have no arterial narrowing greater than 50%. It has been suggested that this difference is the result of the dietary intake of fats (*Essentials of Life and Health*, 1977).

Physical Exercise. Regular physical exercise and high levels of energy expenditure reduce the risk of coronary artery disease (Kannel & Sorlie, 1979), although exercise inappropriate to one's physical condition can be risky (Koplan, 1979). Exercise enhances cardiac efficiency. The heart muscle can be built up like any other muscle. Exercise also increases the network of blood vessels to and in the heart. Thus exercise reduces the heart rate and demand for oxygen at the same time as it provides a more reliable supply of blood to the heart. Exercise is also associated, via changes in metabolism, with lowered levels of low density lipoproteins and with higher levels of high density lipoproteins (Stokes et al., 1981).

Sex. Men are more likely to develop coronary heart disease than women. The exact reason for this is unknown. Women do have higher serum levels of high density lipoproteins. Men often show stronger tendencies toward Type A behavior (see below). It may also be that sex-related differences in hormones or other physiological processes may mediate this difference.

Age. There is an increasing incidence of coronary heart disease with age. Atherosclerosis progresses as a person gets older.

Genetic Predisposition. There is a multifactorial genetic predisposition for the disease. Persons whose close relatives have had coronary artery disease are at greater risk. While it is possible that this relationship is the result of learned behavior (Type A behavior, dietary and exercise patterns, and other health habits), coronary artery disease is influenced by genetic factors independent of environmental and behavioral variables. The mechanism of genetic risk may be mediated by blood pressure or by receptors for low density lipoproteins.

Physiological Risk Factors: A Summary. This list of risk factors is not exhaustive. There are other factors (e.g., diabetes, alcohol consumption, and the use of oral contraceptives) that also enhance the incidence of coronary artery disease. However, it should be clear that the likelihood of the disease is strongly influenced by persons' behavior. Health-impairing habits provide the distal disregulatory forces that foster heart disease.

The traditional risk factors just described, while predictive of coronary artery disease, do not do so with great accuracy. Only about 50% of the incidence of coronary heart disease is accounted for by the best combination of these variables (Keys, 1966). Other risk factors need to be identified before we can more completely understand the etiology of coronary artery disease. The identification of these additional risk factors has focused on psychosocial and behavioral characteristics of individuals. Stress, social support, and Type A behavior have been implicated. We will now turn to a description of these factors.

Psychosocial and Behavioral Risk Factors

As described, health-impairing behaviors play a direct causative role in coronary artery disease. Via the psychophysiological mechanisms described in Chapter 4, persons' appraisal of the environment and the style in which they cope with stress may foster coronary artery disease in an indirect manner.

Stress. Our cardiovascular system is sensitive to how we evaluate and respond to the environment. Under stress, there is an increase in heart rate and force, and the heart must pump against an increased load caused by elevated blood pressure. As a result of this work, the heart is in greater need of oxygen. If there is partial or total occlusion of one or more of the coronary arteries, stress may precipitate angina or a heart attack. The increase in blood pressure may increase lesions in the coronary arteries. This, along with high levels of fats in the blood caused by the release of E and NE from the adrenal medulla as well as glucocorticoids from the adrenal cortex, promotes atherosclerosis. Thus, there is a well-defined biobehavioral connection between stress and coronary artery disease.

The evidence suggests that both chronic and acute stress play a role in the development of coronary heart disease (Jenkins, 1976). The effects of stress on the disease have been studied in three general ways: (1) life dissatisfaction and change, or chronic stress, (2) acute stress, and (3) chronic disturbing emotions. The impact of stress is modulated by the coping skills and social supports available to the individual.

Chronic Stress. The risk of coronary artery disease increases as a person experiences many life changes or dissatisfactions. Coronary artery disease is associated with (1) job dissatisfaction, feelings of work overload, and major changes in occupation and residence; (2) discrepancy between the socioeconomic level and culture of family of origin and those of the current life situation, and (3) loss of significant people and roles. Many of these findings are based on the retrospective reports of individuals who had coronary heart disease and therefore are of questionable validity (Surwitt et al., 1982). However, recent prospective studies have reported similar findings. For example, Dohrenwend and Dohrenwend (1974) found an increased incidence of coronary heart disease for older persons after they became widows or widowers. These data suggest that chronic stress, via the biobehavioral mechanisms described earlier, increases the likelihood of coronary heart disease.

Acute Stress. Acute stress may precipitate angina or a heart attack in persons who are already predisposed. Engel (1971) analyzed over 150 cases of sudden death occurring under extreme stress. While these data are anecdotal and uncontrolled, there was an impressive consistency in the circumstances surrounding these deaths. Most of the deaths occurred soon after persons had received news of the death of a loved one. In each case, the central component was a perception of a great loss or an impending threat over which the person had no control.

Chronic Disturbing Emotions. One of the correlates of stress is disturbing emotions like anxiety or depression. A large number of studies from many social settings have documented the relationship between chronic disturbing emotions and anginal pain. A prospective study done in Israel found that persons who scored high on scales of anxiety and depression had 2 to 2.5 times the risk of developing angina than those who scored low (Multicentre International Study, 1975). High levels of depression and anxiety are also related to increasing levels of atherosclerosis as judged by coronary angiograms (Zyzanski, Jenkins, Ryan, Flessas, & Everest, 1976). As we will see shortly, anxiety and depression after a heart attack influence the recovery of the victim.

Social Support. The impact of stress depends on the resources available to deal with that stress. Social relationships are an important coping resource that mitigates the negative effects of stress. The importance of social networks is nicely demonstrated by a nine-year prospective study of nearly 7,000 people done by Berkman and Syme (1979). They found an increased mortality rate among persons who had few friends or contacts with others. The relationship between social contacts and mortality was linear (as the number of contacts decreased, mortality increased) and was independent of physical status and risk factors (smoking, diet, and exercise) at the beginning of the study. Similarly, Marmot and Syme (1976), in a study of Japanese immigrants to the United States, found a greater incidence of coronary artery disease among those who gave up their traditional Japanese associations with family and friends. Those who retained those associations had a lower rate of the disease. Strong social networks are protective against coronary artery disease, and this effect is independent of traditional risk factors.

A person's education, occupation, housing, and income are also reflective of coping resources. A lack of skill or opportunity may result in more stress and reduce a person's ability to cope with stress. Jenkins (1981) calculated correlations between mortality rates due to coronary artery disease and five socioeconomic variables for persons residing in Massachusetts in 1972 and 1973. Excess mortality from coronary artery disease was related to low education, low occupational status, low income, and substandard housing.

We all experience stress and change in our lives. Stress has its most dramatic effects when we are unable to adapt or to cope successfully with those threats and challenges. Persons who have good resources in terms of social support, socioeconomic opportunity, and stability are less affected. Let us now turn to the effect of various personal modes of evaluating and coping with the environment.

Type A Behavior

Description. Health care professionals have long been aware that certain behavioral features characterize persons who develop coronary heart disease. In 1897, Sir William Osler noted that "in the worry and strain of modern life, arterial degeneration is not only very common but develops at a relatively early age. For this, I believe that the high pressure at which men live, and the habit of working the machine to its maximum capacity are responsible for coronary disease." He went on to suggest that the typical person with coronary heart disease was not "the delicate neurotic" but the "robust, the vigorous in mind and body, the keen and ambitious man, the indicator of whose machine is always at full speed ahead" (Osler, 1910, p. 840).

Friedman, Rosenman, and Rosenman (1959) were the first to systematically assess those behaviors characterizing persons with coronary heart disease. They labeled those behaviors Type A. Type A behavior can be considered a particular style of evaluating and coping with the environment. Jenkins (1971, p. 247) describes Type A as:

> an overt behavioral syndrome or style of living characterized by extremes of competitiveness, striving for achievement, aggressiveness (sometimes stringently repressed), haste, impatience, restlessness, hyperalertness, explosiveness of speech, tenseness of facial musculature, and feelings of being under the pressure of time and under the challenge of responsibility. Persons having this pattern are often so deeply committed to their vocation that other aspects of their lives are relatively neglected.

People who infrequently engage in these behaviors are classified as Type B. Type A behavior has both cognitive and behavioral components. Cognitively, Type A persons create much of their own stress by perceiving challenges and threats where others do not (Glass, 1977). Type A persons emphasize competition and achievement and thus consistently view tasks as challenges to their competency. Behaviorally, they work to exert and maintain control when under stress. They work long hours, complete tasks in a rapid fashion, and often engage in several tasks simultaneously. There appear to be three basic components to coronary-prone behavior: time urgency, achievement striving (competitiveness), and hostility (aggressiveness). Let us look at each of these.

Time Urgency. Type A persons always seem to be in a hurry. They typically do several things at a time. They underestimate the amount of time that has passed (Glass, 1977). They show frustration and impatience when they have to wait, and do more poorly than Type

B persons on tasks that require slow, careful responding (Glass, Snyder, & Hollis, 1974). They exhibit a preoccupation with quantity rather than quality and a tendency to cram as many things as possible into a short period of time. They walk, talk, and eat very quickly (Friedman & Rosenman, 1974).

Achievement Striving. Type A persons have an intense need to succeed. They perceive more situations as competitive than Type B persons. They have to win, even when playing games with young children. Type A students expect higher grades (Glass, 1977) and will work harder without a deadline than Type B students (Burnham, Pennebaker, & Glass, 1975). They self-impose deadlines and view tasks as personal challenges, thereby creating stress. Type A students are involved in more sports in high school and more extracurricular activities in college. They are more likely to achieve academic honors. They ignore or suppress fatigue in order to continue working on a task (Glass, 1977). They frequently feel guilty about "doing nothing" in the evening or on weekends.

Hostility. The third major facet of Type A behavior is hostility and aggressiveness. Type A persons compete with and challenge others. Their speech is judged to carry more rancor and contentiousness (Friedman & Rosenman, 1974). They respond to threat with aggressiveness (Glass, 1977). There is a strong correlation between Type A behavior and hostility as measured by personality tests (Williams, Haney, & Blumenthal, 1981).

Assessment of Type A Behavior. There are two widely accepted modes of measuring Type A behavior: a structured interview (Rosenman, Friedman, Strauss, Wurm, Kositchick, Hahn, & Werthessen, 1964) and a self-administered questionnaire (Jenkins, Rosenman, & Friedman, 1967).

In the structured interview, the classification of a person as Type A or B is based on a clinical judgment of the person's responses to a series of questions designed to elicit Type A behavior. The content of the questions focuses on job involvement, competitiveness, sense of time urgency, and feelings of frustration, anger, and irritation. The manner in which the questions are asked also creates a situation in which Type A behaviors are likely to be displayed. For example, the interviewer will purposefully interrupt the person to elicit anger, ask questions rapidly to encourage quick responding, and slow a question and stumble over words to facilitate interruption. Ratings of Type A or B are based more on the manner in which persons respond to the questions rather than the content of their responses. The features that distinguish Type A and B persons are shown in Table 6-1.

TABLE 6-1 Features of Type A and Type B Behaviors Derived from the Structured Interview

TYPE A BEHAVIOR PATTERN	TYPE B BEHAVIOR PATTERN
1. A general expression of vigor and energy, alertness and confidence	1. A general expression of relaxation, calm and quiet attentiveness
2. A firm handshake and brisk walking pace	2. A general handshake and moderate to slow walking pace
3. Loud and/or vigorous voice	3. A mellow voice usually low in volume
4. Terse speech, abbreviated responses	4. Lengthy, rambling responses
5. Clipped speech (a failure to pronounce the ending sounds of words)	5. No evidence of clipped speech
6. Rapid speech and the acceleration of speech at the end of a longer sentence.	6. Slow to moderate pacing of verbal responses. No acceleration at the end of a sentence.
7. Explosive speech (speech punctuated with certain words spoken emphatically and this is established as the speaker's general pattern) that may contain swear words.	7. Minimum inflection in general speech, almost a monotone with no explosive quality
8. Interruption by frequent rapid responses given before another speaker has completed his question or statement	8. Rarely interrupts another speaker
9. Speech hurrying in the form of saying "yes, yes," or "mm, mm," or "right, right," or by nodding his head in assent while another person speaks	9. No speech hurrying
10. Vehement reactions to questions relating to impedance of time progress (i.e., driving slowly, waiting in lines)	10. No vehement reactions to questions related to impedance of making progress with the utilization of time
11. Use of clenched fists or pointing his finger at you to emphasize his verbalization	11. Never uses clenched fist or the pointing finger gesture to emphasize his speech

(continued)

TABLE 6-1 Continued

TYPE A BEHAVIOR PATTERN	TYPE B BEHAVIOR PATTERN
12. Frequent sighing especially related to questions about his work. It is important to differentiate this from sighs of a depressed person.	12. Rarely sighs unless he is "hyperventilating" and showing nervous anxiety
13. Hostility directed at the interviewer or at the topics of the interview	13. Hostility is rarely, if ever, observed
14. Frequent, abrupt and emphatic one word responses to your questions (i.e., Yes! Never! Definitely! Absolutely!)	14. An absence of emphatic, one word responses

Note: From "Type A Behavior: Assessment and Intervention" (p. 21) by M. A. Chesney, J. R. Eagleston, & R. H. Rosenman, 1981, in C. K. Prokop and L. A. Bradley (Eds.), *Medical Psychology: Contributions to Behavioral Medicine,* New York: Academic Press. Copyright 1981 by Academic Press. Reprinted by permission.

The Jenkins Activity Survey is a self-reported measure of Type A behavior. Persons answer questions concerning their response to waiting, how quickly they do things, their work involvement, and their competitiveness. These responses are used to classify persons along a Type A-B continuum. Three component scores of Type A—hard driving, impatient, and job involvement—can also be derived from the scale.

These two measures of Type A behavior are only modestly related to each other. Each measure is reliable; persons' scores are consistent over time. But the measures that supposedly assess the same thing are not highly related. This suggests that the conceptualization and measurement of Type A behavior require further refinement. As we will see, the lack of care in current definitions and measurement of Type A behavior has led to some confusion.

Association of Type A Behavior and Coronary Artery Disease. Over forty studies have found an association between Type A behavior and atherosclerotic coronary heart disease (Jenkins, 1981). Rather than providing an exhaustive review, two such studies will be considered in detail.

The Western Collaborative Group Study (Rosenman, Brand, Jenkins, Friedman, Strauss, & Wurm, 1975) is a classic. It began in 1960 as a prospective study of the incidence of coronary heart disease in 3,524 men aged thirty-nine to fifty-nine. At the beginning of the study, subjects were given an extensive medical exam and were administered the structured Type A interview. Initially, 113 men had coronary heart disease, 71% of whom displayed Type A behavior. The remaining subjects were followed annually for eight and one-half years. The results of this follow-up are shown in Figure 6-3. Of the 257 men that developed coronary heart disease during this interval, 178 were classified as Type A and 79 as Type B. Type A persons were over twice as likely to develop coronary artery disease. When controlling for age, smoking, blood pressure, and blood cholesterol, Type A persons were still twice as likely to develop coronary artery disease. Recurring heart attacks were observed in 41 subjects, 34 of whom were Type A. Type A persons were five times as likely to have multiple heart attacks. The relationship between Type A behavior and coronary artery disease was linear; the higher the person's Type A score, the greater the risk.

FIGURE 6-3 Association of Type A and Type B Behavior with Coronary Heart Disease (Western Collaborative Group Study)

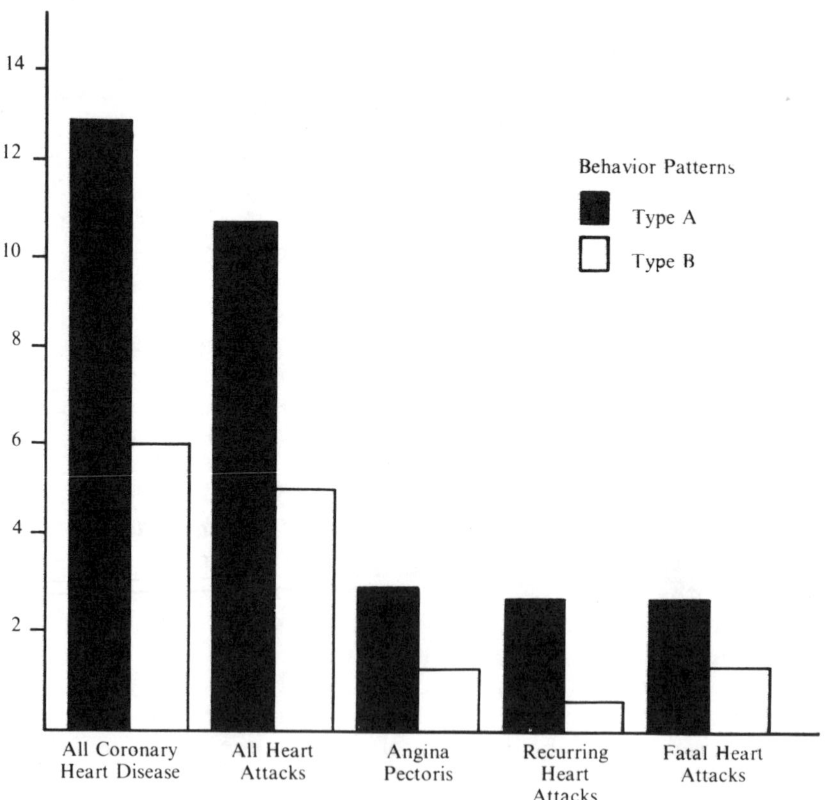

Type A behavior has also been associated with coronary atherosclerosis (Williams, Haney, Lee, Kang, Blumenthal, & Whalen, 1980). Subjects in this study were persons referred for coronary angiography (filming the inside of the coronary arteries). Their angiograms were interpreted by three cardiologists who had no knowledge of the Type A or B status of the subjects. Any subject who had an obstruction of 75% or more in any of the coronary arteries was considered to have a significant disease. In a sample of 307 men and 117 women, 71% of those judged to be Type A had significant atherosclerosis compared to 56% of those judged to be Type B. The findings were as strong for women as men.

More recently, a few studies have failed to find an association between Type A behavior and coronary heart disease (Chesney, 1986). Type A behavior describes a complex cluster of behavioral dispositions, specific actions, and emotional reactions. While these diverse aspects are correlated, it may be that only a subset of the cluster constituting Type A behavior is associated with coronary artery disease. In fact, this seems to be the case. A reanalysis of the data from the Western Collaborative Group Study indicated that, compared to other facets of Type A behavior, hostility and aggression were the best predictors of coronary heart disease (Mathews, Glass, Rosenman, & Bortner, 1977). This has been replicated in prospective studies on other samples (Haynes, Feinleib, & Kannel, 1980). In fact, the data from the work by Williams et al. (1980) just cited suggest that coronary atherosclerosis is positively related to hostility even in individuals who do not display other aspects of Type A behavior.

Clearly, more work is required to define and measure Type A behavior clearly and to ascertain which facets of that behavior pattern enhance the risk of coronary heart disease. At this time, it appears that Type A and coronary-prone behaviors, although related, are not identical. Not all facets of Type A behavior have been convincingly related to coronary heart disease.

The Development of Type A Behavior. Why do some people display high levels of Type A behavior while others display less? Glass (1977) proposed that these patterns are acquired during socialization via direct reinforcement and modeling. Butensky, Farelli, Heebner, and Waldron (1976) found that children from suburban middle class homes displayed more Type A behavior than their age- and sex-matched counterparts from rural working class homes.

Suinn (1977) suggested that Type A behavior is maintained by both positive and negative reinforcement. Type A actions are positively reinforced by the products achieved and the recognition of these accomplishments by others. An advertising executive, for example, who is very aggressive and works long hours to have the highest accounts in the firm, is likely to receive a raise and to be esteemed by coworkers and the boss. However, Type A persons also create a lot of stress for themselves because they perceive their work as a challenge and demand high quantities of work from themselves. Type A behavior is quite effective in meeting these self-imposed demands and thereby reducing the aversive, pressured situation created by the Type A thinking. This reduction in stress negatively reinforces the Type A thinking and behavior. Thus, a vicious circle is set up in which Type A thinking and behavior are promoted and maintained by their success in reducing stress. The ad executive, then, will strive to maintain his number one position in the agency and to increase his accounts because someone might surpass him or because he wants more money and recognition. His hard work and long hours worked before, so all he needs to do is more of the same. Thus he works harder, longer, and more frantically to better his position, leaving less time for recreation and relaxation.

Vicious circles represent a positive feedback system that disrupts homeostasis (which is maintained by negative feedback). It is as if a furnace burns faster and faster as the thermostat registers higher and higher temperatures. Type A behavior, like any negatively reinforced behavior, is particularly hard to extinguish.

Little is known about how Type A behavior develops. Mathews (1980) and Mathews and Siegal (1984) have studied the development of Type A behavior in children, which has similar characterisitics to Type A behavior in adults: time urgency and competitiveness. Mathews and her colleagues have found that the frequency with which children engage in Type A behavior is influenced by their parents. For example, mothers of Type A children give fewer positive evaluations relative to negative evaluations of their children's performance. They encourage Type A children to try harder even while these children are succeeding.

The notion that Type A behavior is learned is also supported by findings that Type A behavior is culture bound. It is highly prevalent in the United States and industrialized Western European societies (Jenkins, 1987), but fewer than 15% of Japanese-Americans living in Hawaii are found to be Type A (Cohen, Syme, Jenkins, & Kagan, 1975).

Psychophysiological Correlates of Type A Behavior. As noted, at least some aspects of Type A behavior are associated with coronary atherosclerosis as well as heart attacks. Type A behavior is associated with hormonal and neural responses that promote atherosclerosis.

Type A persons have higher levels of blood cholesterol than Type Bs, both before and after the emergence of identifiable coronary artery disease (Blumenthal, Williams, Kang, Schanberg, & Thompson, 1978; Friedman, Byers, Rosenman, & Elwitch, 1970). These high levels are caused by the release of E and NE from the adrenal medulla and by the release of glucocorticoids from the adrenal cortex. Type A persons have been shown to excrete more E and NE during a typical day than Type B persons (Friedman, St. George, & Byers, 1960) and to have depleted stores of glucocorticoids as a result of chronic arousal and stress (Friedman, Byers, & Rosenman, 1972). Frequent and sustained arousal of the sympathetic nervous system also increases heart rate and blood pressure (Type A behavior may be similar to the defense and sensory processing reactions described earlier). Increased blood pressure promotes the wear and tear of the lining of the coronary arteries, thus contributing to atherosclerosis (Ross & Glomset, 1976). Sympathetic arousal may also precipitate angina or a heart attack by increasing the heart's need for oxygen beyond the delivery capacity of the coronary arteries.

Type A Behavior: A Summary. We can identify those persons whose biobehavioral response pattern predisposes them to coronary heart disease. Type A persons frequently perceive the environment as threatening, work in a diligent and hostile manner to exert or maintain control, and exhibit a physiological response that may promote coronary atherosclerosis and precipitate angina or a heart attack.

Psychosocial and Behavioral Risk Factors: A Summary

There are multiple risk factors for coronary artery disease. These distal factors are observed at physiological, behavioral, and psychosocial levels. A summary of these factors and their relative impact is shown in Table 6-2.

TABLE 6-2 Risk Factors for Coronary Heart Disease

CHARACTERISTIC	RISK
Age	
Over 65	Strong
45–65	Moderate
Under 45	Not significant
Sex	
Male	Strong
Female	Not significant
Family history	
Heart attack before 55	Strong
Heart attack before 65	Moderate
Other cardiovascular disease	Moderate
None	Not Significant
Cholesterol level (mg%)	
Over 270	Strong

(continued)

TABLE 6-2 Continued

CHARACTERISTIC	RISK
240–269	Moderate
221–239	Weak
Less than 220	Not significant
Triglyceride level (mg%)	
Over 200	Strong
151–199	Moderate
Less than 150	Not significant
Blood pressure (mm Hg)	
Over 160 (systolic) and/or 100 (diastolic)	Strong
140–159 (systolic) and/or 90–99 (diastolic)	Strong
100–139 (systolic) and/or 69–89 (diastolic)	Not significant
Smoking	
Over 1 pack per day	Strong
Less than 1 pack per day	Moderate
Stopped for at least 5 years	Weak
None	Not significant
Behavior pattern	
Type A (symptomatic)	Strong
Type A (asymptomatic)	Moderate
Type B (asymptomatic)	Not significant
Exercise	
None or irregular	Moderate
Regular aerobic	Not significant
Obesity	
Severe	Strong
Moderate	Weak
Mild	Not significant

ILLNESS-RELATED DECISIONS AND ACTIONS IN CORONARY ARTERY DISEASE

Many persons die suddenly each year as a result of heart attacks and subsequent complications. Fifty percent of those who die do so within one hour after the acute symptoms of a heart attack initially occur (Surwitt et al., 1982). Often, these conditions are treatable if individuals seek medical treatment in a timely fashion. Persons' evaluation of and response to their symptoms prior to hospitalization are very important.

Once a person has sought medical treatment, there is typically a two-to-three-week period of hospitalization, a two-to-eight-week convalescent period at home, and a long-term adjustment and rehabilitative period as the person returns to normal roles and activities. The illness-related behaviors of a person during these three periods, including adhering to treatment regimens, adjusting to the treatment environment and procedures, and adapting to a life-threatening illness, play an important role in the person's recovery. In this section, illness-related decisions and actions in response to a heart attack will be described. The impact of these behaviors on prognosis will also be discussed.

Symptom Recognition and Treatment Action

When persons experience chest pain and other symptoms of a heart attack, they are faced with defining the problem and with taking action in response to the symptoms. The most common response to the symptoms of a heart attack is to wait. Persons typically delay seeking medical assistance beyond the one-hour interval associated with sudden cardiac death (Moss & Goldstein, 1970). The average delay in seeking treatment is three hours, but 50% of heart attack victims delay at least twenty-four hours (Gentry & Haney, 1975).

Most of the delay time is spent evaluating the symptoms and attempting self-care. These actions include: (1) a cognitive sequence beginning with the initial perception of the symptoms and ending with the realization that the nature and severity of the symptoms require medical treatment; (2) the use of a variety of patent and prescribed medications; and (3) the communication with spouse, family, and friends about how to cope with the symptoms (Moss, Wynar, & Goldstein, 1969). Seventy percent of those who delay for a long period misinterpret their symptoms and think the pain is due to indigestion, gall bladder problems, an ulcer, or some other disorder. Tjoe and Luria (1972) reported that only twenty-one of seventy-five persons admitted to a coronary care unit thought their symptoms were heart related. Persons who accurately recognize their symptoms are quicker to seek appropriate treatment (Hackett & Cassem, 1969). Misperceiving symptoms involves denial or minimization of their seriousness. Deniers require the impetus of others before seeking treatment. Persons who accurately recognize their own symptoms tend to refer themselves (Williams & Gentry, 1978).

Like any illness-related behavior, the manner in which a person evaluates and responds to the symptoms of a heart attack is complexly determined. The action taken is influenced by a person's history of coronary heart disease. Persons with a history of angina take longer to seek help because the pain does not provide a cue that distinguishes anginal pain from that of a heart attack. Persons who previously had a heart attack are better able to diagnose their symptoms. The social context in which the symptoms occur also influences the action taken. Persons who have a heart attack at work, during a weekday, and in the presence of others are quicker to seek treatment. Other people provide information that assists in the accurate interpretation of the symptoms and cues that elicit appropriate action (Gentry, 1975).

Current education concerning symptom recognition and appropriate action does not appear to be adequate. Surveys of college students have found that only 43% correctly identified heart attack as the problem when given symptoms describing that disorder (Snyder, 1983). Quick and appropriate action is important to successful treatment and recovery. Late compared to quick responders have three times the mortality rate (Moss & Goldstein, 1970).

Adjustment and Adherence During Treatment and Rehabilitation

Persons who experience a heart attack have to adjust to the current and future implications of the event and to the treatment procedures and environment. This adjustment will be discussed in terms of the acute phase, convalescence, and rehabilitation (Keefe & Blumenthal, 1982).

Acute Phase. Acute treatment of a heart attack victim usually occurs in a coronary care unit. During this phase, clients need to give meaning to their heart attack and its consequences and to adjust to the treatment environment.

Treatment in a coronary care unit and realization of having had a heart attack threaten a person's sense of control. A heart attack is often a sudden, unexpected event. At one moment persons are going about their daily routine, and at the next are experiencing severe pain and being taken to the hospital. The usual modes of maintaining control are not functional in these circumstances. The prospect of a sudden death is anxiety provoking. The coronary care unit leads to a loss of control and depersonalization. It is an unfamiliar environment. Sophisticated electronic equipment is attatched to monitor the client's condition. Vital signs are repeatedly taken and medications are administered intravenously. The environment is usually stark. Persons are confined to bed and are literally dependent on the medical staff and equipment for their well-being.

Most studies suggest that clients are stressed and emotionally upset during this acute phase. The most common reactions are anxiety, depression, and anger (Hackett, Cassem, & Winshie, 1968). The initial reaction is usually anxiety or fear, centering on possible death. This anxiety usually dissipates in one or two days (Gentry, Foster, & Haney, 1972). Persons who deny or minimize the seriousness of their condition are less anxious. Even events that objectively indicate recovery may be anxiety provoking. Some clients, for example, display a negative emotional arousal when transferred from the coronary care unit to a general medical ward (Klein, Kliner, Zipes, Troyer, & Wallace, 1968).

As anxiety dissipates, it is often replaced by depression. Once persons realize they have survived their heart attack, the focus is on the potential loss of functioning and ability that may result. The person is concerned with a loss of autonomy, income, sexual functioning, social status, and physical ability. The depression frequently begins after several days in the coronary care unit and may continue when persons are shifted to a nonintensive cardiology unit and when they return home for convalescence (Cassem & Hackett, 1971).

The degree to which clients experience anxiety and depression depends on their coping skills and resources (Doehrman, 1977). Adequate coping during acute care entails: (1) expressing feelings, (2) managing one's own emotional reaction and distress, (3) utilizing adequate perceptual, appraisal, and problem-solving strategies, and (4) cooperating with care (Pranulis, 1975). Different modes of coping are effective at different times in this process. Denial during the recognition of symptoms is not adaptive, but becomes adaptive as an initial coping strategy in the coronary care unit. Later adaptation during convalescence and rehabilitation requires more active coping strategies than denial.

The manner in which clients cope during the acute phase affects their immediate and long-term recovery. Extreme anxiety and depression (hopelessness and helplessness) are associated with psychophysiological responses that may complicate or interfere with recovery. Hypervigilance and anxiety are associated with increased sympathetic arousal, and result in increased metabolic rate, blood pressure, and heart rate as well as changes in body levels of sodium and potassium. Although less clearly documented, helplessness and hopelessness are associated with an autonomic nervous system response that causes the severe depression of heart and metabolic rates (Klein, 1975). Both responses may be life threatening. Persons who exhibit excessive anxiety or depression are more likely to experience another heart attack or to die compared to those who cope more effectively (Cromwell, 1969; Gentry et al., 1972).

Consequently, it is important for clients in the coronary care unit to establish a sense of contol and predictability. During the acute phase, clients also develop perceptions and beliefs about their health state. These perceptions and beliefs influence their mood and guide their recovery-related actions during hospitalization as well as post-hospitalization convalescence and rehabilitation. Clients who view their health as poor and foresee little hope for recovery display lower morale and are less likely to return to normal work and interpersonal roles (Garrity, 1981). They may become cardiac invalids. At the other extreme, clients who minimize, deny, or ignore the seriousness of the problem are likely to ignore medical advice and to fail to engage in rehabilitative actions.

Convalescence. Convalescence is defined as the time from a person's discharge from the hospital through the sixth to eighth week after discharge. It is during this period that successful adaptation consists of beginning to return to normal roles. Care shifts from health professionals to clients and their families. During convalescence, programs are initiated or continued to alter clients' diet and weight, to stop smoking, and to begin physical reconditioning in preparation for return to normal roles. Clients also become responsible for taking medication. During this time, clients need to become more active participants in their own care and recovery, leaving behind a dependency that was more functional during hospitalization. Anxiety and depression again increase as clients return home. They are often confused about what to do, are concerned about their health, their fatigue with exercise, and their ability to return to old roles. The total impact of the illness may now be experienced. Often, these clients were hard driving, aggressive, and impatient persons who were dedicated to their work. Now they are at home all day, face a boring routine, deal with children who fight, follow a complex dietary, exercise, and medication regimen, and worry about work and income. Anxiety and depression may be exacerbated or maintained by family members. Most frequently, this occurs when the family reinforces continued sick role behaviors and discourages well behaviors (Cassem & Hackett, 1971). Recovery and adaptation are influenced by the clients' social support systems.

Clients' responses to the stressors and tasks of convalescence are complexly determined. Their perception of their own health state and potential for recovery, the speed of recovery, the family support, and the quality and nature of communication with health providers all contribute to this response.

Rehabilitation. Rehabilitation refers to the period beginning in the sixth to eighth week after discharge, and represents an ongoing, open-ended process of recovery and treatment. Medical care becomes less frequent and specific. Treatment strategies begun during hospitalization and convalescence (e.g., dietary changes, weight loss, smoking cessation, proper rest, and regular exercise) are continued. Programs to enhance self regulation of these behaviors are initiated or continued.

This is also the period during which persons return to normal social, vocational, and recreational roles. The success of treatment depends not only on persons' biological recovery but also on their successful recovery at behavioral and social levels. The degree to which persons successfully return to normal roles thus depends on biological, social, and behavioral factors. Those persons who have the greatest biological impairment because of the heart attack generally have the greatest difficulty resuming normal roles and activities. Continuing anxiety and depression may also impair adaptation. The context or situation in which persons live, including their sex, age, social status, and occupation, also influence rehabilitation. Three aspects of persons' return to normal roles and activities have received the most attention: work, marital relationship, and recreation.

Eighty to 90% of persons who have had a heart attack return to work within one year of the attack (Williams & Gentry, 1978). Problems in returning to work are greater for persons who are older, more anxious or depressed, have more severe cardiac damage, have physically demanding jobs, and have fewer social and economic resources.

A heart attack also affects the marital relationship. Conflicts may arise because the spouse is too solicitous and takes over too many responsibilities or is perceived as not caring enough (Croog & Levine, 1974). There is a 60 to 80% decrease in sexual activity. This may be the result of continued depression, side effects of medication, fear of another heart attack during coitus, or the spouse's reluctance. In uncomplicated cases in which there has been adequate physical reconditioning, sexual activity is not dangerous. The typical demands of sexual intercourse approximate those of climbing two flights of stairs.

Returning to normal social and recreational activity is difficult in some cases. Forty percent of heart attack victims report being less active. They reduce strenuous activities like playing tennis, cycling, and dancing. Routine household chores like gardening are taken over by other family members. Recreational activities influence clients' mood and self confidence (Croog & Levine, 1974). Successful rehabilitation consists of a reinvestment in roles and activities that are meaningful and enjoyable for clients. It involves a return to feelings of control, hopefulness, and fulfillment.

Illness-Related Decisions and Actions: A Summary

A heart attack poses a series of threats. These include recognizing the symptoms and their meaning, taking prompt and appropriate action, coping with treatment and rehabilitative procedures, and coming to terms with the life-threatening nature of the illness and the limitations implied by its occurrence. How persons cope with these threats importantly influences their biological and psychosocial prognosis and recovery. Successful adaptation entails the flexible use of a variety of illness-related decisions and actions as well as other coping skills. The client plays a critical role in treatment and recovery. Success depends on psychosocial as well as environmental variables.

SUMMARY

Coronary artery disease is a major health problem. Its proximal cause, atherosclerosis of the coronary arteries, is the result of a number of converging and interacting distal risk factors at biological, behavioral, and psychosocial levels: smoking, dietary patterns, exercise, stress, Type A behavior, multifactorial genetic predisposition, high blood pressure, and diabetes. As such, heart disease is the final expression of lifestyle choices as well as biology. Prevention of coronary artery disease and its treatment, once it has developed, entail interventions to change behavior as well as effective medical treatment.

Persons who have developed coronary artery disease are important actors in the treatment process. Illness-related decisions and actions such as symptom recognition, prompt seeking of treatment, alteration of health habits, and adherence to treatment recommendations are a critical part of successful intervention. The experience and treatment of a myocardial infarction also pose a variety of challenges to the client. To negotiate the treatment and rehabilitative process successfully, the client must utilize problem-oriented and palliative forms of coping. Throughout the process, the client is an active and integral agent in his own treatment and recovery.

REFERENCES

Berkman, L. F., & Syme, S. L. (1979). Social networks, host resistance and mortality: A nine-year follow up study of Alemeda County residents. *American Journal of Epidemiology, 104*, 186–204.

Blumenthal, J. A., Williams, R. B., Kang, Y., Schanberg, S. M., & Thompson, L. W. (1978). Type A behavior and angiographically documented coronary disease. *Circulation, 58*, 634–639.

Burnham, M. A., Pennebaker, J. W., & Glass, D. C. (1975). Time consciousness, achievement striving and the Type A coronary prone behavior pattern. *Journal of Abnormal Psychology, 84*, 76–79.

Butensky, A., Farelli, V., Heebner, D., & Waldron, I. (1976). Elements of the coronary prone behavior pattern in children and teenagers. *Journal of Psychosomatic Medicine, 20*, 439–444.

Cassem, N. H., & Hackett, T. P. (1971). Psychiatric consultation in a coronary care unit. *Annals of Internal Medicine, 75*, 9–39.

Chesney, M. A. (1986, November). *Type A behavior: The biobehavioral interface*. Paper presented at the annual meeting of the Association for the Advancement of Behavior Therapy. Chicago.

Cohen, J. B., Syme, S. L., Jenkins, C. D., & Kagan, A. (1975). The cultural context of Type A behavior and the risk of CHD. *American Journal of Epidemiology, 102*, 434.

Cromwell, R. (1969). *Stress, personality and nursing care in myocardial infarction*. Washington, DC: NIMH.

Croog, S. H., & Levine, S. (1974). *The heart patient recovers*. New York: Wiley.

Doehrman, S. R. (1977). Psychosocial aspects of recovery from coronary heart disease: A review. *Social Science and Medicine, 11*, 199–218.

Dohrenwend, B. S., & Dohrenwend, B. P. (1974). *Stressful life events: Their nature and effects*. New York: Wiley.

Engel, G. (1971). Sudden and rapid death following psychologic stress. *Annals of Internal Medicine, 74,* 771.

Essentials of life and health. New York: Random House.

Friedman, M., Byers, S. O., Rosenman, R. H., & Elwitch, F. R. (1970). Coronary prone individuals (Type A behavior pattern): Some biochemical characteristics. *Journal of the American Medical Association, 212,* 1030–1037.

Friedman, M., Byers, S. O., & Rosenman, R. H. (1972). Plasma ACTH and cortisol concentration of coronary prone subjects. *Proceedings of the Society of Experimental Biology and Medicine, 140,* 681–684.

Friedman, M., Rosenman, L., & Rosenman, R. H. (1959). Association of specific overt behavior with blood and cardiovascular findings. *Journal of the American Medical Association, 169,* 1286–1296.

Friedman, M., & Rosenman, R. H. (1974). *Type A behavior and your heart.* New York: Knopf.

Friedman, M., St. George, S., & Byers, S. O. (1960). Excretion of catecholamines, 17-ketosteroids, 17-hydroxycorticoids and 6-hydroxy indole in men exhibiting a particular behavior pattern (A) associated with high incidence coronary heart disease. *Journal of Clinical Investigations, 39,* 758–764.

Garrity, T. F. (1981). Behavioral adjustment after myocardial infarction: A selective review of recent descriptive, correlational and intervention research. In S. M. Weiss, J. A. Herd & B. H. Fox (Eds.), *Perspectives on behavioral medicine,* 67–88. New York: Academic Press.

Gentry, W. D. (1975). Preadmission behavior. In W. D. Gentry & R. B. Williams (Eds.), *Psychological aspects of myocardial infarction and coronary care.* St. Louis: C. V. Mosby.

Gentry, W. D., Foster, S., & Haney, T. (1972). Denial as a determinant of anxiety and perceived health status in the coronary care unit. *Psychosomatic Medicine, 34,* 39–44.

Gentry, W. D., & Haney, T. L. (1975). Emotional and behavioral reaction to acute myocardial infarction. *Heart and Lung, 25,* 738–745.

Glass, D. C. (1977). *Behavior patterns, stress and coronary heart disease.* Hillsdale, NJ: Lawrence Erlbaum.

Glass, D. C., Snyder, M. L., & Hollis, J. F. (1974). Time urgency and Type A coronary prone behavior. *Journal of Applied Social Psychology, 4,* 125–140.

Hackett, T. P., & Cassem, N. H. (1969). Factors contributing to delay in responding to signs and symptoms of acute myocardial infarction. *American Journal of Cardiology, 24,* 651–659.

Hackett, T. P., Cassem, N. H., & Winshie, H. A. (1968). The coronary care unit: An appraisal of its psychological hazards. *New England Journal of Medicine, 279,* 1365–1370.

Hassett, J. (1978). *A primer of psychophysiology.* San Francisco: Freeman.

Haynes, S. G., Feinleib, M., & Kannel, W. B. (1980). The relationship of psychosocial factors to coronary heart disease in the Framingham study. Part II: Eight year incidence of CHD. *American Journal of Epidemiology, 3,* 37–58.

Jenkins, C. D. (1971). Psychologic and social precursors of coronary disease. *New England Journal of Medicine, 284,* 244–255; 307–317.

Jenkins, C. D. (1976). Recent evidence supporting psychologic and social risk factors for coronary heart disease. *New England Journal of Medicine, 249,* 987–944; 1033–1038.

Jenkins, C. D. (1981). Behavioral factors in the etiology and pathogenesis of cardiovascular diseases: Sudden death, hypertension and myocardial infarction. In S. M. Weiss, J. A. Herd & B. H. Fox (Eds.), *Perspectives on behavioral medicine,* 41–54. New York: Academic Press.

Jenkins, C. D. (1987). Behavioral risk factors in coronary heart disease. *Annual Review of Medicine, 29,* 543–562.

Jenkins, C. D., Rosenman, R. H., & Friedman, M. (1967). Development of an objective psychological test for determination of coronary prone behavior in employed men. *Journal of Chronic Disease, 38,* 46–51.

Kannel, W. B., McGee, D., & Gordon, T. (1976). A general cardiovascular risk profile: The Framingham Study. *American Journal of Cardiology, 38,* 46–52.

Kannel, W. B., & Sorlie, P. (1979). Some health benefits of physical activity: The Framingham Study. *Archives of Internal Medicine, 139*, 857–861.

Keefe, F. J., & Blumenthal, J. A. (1982). *Assessment strategies in behavioral medicine*. New York: Grune & Stratton.

Keys, A. (1966). The individual risk of coronary heart disease. *Annals of the New York Academy of Sciences, 134*, 1046–1063.

Klein, R. F. (1975). Relationship between psychological and physiological stress in the coronary cell unit. In W. D. Gentry & R. B. Williams (Eds.), *Psychological aspects of myocardial infarction and coronary care.* St Louis: C. V. Mosby.

Klein, R. F., Kliner, V. A., Zipes, D. P., Troyer, W. G., & Wallace, A. G. (1968). Transfer from a coronary care unit. *Archives of Internal Medicine, 122,* 104–108.

Koplan, J. P. (1979). Cardiovascular deaths while running. *Journal of the American Medical Association, 242*, 2578–2579.

Marmot, M. G., & Syme, S. L. (1976). Acculturation and coronary heart disease in Japanese-Americans. *American Journal of Epidemiology, 104*, 242–243.

Mathews, K. A. (1980). Antecedents of the Type A coronary-prone behavior pattern. In S. S. Brehm, S. M. Kassin, & F. X. Gibbons (Eds.), *Developmental social psychology: Theory and research*, 235–248. New York: Oxford.

Mathews, K. A., Glass, D. C., Rosenman, R. H., & Bortner, R. W. (1977). Competitive drive, pattern A and coronary heart disease: A further analysis of some data from the Western Collaborative Group Study. *Journal of Chronic Diseases, 30*, 489–497.

Mathews, K. A., & Siegal, J. (1984). The Type A behavior pattern in children and adolescents. In A. Baum & J. Singer (Eds.), *Handbook of psychology and health*, 415–431. Hillsdale, NJ: Lawrence Erlbaum.

Moss, A. J., & Goldstein, S. (1970). The prehospital phase of acute myocardial infarction. *Circulation, 41*, 737.

Moss, A. J., Wynar, B., & Goldstein, S. (1969). Delay in hospitalization during the acute coronary period. *American Journal of Cardiology, 24*, 659–664.

Multicentre International Study. (1975). Improvement in the prognosis of myocardial infarction by using practolol. *British Medical Journal, 3*, 735–740.

Osler, W. (1910). The Lumlein Lectures on angina pectoris. *Lancet, 1*, 839–844.

Pranulis, M. F. (1975). Coping with acute myocardial infarction. In W. D. Gentry & R. B. Williams (Eds.), *Psychosocial aspects of myocardial infarction and coronary care*, 65–75. St. Louis: C. V. Mosby.

Rosenman, R. H., Brand, R. J., Jenkins, C. D., Friedman, M., Strauss, R., & Wurm, M. (1975). Coronary heart disease in the Western Collaborative Group Study: Final followup experience of 8 1/2 years. *Journal of the American Medical Association, 233*, 872–877.

Rosenman, R. H., Friedman, M., Strauss, R., Wurm, M., Kositchik, R., Hahn, W., & Werthessen, N. T. (1975). A predictive study of coronary heart disease. *Journal of the American Medical Association, 189*, 152–153.

Ross, R., & Glomset, J. A. (1976). The pathogenesis of atherosclerosis. *New England Journal of Medicine, 295*, 396–420.

Snyder, J. (1983). *Knowledge of symptoms of major illnesses.* Unpublished manuscript, Wichita State University.

Stokes, J., Froelicher, V. F., & Brown, P. (1981). Prevention of cardiovascular disease. In L. J. Schneiderman (Ed.), *The practice of preventative health care*, 213–245. New York: John Wiley & Sons.

Suinn, R. M. (1977). Type A behavior pattern. In R.B. Williams & W.D. Gentry (Eds.), *Behavioral approaches to medical treatment*, 181–199. Cambridge, MA: Ballinger.

Surwitt, R. S., Williams, R. B., & Shapiro, D. (1982). *Behavioral approaches to cardiovascular disease*. New York: Academic Press.

Tjoe, S. L., & Luria, M. H. (1972). Delays in seeking the cardiac care unit. *Chest, 61*, 617–621.

Tsai, S. P., Lee, E. S., & Hardy, R. J. (1978). The effect of a reduction in the leading causes of death: Potential gain in life expectancy. *American Journal of Public Health, 68*, 966–971.

United States Department of Health, Education and Welfare, (1977). *The economic impact of cardiovascular disease: United States, 1975.* Washington, DC: U. S. Government Printing Office.

Williams, R. B., & Gentry, W. D. (1978). Psychological problems inherent in the cardiopathic state. In C. Long (Ed.), *Prevention and rehabilitation in ischemic heart disease*, 87–101. Baltimore: Williams & Wilkins.

Williams, R. B., Haney, T., & Blumenthal, J. A. (1981). Psychological and physiological correlates of Type A behavior pattern. In S. M. Weiss, J. A. Herd & B. H. Fox (Eds.), Perspective on behavioral medicine, 401–406. New York: Academic Press.

Williams, R. B., Haney, T. L., Lee, K. L., Kang, Y., Blumenthal, J. A., & Whalen, R. E. (1980). Type A behavior, hostility and coronary atherosclerosis. *Psychosomatic Medicine 42*, 539–549.

Zyzanski, S. J., Jenkins, C. D., Ryan, T. J., Flessas, A., & Everest, M. (1976). Psychological correlates of coronary angiographic findings. *Archives of Internal Medicine, 136*, 1234–1237.

7
Infectious Diseases

INTRODUCTION

There are hundreds of infectious diseases. Some, although foreign to us, were very familiar to our grandparents and great-grandparents: tuberculosis, whooping cough, tetanus, diphtheria, smallpox, polio, and rubella. Some are common experiences across generations: colds, flu, strep throat, meningitis, bronchitis, syphilis, and gonorrhea. Some are seemingly new scourges: genital herpes and acquired immune deficiency syndrome, or AIDS. Since antiquity people have recognized contagion, even prior to the scientific understanding of its causes and mechanisms. That understanding began in the seventeenth century when Anton van Leeuwenhoek observed bacteria and other microorganisms through his newly developed microscope. In the late nineteenth century, Louis Pasteur and Robert Koch clearly demonstrated that infection was the result of invasion of the body by virulent microorganisms. This led to the development of vaccines that immunize persons against many infectious diseases. With the additional discovery and use of a number of powerful antibiotics, microorganisms came to be viewed as the cause of infectious diseases, and therapy was aimed at their destruction (Norton, 1982). This is known as the germ theory of disease.

The germ theory of disease is a quite limited view, and does not characterize modern medical thinking. Microorganisms are certainly the proximal cause of infectious diseases, but they are not the only important variable in the etiology of such diseases. Infectious diseases have multiple causes, including environmental, behavioral, social, and psychophysiological variables. Although the point is obvious, an individual must come into contact with a virulent organism to become infected. This contact is influenced by the individual's behavior as well as prevailing environmental conditions. On the other side of the coin, immunizations are effective means of preventing some infectious diseases, but only if persons are vaccinated. This depends on seeking health care in a timely fashion. Similarly, antibiotics are only effective if taken properly. Health-impairing and health-promoting behavior and illness-related decisions and actions, as discussed in Chapters 2 and 3, play an important role in infectious diseases.

Another phenomenon, even recognized by Pasteur, is that not all individuals exposed to an infectious agent will develop a disease. Contact with the microorganism is thus a necessary but not sufficient cause of infectious diseases. People have a built-in defense against the invasion of infectious agents: the skin and mucous membranes, the inflammatory response, and nonspecific and specific immune responses. The effectiveness of these mechanisms in resisting pathogens, called host resistance, varies according to diet, age, health state, previous exposure to pathogens, and a number of other variables. Stress also appears to alter host resistance. Recent research suggests that stress, via psychophysiological mechanisms, can influence immune functioning. The study of the influence of stress on immune functioning and resistance to disease is called psychoneuroimmunology (Locke & Colligan, 1986).

In this chapter, we will explore the multiple causes of infectious diseases. The importance of personal and collective behavior in promoting contact with infectious agents will be described. The impact of stress on susceptibility to disease, or psychoimmunology, will be considered. This discussion necessitates an understanding of how the immune system works and how it is reciprocally connected to the nervous system. To make these notions more concrete, we will focus on two infectious diseases: AIDS and infectious mononucleosis.

THE IMMUNE SYSTEM

The body is continually exposed to a variety of potentially harmful agents, including bacteria and viruses, as the result of being an open system. However, the body is capable of resisting most of these pathogens most of the time. This capability is called immunity. There are two types of immunity: nonspecific and specific.

Nonspecific Immune Responses

Nonspecific immunity refers to body defenses that do not require previous exposure to a pathogen in order to react. The mechanisms of nonspecific immunity include body surfaces and the inflammatory response. Body surfaces, including the skin and mucous membranes of the cavities open to the external environment, provide effective barriers to microorganisms. If a pathogen does gain entrance to the body, the second nonspecific response, inflammation, is mobilized.

Inflammation is a short-term response of the body to tissue damage and bacterial invasion. There is an increase in blood flow to the damaged or infected area evoked by the release of chemicals from damaged cells. This causes a local redness and warmth. The blood vessels in the area become more permeable and release fluids, proteins, and white blood cells into the damaged or infected area. This causes swelling. The swelling and chemicals released by damaged cells may also cause pain. Some of the proteins wall off the area to limit the spread of toxins and infectious agents. The white blood cells destroy and ingest the invading pathogens and debris. If the invasion becomes more widespread and enters the circulatory system, white blood cells release a chemical that induces body fever. The fever may enhance the activity of white blood cells and suppress the growth of bacteria and other infectious agents (Spence & Mason, 1987).

Another nonspecific response, especially against viruses, is mediated by a protein, interferon. Cells infected by viruses produce interferon, which then binds to the membranes of uninfected cells and inhibits the invasion of viruses. Interferon may also play a role in protecting the body from some forms of cancer, perhaps by limiting cell division and by mobilizing special lymphocytes (or white blood cells) called natural killer (NK) cells (Spence & Mason, 1987). Natural killer cells have the capacity to recognize, without previous experience, that virally infected and tumor cells are abnormal. They seek out and destroy such cells without harming normal cells.

Specific Immune Responses

There are two types of specific immune responses: humoral and cell-mediated. Humoral (or in the blood) immunity responds to bacterial and extracellular viral infections. Cell-mediated immunity responds to intracellular viral infections. To be most effective, these specific responses require previous exposure to the specific invading microorganism. On first exposure, it takes five to ten days before the specific immune responses can effectively combat a pathogen. On subsequent exposures, the response occurs very quickly and often prevents any clinical symptoms. Overactive specific immune responses are sometimes involved in allergic and autoimmune disorders (Locke & Colligan, 1986).

Specific immune responses require recognition of the presence of foreign molecules, or antigens. An antigen evokes the specific immune response. The immune system does not generate a response to natural body cells. It is programmed to recognize which molecules belong to the body and which are foreigners to be destroyed. The specific immune system also has a "memory." Once exposed to a specific antigen, it produces a biochemical template so that reexposure is met with an immediate immune response.

Humoral Immunity. The humoral immune response is mediated by specialized white blood cells called B-lymphocytes, or B-cells. B-cells are produced by the bone marrow. They circulate throughout the body, but are found in especially large numbers in the lymph nodes and spleen. When a foreign antigen successfully invades the body, some of the B-cells are sensitized and replicate rapidly. Most of the sensitized B-cells develop into plasma cells, which produce chemical antibodies specific to the invading antigen. These antibodies combine with the antigen that stimulated their production. The antibodies neutralize poisons released by the invader and chemically coat the invader. This coat attracts other white blood cells called macrophages, which destroy the invading organism. It has been estimated that B-cells have the capacity to generate over 10 million different antibody molecules (Koshland, 1987). Some of the sensitized B-cells do not develop into plasma cells but rather form memory cells for the specific antigen. Given a subsequent exposure to that antigen, the system is already prepared (Spence & Mason, 1987). An overview of the humoral immune response is shown in Figure 7-1.

Cell-Mediated Immunity. The cell-mediated immune response involves specialized white blood cells called T-lymphocytes, or T-cells. T-cells are also produced by the bone narrow, but are differentiated in the thymus (a gland in the chest) and are thus called T- (for thymus) cells. T-cells are also found in the blood and lymph, but particularly in the lymph nodes and the spleen. There are several kinds of T-cells. Helper T-cells evoke or enhance the aggressive action of other T- and B-cells. Suppressor T-cells dampen the activity of other T- and B-cells and of natural killer cells. Finally, there are killer T-cells that destroy virus-infected and other abnormal cells.

When the antigen of a foreign microorganism is encountered in the body, helper T-cells stimulate the division of other T-cells, which are sensitized to that specific antigen. Some of these T-cells develop into

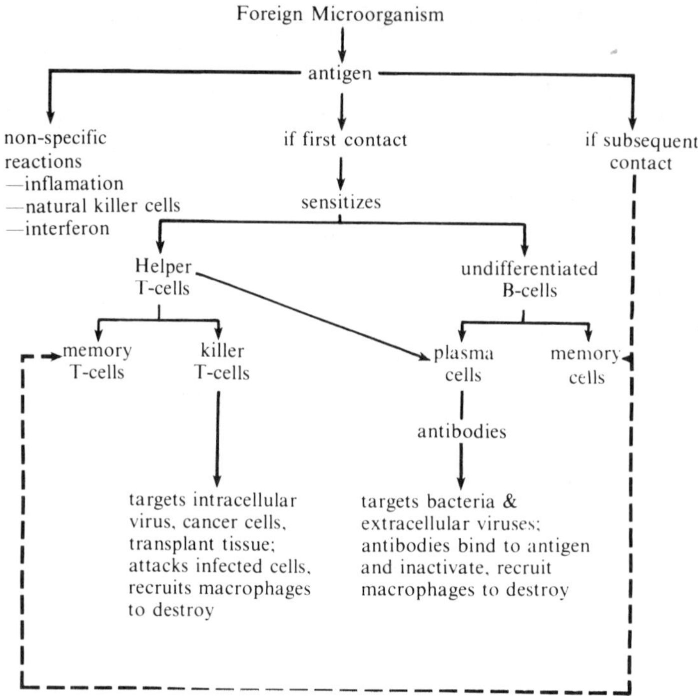

FIGURE 7-1 An Overview of the Specific Immune Response

killer T-cells that attack infected cells and attract macrophages to ingest those cells. The rest of the sensitized cells are reserved as memory T-cells. These cells retain a template for the specific antigen such that, on subsequent exposure, the system is ready to respond immediately to prevent another infection. Once the foreign microorganism is defeated, suppressor T-cells call off the attack (Spence & Mason, 1987; Starr & Taggart, 1984). A schema of cell-mediated immunity is shown in Figure 7-1.

Cell-mediated immunity also plays a role in the surveillance against cancer. Cancer cells are different than normal cells (see the next chapter) and consequently may appear foreign and present antigens to which T-cells can react. Tissue transplants, because they come from another person's body, are foreign and consequently attacked by T-cells. This leads to the rejection of that tissue unless the specific immune response is countered by drugs.

The Immune System: A Summary

The immune system is vital to the maintance of homeostasis in a living, open organism. It recognizes, destroys, and, in the case of the specific immune response, remembers foreign microorganisms, foreign cells, mutant (cancer) cells, and foreign particles and chemicals that enter the body. Without it, we would quickly succumb to these pathogens. However, the immune system must be regulated. It can overreact and underreact to antigens that originate outside or inside the body. If it overreacts to antigens from outside the body such as a bee sting or ragweed pollen, an allergic reaction occurs. If it underreacts to outside antigens such as a virus or bacteria, the result is infection. Overreaction to natural body cells may result in autoimmune disorders like arthritis and lupus. If it is underreactive to abnormal body cells, the result may be cancer (Locke & Colligan, 1986).

The exact mechanisms by which immune regulation occurs are unknown. There is clearly regulation within the immune system, such as suppressor and helper T-cells (Lloyd, 1984). It was long thought that the immune system functioned independent of other physiological systems. However, this is not the case. There is daily variation in its functioning. It is at its strongest around 7:00 A.M. and in the late afternoon and early evening. It is at its weakest around 1:00 P.M. The strength of the immune system also varies with age. It is not fully functional prior to age two and often declines after age sixty. Consequently, very young children are particularly susceptible to infectious diseases and aging individuals to cancer and autoimmune disorders. Immune function also varies according to sex and race and is influenced by diet and drugs.

These observations suggest that the immune system is far from totally independent. It appears to be influenced by other physiological systems, especially the nervous and endocrine systems. These physiological relationships mediate the impact of stress on immune functioning and resistance to disease. Let us consider the connections between the immune, nervous, and endocrine systems.

IMMUNE, NERVOUS, AND ENDOCRINE SYSTEM RELATIONSHIPS

There is a reciprocal relationship between the immune, nervous, and endocrine systems. The effect on the immune system is modulatory rather than regulatory. A number of areas in the brain exert influence on immune functioning. The hypothalamus, centrally involved in the control of the endocrine and autonomic nervous systems (see Chapter 4), is a particularly important site of immune modulation. Lesions to certain parts of the hypothalamus result in suppression of both humoral and cell-mediated immunity. Electrical stimulation of these hypothalamic areas results in enhanced immune functioning (Irwin & Anisman, 1984). But how can neural firing in the brain influence circulating lymphocytes? The cell membranes of lymphocytes have receptors for several types of chemical messengers, including hormones from the endocrine system and neurotransmitters from the nervous system. When these chemical messengers bind with receptors on lymphocytes, lymphocyte development and activity are affected (Irwin & Anisman, 1984). There are several routes by which the hypothalamus and other brain areas may influence the immune response. One route may be via the pituitary and other endocrine glands (see Chapter 4 for a review of the endocrine system) (Rogers, Dubey, & Reich, 1979). Normal levels of several kinds of hormones, including insulin, sex hormones, growth hormone, thyroxin, and glucocorticoids, are required for normal immune functioning. The glucocorticoids appear to be particularly important. An increase in circulating levels of the glucocorticoids, which is often associated with acute stress, suppresses humoral and cell-mediated immunity and, if of long duration, may lead to the atrophy of the thymus. Removal of the adrenal gland often leads to enhanced immune activity (Irwin & Anisman, 1984; Lloyd, 1984).

The second nervous-immune route is the autonomic nervous system. The autonomic nervous system innervates several major immune system structures, including the thymus, spleen, and lymph nodes (Lloyd, 1984). It modulates immune functioning via these connections. For example, the destruction of these connections interferes with immune responses to pathogens (Rogers et al., 1979).

The final brain-immune association may be mediated by the influence of neurotransmitters on lymphocytes. The release of naturally occurring opiate like substances in the brain called endorphins (see Chapter 9) decreases natural killer cell activity and alters T-cell proliferation. Low levels of epinephrine (E) and norepinephrine (NE) from the nervous system and the adrenal medulla are associated with the suppression of immune functioning, whereas high levels of the neurotransmitter dopamine are associated with the enhancement of the immune response (Irwin & Anisman, 1984; Lloyd, 1984).

In summary, there is an array of mechanisms and pathways by which the nervous and endocrine systems modulate immune system functioning. This relationship appears to be reciprocal, for the immune system influences the nervous and endocrine systems. Immunological activation in response to infection is associated with increased electrical activity and norepinephrine (E) and dopamine (D) levels in the hypothalamus. The hormone thymosin, released by the thymus, not only speeds T-cell development but is also circulated to the brain, where it may alter electrical activity (Lloyd, 1984). A summary of these immune, neural, and endocrine connections is shown in Figure 7-2.

These relationships are very complex. The exact effect of neural and hormonal changes depends on which aspect of the immune response is observed. It also depends on the size of the change in the nervous and endocrine systems. Recall that normal levels of glucocorticoids were

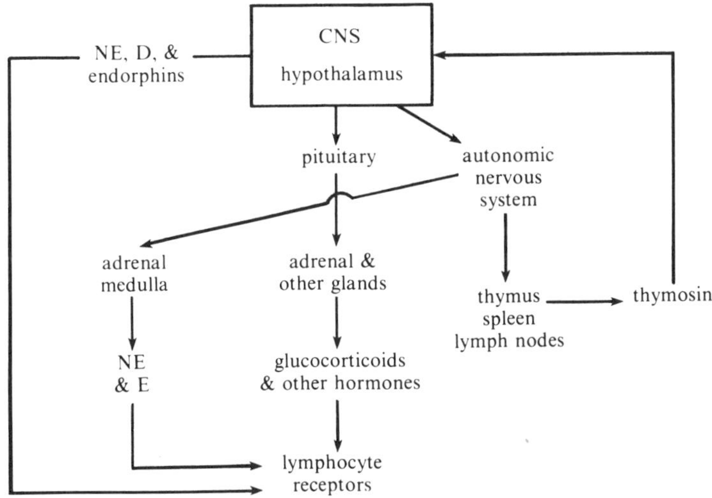

FIGURE 7-2 Relationship of Immune, Nervous, and Endocrine Systems

necessary for good immune functioning but that high levels suppressed its functioning. Further, much of this research has used subhuman species. The degree to which these findings generalize to human beings is not known. It is clear, however, that the connections exist, and may serve as the means by which stress influences immune functioning and resistance to disease, the development of cancer, and the occurrence of allergic and autoimmune disorders. The relationship of stress and other psychosocial events to immune functioning and resistance to disease is called psychoneuroimmunology. Let us explore this in more detail.

PSYCHONEUROIMMUNOLOGY

Conditioning of Immune Responses

One major line of evidence that clearly supports the theory that psychosocial events can influence the immune system and resistance to disease comes from a series of experiments by Adler and his colleagues that demonstrate that immune responses can be classically conditioned (Adler & Cohen, 1975, 1982; Adler, Cohen, & Bovjberg, 1982; Bovjberg, Adler, & Cohen, 1982). In this research, the injection of the drug cyclosphosphamide (CY), which pharmacologically suppresses immune functioning, served as the unconditioned stimulus (US). It was paired with a novel sugar-flavored drinking solution that serves as the conditioned stimulus (CS). In one study, animals were exposed to a foreign antigen three days after the first and only pairing of the CS and US. At the time of this antigen exposure, half of the animals were given the sugar water and half received the plain water. Those given the sugar water showed a reduced immune reaction to the antigen compared to those given the plain water. The sugar water, by its pairing with CY, produced immunosuppression. Subsequent studies have demonstrated that both humoral and cell-mediated immunity can be behaviorally conditioned.

Additional research has shown that conditioned immunosuppression also delays the development of autoimmune disorders in experimental animals. It affects secondary (at reexposure) as well as primary (at first exposure) responses to antigens. It also appears that enhancement as well as suppression of immune responses can be behaviorally conditioned. Gorczynski, Macrae, and Kennedy (1982) used skin grafts as the US. Skin grafts automatically increase T-cell activity. Grafting of skin involves a number of procedures that may serve as the CS. The researchers found that, after an initial skin graft, exposure to the procedure alone (CS) without the skin graft (US) resulted in an increase in T-cells. It also appears that behavioral conditioning of the immune response occurs in humans (Smith & McDaniel, 1983). Individuals who reacted positively to a tuberculin skin test (e.g., delayed hypersensitivity) were given a tuberculin scratch test on one arm and a saline scratch on the other arm once a month for five consecutive months. On the sixth month, unknown to the subjects, the arms to which the scratches were administered were switched. The reaction to the tuberculin on the new arm was significantly reduced.

These conditioning experiments clearly demonstrate that the central nervous and immune systems are closely related. It also suggests that psychosocial events influence immune responses via neural and endocrine connections. At some future time, conditioning may be used to modify immune functioning for therapeutic purposes. There is also evidence that stress can alter immune functioning and susceptibility to disease. Let us review the evidence supporting this relationship.

Stress, Immune Functioning, and Resistance to Disease

Recall that exposure to a pathogen is a necessary but not sufficient condition for the development of an infectious disease. For example, only 20 to 40% of individuals exposed to streptococci develop disease (Cornfield & Hubbard, 1961). Why does the immune system protect some individuals but not others, or an individual at one time but not another? One fascinating possibility is that stress may somehow alter our natural immune defenses against infectious agents. Prior to reviewing evidence supporting this contention, several caveats are in order. Stress is only one, and certainly not necessarily the most important, variable that influences immune functioning or host resistance. Other factors that contribute to host resistance are shown in Figure 7-3. Second, as described in Chapter 4, stress is not a simple phenomenon but rather a complex process entailing cognitive appraisal, coping, and social support. The magnitude and impact of a stressful event are not uniform across individuals and time. Third, the immune system has several facets that may vary somewhat independently. Stress may enhance one aspect while depressing another. Thus, the relationship between stress, immune functioning, and disease is by no means invariant (Adler, 1981; Irwin & Anisman, 1984; Jemmott & Locke, 1984).

To demonstrate definitively that stress influences the occurrence of infectious disease, a systematic relationship between three variables must be established: stress, altered immune functioning, and the expression of clinical symptoms of the disease. Studies typically only look at part of this three-variable problem: either stress and immune functioning, or stress and the occurrence of disease. Rather than attempting

FIGURE 7–3 Variables Contributing to Host Resistance

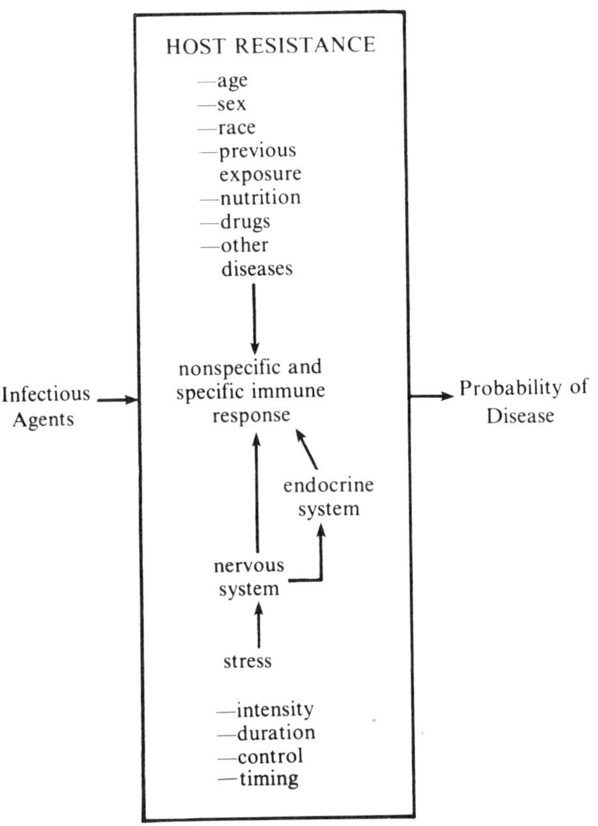

an exhaustive review of these studies, a general summary of the research will first be presented, and then the current status of the evidence will be critically appraised. To facilitate an appreciation of the complexity and difficulty of such research, evidence about the stress-immune-disease relationship will be examined in detail for infectious mononucleosis.

An Overview and Critique of Stress-Immune-Disease Research. Both experimentally and naturally occurring stress have been found to be associated with altered immune functioning. The varieties of stress associated with altered immune functioning include space flight, academic examinations, sleep deprivation and long-duration vigilance tasks, self-reported life change, bereavement, negative mood, and loneliness. Nearly all aspects of immune functioning have been altered by one or more of these stressors: macrophage activity, white blood cell count, antibody responses to antigens, T-cell tranformation and response to viruses, and natural killer cell activity. In the majority of cases, stress has been found to suppress these responses, but in some cases no effect has been found or immune functioning has been enhanced (Irwin & Anisman, 1984; Jemmott & Locke, 1984).

In a similar manner, individuals who experience high levels of stress generally evidence a higher incidence of infectious diseases relative to their lower stress counterparts. These diseases include tuberculosis, streptococcal infections, upper respiratory infections, mononucleosis, oral herpes, and genital herpes (Irwin & Anisman, 1984; Jemmott & Locke, 1984). However, there are also reports in which stress has not affected the incidence of disease.

The impact of stress on immune functioning and resistance to disease depends on a number of accompanying variables: the severity and duration of stress, the degree of control over stress, and the timing of the stress in reference to exposure to the infectious organism. While not firmly established, it appears that acute stress and a lack of control are particularly associated with immune suppression. Under these conditions, there are also the greatest release of glucocorticoids and the greatest reduction in central nervous system norepinephrine and dopamine. Recall from our previous discussion that these chemical changes are associated with depression of the immune system. It is, of course, likely that stress can indirectly lead to alteration in immune responses. Individuals under stress may ingest alcohol, tranquilizers, and tobacco or alter their diets. These activities may affect immune functioning. Persons may also respond to stress in a manner that increases their exposure to pathogens (Adler, 1981).

To this point, our discussion of stress, immune functioning, and resistance to disease has been very general. These broad brush strokes will now be complemented with an exhaustive review of the psychoneuroimmunology of mononucleosis. A further discussion of psychoneuroimmunology in relation to cancer is presented in the next chapter.

Infectious Mononucleosis

Infectious mononucleosis is a prevalent disease, particularly among adolescents and young adults. It occurs in 45 to 200 out of every 100,000 college students, and in 150 to 250 out of every 100,000 persons in the armed forces (Evans, 1978). It is caused by a herpes-type virus called Epstein-Barr, which typically enters the body through the mouth and respiratory tract, often during salivary exchange in kissing. After contact, the virus finds its way into the blood and lymph, where it infects B-lymphocytes. Onset of the clinical symptoms usually occurs in four to seven days. Initial symptoms are lethargy and malaise, followed by a sore throat, swollen glands, fever, and chills, and in some cases an enlarged spleen. The disease usually lasts one to two weeks. Not all individuals exposed to the virus develop mononucleosis. But once exposed, the person develops life-long antibodies that guard against reinfection. However, the virus often persists in an inactive or latent form in B-lymphocytes.

Being "run-down" or "stressed out" has been popularly associated with "getting" infectious mononucleosis. There is some evidence to support this notion. In an early study, Roark (1971) compared the self-reported stress experienced by fifty college students who had infectious mononucleosis with that of fifty students who did not have the disease. Men with the disease retrospectively reported more academic stress and more worry about being drafted into the armed forces than those without the disease. There was no difference in the stress reported by women with and without the disease. Another study of similar design failed to find any relationship between stress and mononucleosis (Wilder, Hubble, & Kennedy, 1971).

Stronger evidence comes from a four-year prospective study of the role of stress on the occurrence of infectious mononucleosis in one class of 1,400 cadets at West Point (Kasl, Evans, & Niederman, 1979). At entry to West Point, two-thirds of the cadets were already immune, for they showed an antibody for the Epstein-Barr virus. Over the following four years, approximately 50% of the men who were susceptible on admission had become infected, but only 25% of those infected developed clinical symptoms. What differentiated those who were exposed and did not develop the disease from those who were exposed and became diseased? Clinical expression of the infection was greatest in those who very much wanted to succeed at West Point but were performing very poorly academically (44%). It was relatively unlikely in individuals who were performing well academically or who were performing poorly but did not care (17%). Thus, individuals who were maximally stressed (greatest discrepancy between the desired and real state of affairs) were most at risk for developing infectious mononucleosis when exposed to the Epstein-Barr virus. They were also most likely to be exposed to the virus and took longer to recover. These data on recovery are very similar to those of Greenfield, Roessler, and Crosby (1959). They found that those individuals who recovered most quickly from mononucleosis had better coping skills than those who recovered slowly. Thus, there is some evidence that stress increases the probability of mononucleosis when persons come into contact with the causative virus. But is this effect mediated by the immune system?

Two studies support the hypothesis that stress enhances the likelihood of infectious mononucleosis by altering immune functioning. Both studies focused on examination stress in medical school students. In the first study, students already having antibodies for Epstein-Barr were studied. Their antibody response to the dormant virus was elevated at times of high stress (before and during final examinations) compared to times of low stress (on return from summer vacation). Social support was an important moderating variable. Those who were lonely showed a greater antibody response than their less lonely counterparts. The elevated antibody reaction reflects decreased immune control over the latent virus (Glaser, Kiecolt-Glaser, Holliday, & Speicher, 1986). In the second study, the transformation of B-lymphocytes by the Epstein-Barr virus was assessed three times: one month prior to finals, during finals, and after return from summer vacation. Self-reports of stress were also obtained at each of these times. All subjects had been previously exposed to the virus. The examination period was reported to be more stressful than the other two. There was less B-lymphocyte response to the virus during this high stress exam period than at the other times. This stress-immune effect was also moderated by social support. Students who were lonely showed less B-cell response (Kiecolt-Glaser, Speicher, Holliday, & Glaser, 1984).

Psychoneuroimmunology: A Summary

Research in the area of psychoneuroimmunology is relatively new. It suggests that stress can influence immune functioning and consequently resistance to disease. However, the causal nature of these relationships is quite tentative at this time. Psychoneuroimmunology focuses on a very complex puzzle. Stress is only one of a number of variables, assuming contact with infectious agents, that influence resistance to disease. We have seen that age, gender, diet, race, and health habits all interact with stress to affect host resistance. The relationship of stress to disease is further complicated by a number of other factors: the frequency, severity, and timing of stress; the degree of control exercised by the individual; and the social support and coping skills available to the individual. The immune system itself is very complex. A stressor may depress one aspect of immune functioning while enhancing a different aspect.

Existing research does not provide definitive answers about the relationship between stress and infectious disease. Much of the research lacks methodological sophistication. In our in-depth review of the research on infectious mononucleosis, we saw that many studies used retrospective reports of stress. Such reports are notoriously unreliable. Many of the studies are cross-sectional. As a consequence, it is not possible to ascertain whether stress is causing disease or disease is causing stress. Many studies use self-reports of disease as the dependent variable without establishing the reliability of such reports. The stress-immune-disease connection is tantalizing and promising. It has important theoretical and practical implications, but before these implications can be realized, much additional research is required.

A number of other psychosocial variables are important in understanding infectious diseases. To "catch" an infection, we must come into contact with the infectious agent. This contact is often not serendipitous. It is strongly influenced by our behavior. Let us turn to the role of behavior in contact with infectious agents.

CONTACT WITH INFECTIOUS AGENTS: THE ROLE OF BEHAVIORAL AND ENVIRONMENTAL VARIABLES

Up to this point, we have considered how the immune system protects individuals from infectious agents and have identified genetic, biological, developmental, and psychosocial factors that alter the response of the immune system to contact with such pathogens. In this section, we will focus on behavioral and environmental factors that affect contact with infectious agents.

Various disease-causing agents, such as bacteria and viruses, gain entry to the body in different ways. Some enter through the skin, especially if its integrity is compromised by a sore, cut, or puncture. Most agents typically enter through natural body openings: the gastrointestinal, respiratory, genital, and urinary tracts. Viruses and bacteria can be carried and discharged in any natural body product, including blood, saliva, mucus, feces, urine, and semen. Some bacteria and viruses can survive outside of the body in food, water, dirt, and other media. Contact with the agent can thus occur in an indirect manner by ingesting these media. Other infectious agents cannot survive outside of the body; infection by these agents requires direct contact with another organism. There are four principle modes of transmission of pathogens: (1) direct physical contact with an infected person; (2) contact with airborne agents; (3) indirect contact through food, water, and other materials; and (4) insect transmission (Sheldon, 1984).

Transmission via direct physical contact with an infected person is especially important for those bacteria and viruses that cannot survive outside of the body. This includes a number of venereal diseases, such as genital herpes and gonorrhea, as well as hepatitis and infectious mononucleosis. Other bacteria and viruses can be carried by materials handled by an infected person, such as clothing, food, and eating utensils. Bacteria and viruses that can exist in food and water are of special concern to community health agencies, and are responsible for diseases such as food poisoning, typhoid, cholera, and dysentery. Infectious agents can also be transmitted by airborne particles in the form of dust or droplets. For example, dried mucus attached to dust particles is an important transmission route for tuberculosis. One sneeze may contain up to 20,000 virus-filled droplets, often propelled up to fifteen feet. Finally, some infectious agents can be carried and transmitted by insects, including ticks, fleas, lice, and mosquitoes. Insect-transmitted diseases include plague, typhus, yellow fever, and malaria.

There are two principle strategies for limiting contact with infectious agents. The first entails social planning and regulation that focus on altering general environmental conditions to reduce the occurrence and transmission of infectious organisms. This includes developing sewage disposal systems, providing pure drinking water, regulating of food preparation and storage, spraying to reduce insect carriers, and establishing legal requirements for the vaccination of children before entering school. These actions and policies have nearly eliminated many of the major infectious diseases that were the primary causes of death a century ago.

The second strategy focuses on educating and motivating individuals to alter their personal behavior to prevent the contact with and spread of infectious microorganisms. This strategy is more costly and less efficient, but is necessitated when infectious agents are transmitted by direct, personal, and often private contact between individuals. Venereal diseases, including genital herpes, syphilis, gonorrhea, and AIDS, are exemplars of this class. Our examination will focus on altering individuals' behavior and will use AIDS as a vehicle for discussion.

Acquired Immune Deficiency Syndrome (AIDS)

Some knowledge about AIDS is required to understand the role of behavior in the transmission of the disease. AIDS is a syndrome caused by a virus called the human immunodeficiency virus (HIV), also known as the human T-cell lymphocytic virus III (HTLV-III). Upon initial infection with the virus, the individual may experience flulike symptoms: malaise, fever, and swollen glands. The virus may then go into a dormant stage during which the person is infected and capable of infecting others but lacking clinical symptoms. This dormant stage may last for several years. When the virus becomes clinically active, it attacks the immune system and results in a decreased number of helper T-cells, a reversal of the normal ratio of helper to suppressor T-cells, and a reduction in natural killer cell activity and in the proliferation of lymphocytes. Consequently, it interferes with adequate humoral and cell-mediated immunity. The immune system does develop antibodies in response to HIV, but these antibodies do not eliminate the virus. The presence of antibodies does provide the means to test individuals for AIDS (Peterman & Curran, 1986; Sheldon, 1984; U.S. Department of Health and Human Services [U.S. DHHS], 1986).

The full-blown clinical expression of AIDS involves the appearance of multiple, often unusual opportunistic infections. "Opportunistic" refers to those diseases that are usually resisted but have the opportunity to thrive because the immune response is compromised. These diseases include certain types of pneumonia, herpes, tuberculosis, and a rare form of cancer called Karposi's sarcoma. These diseases are difficult to control medically given clients' lowered immune defenses and usually result in death. The estimated mean survival time after the onset of this classic syndrome is a little over a year (Hardy, Rauch, Echenberg, Morgan, & Curran, 1986).

Some persons infected with HIV develop AIDS related complex (ARC) rather than full-blown AIDS. ARC has a different and less severe set of symptoms, including a loss of appetite, weight loss, fever, night sweats, skin rashes, diarrhea, tiredness, swollen lymph nodes, and a lowered resistance to infections. ARC may progress to classic AIDS (U.S. DHHS, 1986).

HIV is transmitted by direct physical contact with natural body fluids of an infected person, especially blood, semen and vaginal secretions. This contact occurs in one of three ways. The primary route of contact is during intimate sexual interaction with a person of the same or opposite sex. Semen and, to a lesser degree, vaginal secretions carry the virus. This mode accounts for about 75% of the current AIDS cases. The second route entails transmission by contact with the blood of an infected person when sharing an unsterilized hypodermic needle and syringe, typically associated with illegal intravenous drug use. This accounts for about 20% of the current AIDS cases. The third mode of transmission has occurred when persons received blood or blood-product transfusions carrying HIV. Although this route accounted for about 2 to 3% of past AIDS cases, all donated blood has been tested for AIDS antibodies since 1985. Consequently, transmission of AIDS via this route has not occurred since that time. Giving and receiving blood are safe. HIV is also found in saliva, but is not likely to be transmitted by this medium. The virus is not transmitted by insects or air. It does not usually cross intact skin, but more easily crosses mucous membranes in the mouth, penis, vagina, and rectum. It is not indirectly transmitted through food, water, clothing, or other materials handled by an infected person (Peterman & Curran, 1986; U.S. DHHS, 1986).

The risk of direct contact with AIDS for persons other than illegal intravenous drug users is greatest during intimate sexual interaction. Such interactions with males or females in gay or heterosexual contexts are risky. The exact risk is unknown, but in most cases depends on a number of distinct but correlated parameters of sexual behavior: the number of partners, the number of sexual acts, the type of sexual acts, and the characteristics and histories of the partners. Although one contact with an infected person is sufficient for transmission, the probability of acquiring HIV increases with the number of partners, the number of sexual acts, and the sexual interaction of partners who have had an active sexual history with a number of individuals. Contact with infectious body fluids is more likely when there is rectal-genital, genital-genital, oral-genital, and oral-rectal contact (Martin & Vance, 1984; Peterman & Curran, 1986; U.S. DHHS, 1986).

It is helpful to think about the transmission, infection, and clinical expression of HIV as a series of transitive events: contact with the virus, successful invasion of the body, unapparent (dormant) expression, ARC, and classic AIDS (i.e., opportunistic infections). Progression in this series depends on an array of factors, many of which are not clearly identified or understood at the present time. These factors include the number of contacts with HIV, contact with and expression of other infectious diseases, and variables that influence host resistance like diet, genetics, age, sex, and stress (Martin & Vance, 1984; Peterman & Curran, 1986).

AIDS is a genuine national health problem. The first official cases were recorded in 1981. Since that time, the number of persons diagnosed with AIDS has increased to over 56,000 at the end of 1987. It is estimated that between one to one and one-half million people are currently infected in the United States (Centers for Disease Control, 1988). In addition to the personal suffering, agony, and death, the health care costs of AIDS are and will be staggering. By 1990, the annual medical costs of AIDS are estimated to be between $8 and $16 billion (Hardy et al., 1986; U.S. DHHS, 1986).

At the present time, there is no vaccine to protect individuals from AIDS and no cure once it is acquired. A new drug, azidothymidine (AZT), has been used to treat AIDS since 1986. This drug appears to inhibit the replication of HIV, reduce the number of opportunistic infections, and increase survival time. It is not a cure (Douglas, 1987). Other approaches to the treatment of AIDS are being pursued. Recently, one of these avenues focused on the development of synthetic antigens like CD4, which bind to and neutralize the AIDS virus (Smith, Byrn, Marsters, Gregory, Groopman, & Capon, 1987). Consequently, the current primary health care strategy is to prevent the further spread of AIDS. This requires the means to alter the behavior of persons who are and who are not infected.

To effectively prevent the spread of AIDS, a number of issues must be addressed. For those not currently infected, the means to educate and motivate individuals to engage in sexual practices that effectively reduce the risk of contact with the AIDS virus must be developed and implemented. Some individuals may be infected but not know it. To prevent the spread of AIDS, persons who are at high risk for having the virus must be motivated to get blood tests. This will allow them to communicate with others and to behave in a responsible manner. This is no easy task. The diagnosis of AIDS is catastrophic, and carries with it a stigma and social ramifications that tax even the best-adjusted individual's coping repertoire. Cheap and convenient access to confidential diagnostic testing is essential. In addition, efforts at motivating individuals to utilize these services are required. Efforts must also be directed at encouraging timely and appropriate health care utilization and health-promoting actions by persons already infected. Targets may include enhancing the ability to communicate with health providers and others, to express one's sexuality in a manner that does not compromise others, and to cope with the severe social, personal, and biological challenges of AIDS. Such behaviors not only prevent the spread of AIDS, but may also limit or prevent the progression of the disease from dormant to ARC or full-blown expression (Coates, Temoshok, & Mandel, 1984).

These preventative and clinical targets require the application of the principles of health-related behaviors described in Chapters 2 and 3. Their application to AIDS will be detailed and evaluated in Chapter 16. It should be emphasized that the risk of acquiring a number of other infectious diseases is strongly influenced by personal behavior and that a number of these diseases also have very serious health and adjustment consequences, including genital herpes, gonorrhea, syphilis, and hepatitis B. Some of these are highly resistant to antibiotic and other forms of medical treatment. Altering health behaviors associated with these infectious diseases is also important.

INFECTIOUS DISEASES: IMPACT AND COPING

Our usual experience with infectious diseases promotes schemata suggesting that they are time limited, treatable, and circumscribed in their impact on our lives. As evidenced by AIDS, this is not necessarily the case. As with all diseases, AIDS has an impact at all levels within the system. At times, this impact can be pervasive and powerful. Rather than attempting a broad review of the impact of a number of infectious diseases, our discussion will continue to use AIDS as an example. AIDS presents infected and high risk but uninfected individuals with a range of stressful issues that elicit discomfort and distress. The manner in which individuals attempt to cope with these stressors influences the quality of their lives and, for those with the disease, the expression and progression of the disease.

Because of its recent occurrence, our knowledge of the impact of AIDS is barely at a descriptive stage. Let us first consider individuals who are at high risk for AIDS but to their knowledge are not infected. Many of these individuals have been found to manifest excessive anxiety and multiple somatic complaints, many of which may be similar to ARC. These individuals are the "worried well." They may obsess about the possibility of the disease, about getting a blood test, and about the results of the test. This distress varies in severity and duration, but often interferes with social and occupational functioning. These individuals may alter their lifestyle, including their social and sexual behavior, to prevent infection. But the ensuing lack of social support and change in routine also can become a significant source of stress (Marin, Charles, & Malyan, 1984).

A larger and more challenging set of problems confronts individuals infected with AIDS. The impact of receiving the diagnosis of AIDS is, by itself, catastrophic. These individuals have already not been feeling well physically or psychologically. Confirmation of the diagnosis evokes a number of realistic reactions including fear of suffering, death, and dying; of the loss of financial, physical, and social independence; of contagion; and of the loss of social support and outright ostracism. There is a loss of self-esteem and increased guilt, depression, and anxiety. There is confusion about the options for medical treatment and the cost of that treatment (Marin & Batchelor, 1984).

Even less is known at a descriptive level about modes of coping with these multiple and often contradictory stressors and tasks. Practically nothing is known about the effectiveness of different coping strategies (Joseph, Emmons, Kessler, Wortman, O'Brien, Hacker, & Schaefer, 1984). It is clear that the psychosocial as well as medical needs of these individuals must be addressed. Some suggestions and strategies will be described in Chapter 16.

SUMMARY

We usually think of infectious diseases in relatively simple terms. They are caused by bacteria, viruses, or other organisms. They are self-limited and easily treated. This is somewhat inaccurate and limited. We have a built-in defense against pathogens, the immune system. Whether a "germ" causes disease depends on how well the immune system is functioning, or host resistance. Host resistance is subject to a number of variables including stress. Via the nervous and endocrine systems, stress has psychophysiological effects that often alter immune response and resistance to disease. Once infection has occurred, stress may influence the course of the disease and the speed of recovery. Not all infections are time limited. Some have very serious, lasting, and lethal consequences. Thus infectious diseases present individuals with a variety of sometimes severe challenges requiring adaptation. Infection requires contact with pathogenic agents. This contact is not a random event. It depends on our health-impairing and health-promoting habits and our collective social and economic decisions and actions. Recovery from infection often requires seeking health services in a timely fashion and adhering to treatment recommendations.

REFERENCES

Adler, R. (1981). Behavioral influences on immune responses. In S. M. Weiss, J. A. Herd, & B. H. Fox (Eds.), *Perspectives in behavioral medicine*, 163–182. New York: Academic Press.

Adler, R., & Cohen, N. (1975). Behaviorally conditioned immunosuppression. *Psychosomatic Medicine, 37*, 333–340.

Adler, R., & Cohen, N. (1982). Behaviorally conditioned immunosuppression and murine systemic lupus erythematosis. *Science, 215*, 1534–1535.

Adler, R., Cohen, N., & Bovjberg, D. (1982). Conditioned suppression of humoral immunity in the rat. *Journal of Comparative and Physiological Psychology, 96*, 517–520.

Bovjberg, D., Adler, R., & Cohen, N. (1982). Behaviorally conditioned suppression of a graft-vs-host response. *Proceedings of the National Academy of Sciences, 79*, 583–585.

Centers for Disease Control. (1988). Human immunodeficiency virus infection in the United States. *Morbidity and Mortality Weekly Report, 77*, 801–804.

Coates, T. J., Temoshok, L., & Mandel, J. (1984). Psychosocial research is essential to understanding and treating AIDS. *American Psychologist, 39*, 1309–1314.

Cornfield, D., & Hubbard, J. P. (1961). A four-year study of the occurrence of beta-hemolytic streptococci in 64 school children. *New England Journal of Medicine, 264*, 211.

Douglas, R. G. (1987). Infectious disease. *Journal of the American Medical Association, 258*, 2252–2254.

Evans, A. S. (1978). Infectious mononucleosis and related syndromes. *American Journal of Medical Science, 276*, 325–339.

Glaser, R., Kiecolt-Glaser, J. K., Holliday, J., & Speicher, C. (1986). *The relationship of stress and loneliness to herpesvirus antibody titers*. Unpublished manuscript, Ohio State University, Department of Psychiatry, Columbus.

Gorczynski, R. M., Macrae, S., & Kennedy, M. (1982). Conditioned immune response associated with allogenic skin grafts in mice. *Journal of Immunology, 129*, 704–709.

Greenfield, N. S., Roessler, R., & Crosby, A. D. (1959). Ego strength and length of recovery from infectious mononucleosis. *Journal of Nervous and Mental Disease, 128*, 125–128.

Hardy, A. M., Rauch, K., Echenberg, D., Morgan, W. M., & Curran, J. W. (1986). The economic impact of the first 10,000 cases of acquired immune deficiency syndrome in the United States. *Journal of the American Medical Association, 255*, 209–211.

Irwin, J., & Anisman, H. (1984). Stress and pathology: Immunological and central nervous system interaction. In C. L. Cooper (Ed.), *Psychosocial stress and cancer*, 93–148. New York: John Wiley & Sons.

Jemmott, J. B., & Locke, S. E. (1984). Psychosocial factors, immunologic mediation, and human susceptibility to infectious diseases: How much do we know? *Psychological Bulletin, 75*, 78–108.

Joseph, J. G., Emmons, C. A., Kessler, R. C., Wortman, C. B., O'Brien, K., Hacker, W. T., & Schaefer, C. (1984). Coping with the threat of AIDS: An approach to psychosocial assessment. *American Psychologist, 39*, 1297–1302.

Kasl, S. V., Evans, A. S., & Niederman, J. C. (1979). Psychosocial risk factors in the development of infectious mononucleosis. *Psychosomatic Medicine, 41*, 445–466.

Kiecolt-Glaser, J. K., Speicher, C. E., Holliday, J. C., & Glaser, R. (1984). Stress and the transformation of lymphocyte for Epstein-Barr virus. *Journal of Behavioral Medicine, 7*, 1–12.

Koshland, D. E. (1987). Frontiers in immunology. *Science, 238*, 1023.

Lloyd, R. (1984). Mechanisms of psychoneuroimmunological response. In B. H. Fox & B. H. Newberry (Eds.), *Impact of psychoendocrine systems on cancer and immunity*, 321–336. Lewiston, NY: C. J. Hogrefe.

Locke, S., & Colligan, D. (1986). *The healer within: The new medicine of mind and body*. New York: Free Press.

Marin, S. F., & Batchelor, W. F. (1984). Responding to the psychological crisis of AIDS. *Public Health Reports, 99*, 4–9.

Marin, S. F., Charles, K. A., & Malyan, A. K. (1984). The psychological impact of AIDS on gay men. *American Psychologist, 39*, 1288–1293.

Martin, J. L., & Vance, C. S. (1984). Behavioral and psychosocial factors in AIDS: Methodological and substantive issues. *American Psychologist, 39*, 1303–1308.

Norton, J. C. (1982). *An introduction to medical psychology*. New York: Free Press.

Peterman, T. A., & Curran, J. W. (1986). Sexual transmission of human immunodeficiency virus. *Journal of the American Medical Association, 256*, 2222–2225.

Roark, G. E. (1971). Psychosomatic factors in the epidemiology of infectious mononucleosis. *Psychosomatics, 12*, 402–412.

Rogers, M. P., Dubey, D., & Reich, P. (1979). The influence of the psyche and the brain on immunity and disease susceptibility: A critical review. *Psychosomatic Medicine, 41*, 147–164.

Sheldon, H. (1984). *Boyd's introduction to the study of disease* (9th ed.). Philadelphia: Lea & Febiger.

Smith, D. H., Byrn, R. A., Marsters, S. A., Gregory, T., Groopman, J. E., & Capon, D. J. (1987). Blocking of HIV-I infectivity by a soluble, secreted form of CD4 antigen. *Science, 238*, 1704–1707.

Smith, G. R., & McDaniel, S. M. (1983). Psychologically mediated effects on the delayed hypersensitivity reaction to tuberculin in humans. *Psychosomatic Medicine, 45*, 65–70.

Spence, A. P., & Mason, E. B. (1987). Human anatomy and physiology (3rd ed.). Menlo Park, CA: Benjamin/Cummings.

Starr, C., & Taggart, R. (1984). *Biology: The unity and diversity of life*. Belmont, CA: Wadsworth.

U.S. Department of Health and Human Services, U.S. Public Health Service (1986). *Surgeon General's Report on Acquired Immune Deficiency Syndrome*. Washington, DC: U.S. Government Printing Office.

Wilder, R. M., Hubble, J., & Kennedy, C. E. (1971). Life change and infectious mononucleosis. *Journal of the American College Health Association, 20*, 115–119.

8

Cancer

INTRODUCTION

> To grow old and to die is universally accepted as part of the natural order of things. But to die of cancer at old age, or at any other time, is not considered natural but a tragedy (Miller, 1980).

> When we think of cancer in general terms we are apt to conjure up a process characterized by a steady, remorseless and inexorable progress in which the disease is all conquering, and none of the immunological and other defensive forces which help us to survive the onslaught of bacteria and viral infections can serve to halt the faltering footsteps to the grave (Boyd, 1966).

The word *cancer* strikes fear into the hearts and minds of many people, laypersons and health providers alike. There are several prevalent but inaccurate generalizations about cancer that cause fear: (1) cancer can occur without warning so that it is too late for medical intervention; (2) medical intervention is not very effective in stopping cancer; (3) because cancer uses most of the body's nutrients, the body wastes away while the cancer thrives; (4) advanced cancer causes unmanageable pain that is not responsive to pain killing medication; (5) persons with cancer are often abandoned because family, friends, and health providers feel there is little hope; (6) the diagnosis of cancer is difficult and effective treatment cannot be implemented until the cancer is far along; (7) treatment of cancer is painful and mutilating; (8) the cause of cancer is unknown and persons have little control over whether they will get cancer; and (9) persons have little control over cancer once they get it; even if they cooperate fully with health providers, treatment is unsuccessful (Clark, 1976; Miller, 1980).

In this chapter, the causes and course of cancer and its treatment will be explored. The role of environmental, behavioral, and psychosocial factors in the etiology and course of cancer will be examined. The impact of cancer and its diagnosis and treatment will also be described. Let us begin by defining cancer and its manifestations.

WHAT IS CANCER?

Cancer does not have uniform symptoms. It is not one disease. Over one hundred different types of cancer have been identified. However, all cancers have some common characteristics. Cancer involves an alteration in a normal cell or group of cells such that they proliferate rapidly because normal mechanisms that inhibit cellular growth are impaired. With time, cancer cells may spread from their original site to adjacent tissue by infiltration, often via the lymphatic and circulatory systems. Some cancer cells may break off their original site and circulate until they lodge in other tissues in the body. If these tissues provide a suitable environment, the cancer cells may invade them and proliferate, a process called metastasis (Baldanado & Stahl, 1978; Poste, 1977).

Cancer cells are not compatible with normal cells and do not have any function. A neoplastic tumor can be thought of as a factory and as a growth. As a factory, a tumor manufactures increased normal tissue products, like hormones or enzymes. As a growth, a tumor can compress and replace normal cells and produce symptoms of obstruction (Ultman & Golomb, 1977). Cancer cells can appear anywhere in the body. These characteristics of cancer cells make the symptoms of cancer difficult to recognize and highly variable. A tumor at any one body site can cause a number of disruptions in body functioning. They can mimic the natural function of the tissue from which they originate. They can disrupt the functioning of that tissue and of nearby tissues. The symptoms vary depending on the sites to which cancer cells metastasize (Fox, 1981).

WHO GETS CANCER?

Cancer is a major health problem. It is estimated that one out of every four people will have cancer in their lifetime. Approximately 15% of all deaths are due to cancer (Fox, 1981). There are over a half-million new cases of cancer in the United States every year (Baldanado & Stahl, 1978). In 1976, there were more than 1.5 million hospital admissions for cancer, costing approximately 3.5 billion dollars. Total medical costs for treating cancer in the United States in 1976 were over 6 billion dollars (Eisenberg, 1979).

Recent incidence rates for common forms of cancer are shown in Table 8-1. This table also shows the incidence of these cancers in 1947–50. The incidence of many cancers (breast, prostate, colon, and rectum) have been steady or rising slowly over the last two decades. The in-

TABLE 8-1 Trends in Cancer Incidence[a]

		INCIDENCE	
CANCER	GENDER	1947–50	1983–84
Mouth and pharynx	Male	12.5	13.5
	Female	3.4	5.3
Esophagus	Male	6.5	5.2
	Female	1.6	1.5
Stomach	Male	34.7	10.9
	Female	19.3	5.0
Colon	Male	24.6	44.4
	Female	30.3	33.3
Rectum	Male	20.8	19.9
	Female	14.1	12.4
Lung	Male	27.1	87.1
	Female	6.8	35.0
Melanoma (skin)	Male	2.8	11.1
	Female	2.8	8.1
Breast	Male	—	—
	Female	74.6	97.4
Uterus	Male	—	—
	Female	55.8	32.2
Prostate	Male	45.0	75.3
	Female	—	—
Hodgkin's disease	Male	3.2	4.0
	Female	2.2	2.8
Leukemias	Male	11.1	13.0
	Female	7.8	7.8

Note: From U.S. Department of Health and Human Services, Public Health Service, National Institute of Health, *Incidence and Mortality Trends among Whites in the United States*, 1987. Washington, DC: U.S. Government Printing Office.

[a]Rates per 100,000, age adjusted.

cidence of stomach cancer has decreased steadily since 1950. Lung cancer, as a result of trends in tobacco use, has increased. This increase is expected to continue, especially for women. These figures may be inflated due to changes in the methods used to report cancer (Henderson, 1981). The increasing incidence of cancer may also reflect the successful medical control of other diseases. Health care costs for cancer can be expected to increase even faster than its incidence because improved treatment of cancer will prolong survival and thus treatment time (Eisenberg, 1979).

BEHAVIORAL AND PSYCHOLOGICAL FACTORS IN THE ETIOLOGY OF CANCER

In relation to psychological and behavioral variables, cancer can be viewed as either an independent or a dependent variable. As an independent variable, cancer and its diagnosis and treatment have a strong impact on behavior and psychological well-being. As a dependent variable, behavioral and psychological variables have an impact on the appearance, growth, and metastases of cancer cells. In this section, we will focus on the manner and degree to which behavior and environment influence the incidence of cancer.

Behavioral and psychosocial variables influence the appearance and course of cancer in a complex fashion. For an overview of this relationship, we will use the environment-person-behavior model shown in Figure 8-1. In the environmental portion of this figure, exogenous agents are substances to which persons are exposed that influence cancer by direct action on body tissue (e.g., cigarette smoke and asbestos). Psychosocial stimuli refer to aspects of the environment perceived and appraised by the person as stressful. Other people are persons with whom an individual has contact and whose behavior influences the individual's environment. Within the individual, host characteristics refer to a person's biological structure and functioning. This structure and functioning are the result of genetic factors and of past and current interaction with the environment (e.g., diet, exercise, and disease). Neoplastic process refers to the development of cancer cells and is the variable we wish to predict. Behavior refers to all overt responses made by the individual. Each of these variables is related to the others as suggested by the arrows. The effect of behavior and psychosocial variables on the development of cancer will be described using these relationships.

The Neoplastic Process

To understand the causes of cancer, it is first necessary to understand more completely the neoplastic process. All cancer cells are derived from normal cells. Alteration of a normal cell into a malignant cell

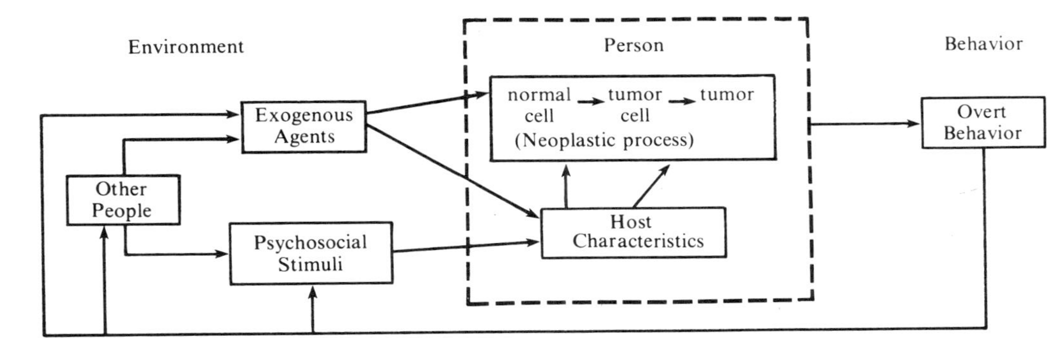

FIGURE 8-1 The Impact of Behavior and Psychosocial Stimuli on Cancer. (From "Variables in Behavioral Oncology: Overview and Assessment of Current Issues" (p. 88) by B. H. Newberry, A. G. Liebelt, and D. A. Boyle, 1984, in B. H. Fox and B. H. Newberry (Eds.), *Impact of Psychoendocrine Systems in Cancer and Immunity*, Lewiston, NY: C. J. Hogrefe. Copyright 1984 by C. J. Hogrefe. Reprinted by permission.)

is a multistage process that takes place over a long period of time. The alteration does not have one cause. It is the result of a number of insults, or "hits," that alter normal cellular structure or function (Miller, 1980). A wide variety of stimuli can serve as "hits." This process is constantly occurring within the body. Once a cell is altered by "hits," several things can happen. Many altered cells die or are destroyed. Of those that survive, only a few have the potential to become malignant. Altered cells with such a potential are called precursor cells. Precusor cells often have to be further altered by additional "hits" before they become malignant, a process estimated to take ten to twenty years, depending on the type of cancer (Fox, 1978). Once a malignant cell appears, it does not necessarily survive. Its survival and growth are further determined by the number and type of "hits" experienced. The arrows pointing to the neoplastic process in Figure 8-1 represent the sources of those hits, which involve a complex interaction of exogenous agents, host characteristics, psychosocial stimuli, and behavior.

The following analogy may be useful in understanding the neoplastic process. Suppose you see a 1968 Ford Mustang in a parking lot. The body of the car is badly rusted, but in 1968 it was a bright and shiny red. The appearance and spread of rust were the result of years of exposure to road salt, grime, rain, and snow. This exposure in turn was dependent on the driving habits of the owner. The appearance and spread of rust were also dependent on the care of the car by the owner, such as washing and waxing the car and repairing small dents. The appearance and spread of rust (cancer) were dependent on the conditions to which the car was exposed ("hits") and the manner in which the car was cared for (host characteristics) and driven (behavior).

The inception and course of cancer, then, are the result of "hits" coming from a variety of sources over a long time. There are two primary ways in which psychosocial stimuli and behavior influence the occurrence of these "hits." The first is the direct route. In this case, the behavior of the individual or of others brings the individual into contact with exogenous carcinogenic agents (see the behavior of other people to exogenous agents to neoplastic process arrows in Figure 8-1). The second is the indirect route. In this case, the behavior of the individual and of others influences the amount of stress experienced by the individual. Stress influences host resistance (see the behavior and other people to psychosocial stimuli to host characteristics to neoplastic process arrows in Figure 8-1). We will first examine the direct route.

The Direct Influence of Behavior on Cancer

Contact with Carcinogenic Agents. A number of environmental agents increase the likelihood of cancer. A partial list of these agents, the degree of risk they pose, and the type of cancer with which they are associated is shown in Table 8-2.

TABLE 8-2 Conditions Associated with an Altered Risk of Cancer

BEHAVIOR	AGENT	RISK LEVEL	CANCER SITE
Habits	Tobacco	Certain	Lung, mouth, throat
	Alcohol	Probable	Mouth, throat, liver
	Coffee, tea	Speculative	Nonspecific
Customs	Sunbathing	Certain to probable	Skin
	Age at marriage (female)	Probable to speculative	Breast, cervix
	Age at first intercourse	Certain to probable	Cervix
	Number of sexual partners (female)	Probable to speculative	Cervix
	Circumcision (male)	Probable to speculative	Penis
Diet	Amount	Probable to speculative	Nonspecific
	Fats	Speculative	Colon, rectum, breast
	Vitamin deficiency	Probable to speculative	Various
	Dietary carcinogens	Probable to speculative	Various
	Refined foods	Speculative	Colon, rectum
	Food additives and preservatives	Speculative	Nonspecific
Environmental pollution	Pesticides, herbicides	Speculative	Liver, nonspecific
	Air pollution	Probable to speculative	Lung, nonspecific
	Water pollution	Speculative	Nonspecific
	Ionizing radiation	Speculative	Nonspecific
Occupational contact	X-ray, uranium, asbestos, arsenic, polyvinyl chloride, benzene (plus failure to take protective measures)	Certain	Various

(continued)

TABLE 8-2 Continued

BEHAVIOR	AGENT	RISK LEVEL	CANCER SITE
Iatrogenic (medically caused)	Some types of drugs (chemotherapy, hormones, immunosupressants)	Certain to speculative depending on type	Various
	X-ray therapy or diagnosis	Certain to speculative	Various

Note: From "The Psychosocial Epidemiology of Cancer," (p. 12) by B. H. Fox, 1976, in J. W. Cullen, B. H. Fox, and R. N. Isom (Eds.), *Cancer: The Behavioral Dimensions*, New York: Raven Press. Copyright 1976, by Raven Press. Reprinted by permission.

In the top portion of the table is a list of carcinogenic agents whose exposure is dependent on the individual's own behavior. Smoking, for example, is strongly associated with cancer. Smoking is under the individual's control and is definitively related to the incidence of lung cancer. A smoker, by middle age, has ten times the risk of lung cancer as a nonsmoker. If all persons refrained from smoking during their lifetime, the number of deaths due to cancer in 1978 would have been reduced by 30%, or 115,000 (Doll & Petro, 1981). Other personal behaviors such as sunbathing and diet also influence the incidence of cancer.

Cancer is also associated with environmental agents over which we have minimal personal control but which are the result of collective socioeconomic decisions. A partial list of these agents is shown in the bottom portion of Table 8-2. For example, asbestos is strongly associated with the incidence of cancer. It has been estimated that industrial exposure to asbestos prior to 1978 will account for 10 to 20% of all cancer deaths in the coming decades (Bridbord, et al., 1978). Cancer is also associated with various medical treatments, such as drugs used in chemotherapy for cancer itself, drugs used to minimize rejection of transplanted organs, and drugs used to maintain pregnancy. Changes in social and economic policy could reduce contact with some of these agents and consequently reduce the incidence of cancer.

The variety and ubiquity of these carcinogenic agents do *not* mean that everything causes cancer. It should *not* be taken to mean we have no control. Doll and Petro (1981) estimate that several simple changes in personal behavior (not smoking, drinking alcohol in moderate amounts, and showing prudence in the amount and type of food eaten) could substantially reduce the risk of cancer. Changes in social and economic policies could similarly reduce the incidence of cancer.

Exposure to carcinogenic agents does *not* mean that a person will invariably get cancer. These agents are one type of "hit," and whether these "hits" contribute to the development of cancer depends on the dose and length of exposure. For example, the risk of lung cancer due to smoking varies with the number of cigarettes smoked daily and the number of years a person has smoked. A combination of carcinogenic agents may have a multiplicative effect. The carcinogenic risk engendered by alcohol consumption in nonsmokers is small, but the consumption of an equal amount of alcohol by smokers potentiates the carcinogenic risk of alcohol consumption (Doll & Petro, 1981).

Host Resistance. The likelihood that environmental "hits" will result in cancer also depends on host characteristics. Biological structure and function can increase or decrease resistance to these "hits." Host characteristics that influence the risk of cancer, the certainty of their effect, and the types of cancer affected are shown in Table 8-3. Possession of these host characteristics does not cause cancer but is statistically associated with an increased likelihood of cancer. Host characteristics represent the physiological milieu in which the neoplastic process takes place. The endocrine and immune systems mediate the host's resistance to abnormal cells and influence cellular growth rates. A number of host factors that influence the likelihood of cancer have been identified. The exact mechanisms by which host characteristics influence susceptibility to cancer are not well understood. Nevertheless, let us consider a few examples.

The incidence of cancer increases with age. With each five-year increase in age after twenty-five, there is an approximate doubling in the incidence of cancer. However, not all specific types of cancer show this age trend (e.g., cancer of the testis, uterus, and cervix). Aging does not cause cancer. Rather, aging and cancer are associated because more "hits" accumulate as the person gets older; age provides the necessary time for the multistage process of neoplastic development to occur (Miller, 1980). A number of genetic disorders are associated with an increased risk for cancer (e.g., inherited immune deficiency), and certain types of cancer tend to run in families (e.g., breast cancer). Cancer is not certain in these cases; genetic factors only serve as a predisposition that increases the risk of cancer. It is another "hit." It has been estimated that there are many billion cell divisions in a person's lifetime, and that one in a million of these divisions results in cell transformations. Most of these transformed cells are not viable. Of those that are viable, most are not malignant. Natural repair to the disrupted chromosomal material in these cells may be influenced by genetics (Miller, 1980).

External agents can influence cancer development by altering host characteristics. For example, the clinical use of sex hormones (e.g., in birth control pills and in medication used to maintain pregnancy) alters

TABLE 8-3 Host Characteristics Associated with an Altered Risk of Cancer

HOST CHARAC-TERISTIC	RISK FACTOR	RISK LEVEL	CANCER SITE
Physical characteristics	Obesity	Probable to speculative	Uterus
	Complexion and eye color	Certain to probable	Skin
Congenital and genetic	Age at menarche	Probable to speculative	Cervix, breast
	Family history of cancer	Certain to speculative (depending on type)	Breast, various
	Congenital deformity or abnormality	Certain to speculative (depending on type)	Various
Other diseases	Cirrhosis (liver, kidney stones)	Certain to speculative (depending on type)	Various
	Scars or burns	Certain to speculative	Skin, esophagus
	Communicable diseases, AIDS	Certain to speculative	Bladder, blood, skin
Personal characteristics	Sex	Certain	Various
	Age	Certain	Nonspecific
	Race	Certain to speculative	Nonspecific
	Geographic location	Certain to speculative	Various

Note: From "The Psychosocial Epidemiology of Cancer" (p. 13), by B. H. Fox, 1976, in J. W. Cullen, B. H. Fox, and R. N. Isom (Eds.), *Cancer: The Behavioral Dimensions,* New York: Raven Press. Copyright 1976 by Raven Press. Reprinted by permission.

hormonal balance, which may increase the risk of cancer. Nonmalignant infections may alter immune functioning, raise body temperature, and enhance cell division, thus affecting a person's susceptibility to cancer. Alteration of host characteristics by exogenous agents serves as another "hit," increasing the susceptibility to cancer.

The behavioral and environmental influences described by the direct route have been reliably and convincingly associated with the neoplastic process. Our individual and collective decisions and actions expose us to agents that are implicated in the development of cancer.

The Indirect Influence of Behavior on Cancer

Behavioral variables can also influence the likelihood of cancer in a manner less direct than exposure to carcinogens. Psychosocial stimuli appraised as stressful alter the individual's physiology (see the endocrine, nervous, and immune system changes associated with stress described in Chapters 4 and 7). These alterations in physiology provide a milieu that is more or less resistant to the development of cancer (Rogers, Dubey, & Reich, 1979) as well as bacterial and viral infections (Jemmott & Locke, 1984).

The degree to which stress alters a person's susceptibility to cancer is not clearly known (Fox, 1978; Morrison & Paffenbarger, 1981; Newberry et al., 1984). Research on the stress-cancer connection is like a very intricate detective story. Several research strategies are available to gather evidence concerning this relationship. One strategy is to determine those physiological changes associated with stress, and then to determine whether these changes are associated with an increased incidence of cancer. (This is a two-step process: finding that stress results in physiological changes x, y, and z, and that x, y, and z increase cancer risk.) Another strategy assesses the correlation between stress and cancer without worrying about the physiological mechanisms. Several other requirements must be met before data from these strategies could be used to demonstrate convincingly that stress influences cancer. Stress must occur before the cancer (cause must precede effect); the incidence of cancer should increase as stress increases (a dose-effect relationship); and stress and cancer should not both be caused by some third variable like smoking or exposure to asbestos (Morrison & Paffenbarger, 1981).

We will first examine the evidence for the stress-cancer connection obtained from the two-step strategy: stress to physiology and physiology to cancer. From our discussion in Chapters 4 and 7, we know that stress alters immune functioning. Stress has been shown both to enhance and inhibit the functioning of the immune system. The specific effect depends on the type of stress, the amount of control over stress, the aspect of the immune system being assessed, and the temporal relationship between the stressor and the assessment of immune functioning (Jemmott & Locke, 1984).

The immune system fosters homeostasis by identifying and destroying foreign molecules. Cancer cells, because they are mutants, may be identified and destroyed by the immune system. Evidence suggests that both nonspecific and specific immune responses may play a surveillance role against cancer. Many cancer cells are not foreign in appearance and thus slip by the specific immune system. The specific immune response only seems to guard against certain types of cancers. In some cases, the specific immune system has been found to enhance rather than inhibit cancer growth (Prehn, 1976). The specific immune response is now thought to play a stronger role in inhibiting tumor growth and metastasis than in inhibiting the inception of cancer (Alexander, 1977). The nonspecific immune response plays a more important role in guarding against the initial appearance and viability of cancer cells. Macrophages and natural killer cells are thought to be the body's first line of defense against precursor and malignant cells (Alexander, 1977; Herberman & Holden, 1979). Suppression of the immune system may increase susceptibility to cancer. But because stress can both enhance and suppress the immune response, the stress-cancer connection via the immune system is quite tentative and unclear.

What can we say about the evidence for the two-step connection between stress and cancer? Stress alters endocrine and immune functioning, but the nature and degree of this alteration are quite variable. Such changes in endocrine and immune functioning have been associated with both increased susceptibility and increased resistance to cancer. The evidence for both steps is tentative. It would not convince an unbiased judge and jury.

The second research strategy is to determine whether persons who experience a lot of stress are more likely to get cancer. Evidence using this approach comes from retrospective and prospective studies. Retrospective studies ask individuals who have cancer to recall how much stress they experienced over some previous period. These responses are compared to those of persons who do not have cancer. Retrospective studies generally support the stress-cancer connection. Persons with cancer report having experienced more stress. They are more likely to have been widowed, divorced, or separated and to have lost a significant other. The connection of stress with cancer is more marked when coping ability and control are also assessed. A sense of hopelessness, a lack of social support, and inadequate behavioral coping skills (e.g., an inability to express emotions or to deal with conflict) potentiate the relationship between stress and cancer (Sklar & Anisman, 1981). Although this evidence may appear rather convincing, retrospective studies are plagued with problems that make the evidence suggestive rather than conclusive. The clinical diagnosis of cancer occurs years after the first cancer cells appear; the disease may have begun before the time of the stressors reported (the effect precedes the cause). While stress may influence the growth and metastases of the cancer, we cannot be sure that it has a role in its inception. The validity of the cancer patients' recall is also suspect. Their knowledge of having cancer may influence their memory of past events. The physiological effects of having cancer (e.g., brain metastases and changes in hormone levels) may interfere with a person's coping ability; cancer is causing stress rather than stress causing cancer (Fox, 1978). Evidence from retrospective studies is thus not very convincing.

Prospective studies are a better test of the stress-cancer connection. In prospective studies, stress is assessed prior to the development of cancer. The stress levels of persons who ultimately develop cancer are then compared to those who do not develop cancer. Only a handful of prospective studies have been done. These studies tend to support the stress-cancer connection. Persons who get cancer experience more stress (e.g., unemployment, loss of a significant relationship, or little stability in their lives) and have poor coping resources (e.g., have few close relationships or do less planning). While prospective studies provide more convincing evidence, they still present problems. Most of these studies use a small number of subjects and do not control for the possibility that stress and cancer are both related to some third variable like smoking. Even though stress is assessed prior to the diagnosis of cancer, the stress being assessed may have occurred after the cancer initially appeared; a lengthy period is required for a neoplastic cell to proliferate to a clinically detectable size (Fox, 1978).

In summary, evidence concerning the indirect influence of stress on cancer supports the possibility of a connection, but that evidence is far from conclusive. Stress may increase or decrease susceptibility to cancer via alteration of immune and endocrine functioning. Its effect varies from individual to individual and from cancer to cancer. The modification of host characteristics by stress is best conceptualized as another "hit" in the multistage neoplastic process. It does not cause cancer but is another insult. Along with other insults, stress increases the likelihood of cancer. Cancer is not serendipitous; it is partially predictable and under our control.

Behavioral and Psychological Factors and the Etiology of Cancer: A Summary

The model presented in Figure 8-1 nicely depicts the person as a system. The effect of behavioral and psychophysiological variables on cancer demonstrates the dynamic interplay of the elements in that system. Exposure to carcinogens and stressful transactions with the environment alter the physiological milieu and play a role in the development of cancer. The body attempts to adapt to these "hits" to maintain homeostasis. But when a certain number of "hits" occur over a period of time, the body is unable to keep up with this process and cancer occurs.

We have examined how behavior and the psychosocial environment affect the development of cancer. Let us turn to how cancer, its diagnosis, and its treatment influence behavioral and psychosocial adaptation.

THE EFFECT OF CANCER ON THE PERSON

Cancer, as an independent variable, has strong indirect and direct behavioral and psychosocial consequences. An overview of the impact of cancer on the person is shown in Figure 8-2. Note that while many of the variables are the same as those shown in Figure 8-1, there are additional variables and new relationships. The arrow from neoplastic process to host characteristics suggests that tumor growth and metastases alter appearance and disrupt normal physiology, and may consequently affect behavior. As these symptoms become perceptible, they lead to recognition that something is wrong (neoplastic process to behavior to psychosocial stimuli) and to seeking health care (neoplastic process to behavior to other people). The diagnosis and treatment of cancer may slow or eradicate the problem (diagnosis and treatment to neoplastic process) but also may be quite stressful for the individual (diagnosis and treatment to psychosocial stimuli). These stressors can be mitigated or exacerbated by support from family, friends, and health providers (other people to psychosocial stimuli). Let us now consider these effects in more detail, beginning with initial symptom recognition by the client.

Detection

In most cases, cancer victims first notice their own symptoms. The person may not be sure the symptom is associated with cancer. Recall that the symptoms of cancer are often vague, diffuse, and easily ascribed to other diseases. Several variables, as detailed in Chapter 3, contribute to symptom recognition and corrective health action: salience of the symptom relative to other competing stimuli, the meaning given to the symptom, social supports, and the relative payoffs and costs of the various health actions. The operation of these variables is apparent in the initial recognition by a thirty-eight-year-old woman of a change in a mole (later diagnosed as malignant melanoma, a form of skin cancer):

> I really didn't discover it. My husband is a real nit-picker about things. When he was fastening my swimming suit, he said, "I think there's a difference in this mole." I had to look over my shoulder in the mirror to see it. I really couldn't see that much of a difference. Because he kept after me and because I'd heard all my life in terms of skin cancer and people who have freckles and moles, I had the doctor look at it when I had my kids in for their physicals.

Early detection is important because it increases the likelihood of treatment success for many types of cancer (Levy, 1983). The length of delay in seeking medical assistance is quite variable. Worden and Weisman (1975), for example, found that the average delay in seeking treatment for lung cancer was 3.1 months, for colon-rectum cancer was 3.5

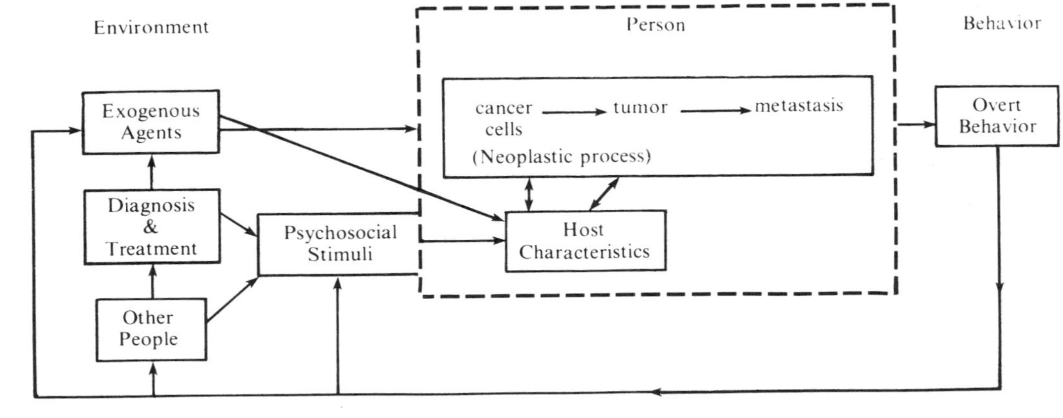

FIGURE 8-2 The Impact of Cancer on Persons and Their Environment. (From "Variables in Behavioral Oncology: Overview and Assessment of Current Issues" (p. 88) by B. H. Newberry, A. G. Liebelt, and D. A. Boyle, 1984, in B. H. Fox and B. H. Newberry (Eds.), *Impact of Psychoendocrine Systems in Cancer and Immunity*, Lewiston, NY: C. J. Hogrefe. Copyright 1984 by C. J. Hogrefe. Reprinted by permission.)

months, for breast cancer was 4.7 months, and for melanoma was 6.0 months. While most people delay about only 1 month, the delay range was very broad, from 0 to 48 months.

Recognition and delay depend on health-protective behavior like breast self-examinations and Pap smears (Levy, 1983; Stephenson, Adams, Hall, & Pennypacker, 1979). Recognition and delay also depend on knowledge of cancer symptoms and on the location and severity of the symptoms (Temoshok & Fox, 1984; Worden & Weisman, 1975). Delay in seeking treatment is influenced by the amount of fear engendered by recognition of the symptom. Very high and very low fear levels are associated with greater delay. Persons who have good social support systems and who have an internal locus of control delay less (Fox, 1981; Worden & Weisman, 1975).

Diagnosis

Unlike many illnesses in which the person feels relieved when a diagnosis is made and treatment is outlined, the diagnosis of cancer increases anxiety and distress. Because cancer is perceived as a mysterious, silent, and deadly disease, the communication of the diagnosis is a very stressful event. In addition, many diagnostic procedures for cancer are stressful (e.g., biopsy, surgical excision, and bone marrow aspiration). These procedures and the diagnosis of cancer challenge the person's adaptive resources and result in a variety of emotional (e.g., anxiety and depression), cognitive (e.g., denial and intellectualization), and behavioral (e.g., crying, asking for information, and seeking out a loved one for support) responses.

To get a feeling of this diagnostic period, let us return to the experience of the melanoma client:

> And I thought that I probably sensed there was some urgency in the way my physician said, "I want a plastic surgeon to do this and I want to have it removed immediately." But I kept thinking, "It probably isn't anything, and if it is, it will be a simple skin cancer." I went in for the excision and the plastic surgeon did that. He came in and said very matter of factly, "I want to tell you you have a melanoma malignancy." At that point everything went into a sort of transition state. I could hear the words, "the good points are and the bad points are ...," but I really couldn't have told you after the word cancer what he said. I thought, "I don't want to die."

Individuals' response to the diagnosis of cancer is dependent on their characteristics, coping styles, and social support systems and on the timing and manner in which the diagnosis is communicated by health providers. Most clients want complete and accurate information about the diagnosis and prognosis of their cancer (McIntosh, 1974). In the United States, nearly all physicians communicate the diagnosis of cancer to their clients (Fox, 1981). The timing and amount of information given to clients are quite variable. Providers try to communicate in a manner that is best, given their clients' ability to digest and handle the information. Communication about cancer is difficult for the health professionals. Prognosis and optimal treatment for a given case are a matter of probabilities rather than certainties. Communication of this uncertainty may challenge the providers' expert status and weaken the clients' faith in their ability. Health professionals do not like to communicate bad news; like everyone else, they do not like to distress others. Consequently, they often tell as little as possible as late as possible (McIntosh, 1974).

While there is no uniformly correct manner to communicate the diagnosis and prognosis of cancer to all clients, most clients benefit from accurate information provided in a sensitive manner. Persons who are told they have cancer are distressed. Those who have cancer but are not told in a timely fashion are even more distressed. Even without direct communication, noninformed clients are usually aware that something is seriously wrong (McIntosh, 1974).

Providing clients with accurate information in a sensitive manner results in less client distress in the long run. Information provides the client with some predictability and control. Accurate information fosters the collaboration of the client in treatment. This is important because additional diagnostic and treatment strategies are often aversive and require active cooperation by the client. Clients are more likely to cooperate and to tolerate these procedures if they feel actively involved. Communicating in a sensitive fashion about cancer is not an easy task, but it is an essential facet of effective treatment at both the psychological and physical levels (Levy, 1983).

Treatment

Cancer is treated using several methods either singly or in combination: surgical resection, chemotherapy, and radiation therapy. The treatment of cancer is not discrete and time limited like that of most other diseases. It often lasts for months and sometimes years. These treatments extend persons' lives but have a tremendous impact physiologically, psychologically, socially, and financially. Cancer and its treatment disrupt personal and vocational routines, family and social relationships, lifestyles, and values. The treatment of cancer is often as frightening as cancer itself. Let us look at the impact of the various cancer treatment modalities.

Surgery. Surgery may be used to determine whether a tumor is malignant, to determine the location and spread of cancer, to remove the cancerous tissue, and to prevent its further growth and metastasis. Any type of surgery is stressful for most people. It is especially so in the case of cancer. Diagnostic surgery provides information about the status of the cancer and about the possibility of effective treatment. Surgical removal of the cancer tissue may dramatically alter physical appearance (e.g., loss of a breast or a leg or mutilation of the face or jaw) and disrupt normal functioning and capabilities (e.g., loss of independent toileting, mobility, and reproductive capacity). The client is faced with major readjustments. The outcome of surgery often strongly influences chances for recovery and survival time (Fox, 1981).

The capacity to cope with threats resulting from surgery is influenced by information and preparation provided by health providers. In providing information and preparation, providers need to strike a balance between enumerating every possible detail and risk and withholding information in the clients' "best interest." They need to be honest, to help clients anticipate likely outcomes, to describe the meaning of those outcomes, and to help clients make the adjustments required by those outcomes (Lazarus, 1982). Providing information and assistance is a complex and time-consuming task. Quite often, the information needs to be provided in small pieces, at a level the client can understand, and timed according to the client's ability to listen and comprehend (Fox, 1981).

The importance of offering information and preparation is evident in the experience of the woman with melanoma:

> None of the hospital staff seemed to know what I was in the hospital for. We were referred to a tremendous surgeon. I never saw him before the surgery and I seldom saw him after. If I went to the bathroom, that's when he made rounds. This surgery was the one thing I knew meant how serious it [the cancer] was. The evening before surgery, I stopped the resident and said, "I really have some questions and no one is answering the questions about what this means." He started to leave, came back, sat down on the bed and talked. Before, no one was recognizing that this was a trauma; it was all treated very matter of factly. Nobody said, "You must be going through some hard times."

This woman's report leads to two further observations. First, what is behind health providers' occasional use of a depersonalized, detatched approach to cancer clients? Treating individuals with cancer is hard on health providers. Rather than indicating a lack of caring, a detached approach may be a defense against the burnout and emotional exhaustion that result from working with clients with life-threatening diseases (Fox, 1981). Second, the client plays an active part in eliciting information and in finding methods to manage the distress caused by surgery (Lazarus, 1982). A collaborative interaction of health professionals and the client is useful in this regard.

Chemotherapy. Chemotherapy has been used in the treatment of cancer for over forty years and is becoming the treatment of choice for many types of cancer. It introduces into the body substances that are toxic to cancer cells. Several courses of chemotherapy are typically given, lasting from a few months to a couple of years. As well as having a toxic effect on cancer cells, chemotherapeutic agents also have toxic effects on normal cells. This results in a number of side effects whose severity and nature depend on the client and the type of drug used. Common side effects are nausea, vomiting, hair loss, skin rashes, diarrhea, loss of appetite, neurological symptoms, and immunosuppression. Nausea and vomiting typically begin one to two hours after the chemotherapy session and persist for several days (Burish & Carey, 1984; Redd & Andrykowski, 1982).

After several sessions of chemotherapy, clients may experience side effects prior to a treatment session or between treatment sessions. These side effects are not directly due to the toxic effects of the drugs but are the result of a classical conditioning process. How does this conditioning take place? The unconditioned stimulus (the chemotherapy drug), which naturally elicits the unconditioned response (nausea and vomiting), is incidentally paired with a number of stimuli that may serve as conditioned stimuli (e.g., the physician's office, the chemotherapy apparatus, thoughts about the chemotherapy, and the staff who administer chemotherapy) such that, after several pairings, the conditioned stimulus alone elicits the response. There are anecdotal reports, for example, of clients who get nauseous at seeing their chemotherapy nurse at a grocery store. Twenty to 65% of all chemotherapy clients experience these conditioned side effects. The development of conditioned side effects depends on the drug used, the number of chemotherapy sessions, and the clients' coping abilities. Clients who are highly anxious and have few coping skills and little social support are more likely to develop conditioned side effects (Burish & Carey, 1984; Redd & Andrykowski, 1982).

The side effects of chemotherapy are quite aversive and pose a challenge to clients. The number and severity of side effects and client coping strategies are good predictors of the amount of distress experienced during treatment (Nerenz, Leventhal, & Love, 1982). It is not only the side effects that are stressful as again the melanoma client relates:

> I didn't know whether it was doing any good, whether there was really any reason to take it. I was really sick! I found chemotherapy discouraging because it went on for a long period of time and I knew it was going to continue. It kept me aware all that time that I had cancer. If I had stopped with the surgeries, I could have put that all behind me. There were a lot of things I had to face because of the chemotherapy.

The length of chemotherapy is a constant reminder of having cancer. It is easier to accept an aversive treatment if there is evidence that treatment is having a beneficial effect. Most often, however, clients have very little evidence that chemotherapy is really working. There are no clear physiological cues, with the exception of a reduction in the size of a palpable tumor, that improvement has occurred (Nerenz et al., 1982). Successful adaptation to chemotherapy is influenced by the information and preparation provided by providers and by clients' coping skills and social supports. The melanoma client states:

> The chemotherapy staff were really neat people. You had to get to know them because you go every week for blood tests and one week of every month for daily chemotherapy. I got over being afraid of people with cancer. The staff encouraged you, if you had been coming for a while, to help other people in their initial times in chemotherapy. Toward the end of chemotherapy, I thought I had the cycle all figured out: "On Friday nights I'm not so sick." My family brought home chicken one Friday night and I figured there was no reason why I couldn't eat it. But I got really sick. The next round was the last round of chemotherapy. I had promised that when I finished, we'd have champagne in the office to celebrate. So I went up with my bottle of champagne on Friday, and my husband said, "Again!!" I said, "I don't care, we really need to celebrate." So we had champagne, drank to everybody's health, and then I went home and got sick. But it was worth it.

Radiation Therapy. The course of radiation therapy is generally shorter than that of chemotherapy. There are similar toxic side effects with radiation, but most of these subside after a month. The side effects of radiation therapy are nausea, vomiting, hair loss, sore throat, dry mouth, and skin rashes. Information and preparation of the client for radiation therapy are important. Prior to radiation, clients have numerous concerns about the treatment: what the machine will look like, what kind of sounds it will make, being alone in the room, undressing, how long a treatment will last, how many treatments are scheduled, and whether they can move, cough, or breath during exposure to radiation (Peck & Boland, 1977). Clients who are given information and who are prepared for the treatment develop better coping skills and are less anxious and more cooperative.

Rehabilitation and Convalescence

The success of cancer treatment depends on many factors, including the type of cancer and its progression when first diagnosed. In 1980, 40% of cancer clients in initial treatment were expected to survive five years. The comparable estimates for specific types of cancer vary. About 20% of lung cancer clients survive for five years, about 70% of leukemia clients survive for five years.

When primary treatment eradicates detectable cancer, clients have additional adaptational tasks. They face the possibility of a recurrence of the disease. This fear is greatest just after primary treatment and diminishes with time (Mages & Mendelsohn, 1979). It is common for clients, during this period, to think about their death as less remote and to adjust their life priorities. These concerns are apparent in the client with melanoma:

> I began to look at it and realize, "I'm not immortal." Before I'd always refused to look at myself as dying very soon. I could see myself dying at 92 in my rocking chair with a full calendar of events for the next day, but not soon. I began to look at things with a kind of urgency, at the kind of things I really wanted to get done in my life.

Very little research is available about this period. Clients continue to experience anxiety and depression. A flexible denial appears to be a very adaptive approach. This consists of "forgetting" about the cancer and its possible recurrence most of the time, but maintaining an underlying sensitivity that promotes appropriate health actions (Lazarus, 1982).

In cases in which cancer and its treatment result in physiological disruption or altered appearance, clients have to develop a new self-image and have to learn new self-care and vocational skills in order to optimize their independence within the limitations imposed. These physical changes impact on social relationships; the client may have to deal with reactions ranging from overprotection and overconcern to rejection, fear, and avoidance (Fox, 1981). Clients' adjustment can be facilitated by medical rehabilitation. This includes the use of prostheses, rehabilitative exercises, new modes of self-care, and vocational rehabilitation. The rehabilitation should not only restore clients to their fullest physiological independence but also promote clients' psychosocial adjustment. Rehabilitation efforts should be planned and communicated at the same time that primary treatment strategies are being developed (Leopold & Ramsden, 1979).

Recurrence and Terminal Illness

The course of cancer is unpredictable. If primary treatment eradicates the cancer, the length of remission is variable. If the cancer is not eradicated by primary treatment, the cancer may grow rapidly or slowly, it may become dormant, or it may even regress. Relapse after primary treatment is an extremely difficult time for clients. Relapse often indicates a poor prognosis. There will be another course of surgery, chemotherapy, or radiation. Clients are faced with the prospect of increasing infirmity and disability. Clients again experience fear, depression, and anger. The adaptive task is to maintain a sense of self-control and self-sufficiency when events indicate an increasing powerlessness. If another remission is not effected, the goal of treatment is to control the cancer so that clients can continue to lead as productive and comfortable lives as possible (Fox, 1981; Mages & Mendelsohn, 1979).

Pain may occur during the later stages of cancer. About 50% of all persons with cancer experience no cancer related pain. Ten percent experience modest pain, and about 40% experience severe pain. Pain is the result of the compression or obstruction of tissue by a tumor. Cancer pain is chronic; it is ongoing and nonfunctional, and often becomes the focal point of clients' lives. It causes additional anxiety, depression, and hopelessness (see Chapter 9 for an extended discussion of chronic pain). The treatment of pain may involve further surgery, chemotherapy, or radiation to reduce the size and invasion of the cancer on normal tissue. Pain may also be treated symptomatically by analgesics. Nonnarcotic substances are used initially. When they become ineffective, there is a shift to narcotic painkillers in combination with tranquilizers and antidepressants. The use of painkilling medication is effective but can result in several problems. Tolerance often develops to such medication so that increasingly large doses are required to control the pain. As dosage increases, narcotic drugs have increasingly aversive side effects, including clouding clients' cognitive and affective capacities. Cognitive-behavioral interventions, including biofeedback, relaxation, and coping strategies, are adjuncts to more traditional methods of pain control. When begun before the pain is severe, these cognitive-behavioral interventions may ultimately reduce the amount of medication needed to control pain effectively (Turk & Rennert, 1981).

Successful treatment and adaptation during the recurrence of cancer are fostered by a collaboration between the client and the health provider. The extent of treatment to combat the disease must be balanced with the overall quality of clients' lives.

The terminal phase of cancer, when death is imminent, is often the most fearsome. Each client approaches death in unique ways, using those coping strategies that are personally meaningful. Anxiety and depression are often experienced by clients during the terminal phase. These feelings are related to specific medical, financial, familial, and social concerns as well as to the prospect of death. Support and assistance help clients address specific concerns, but dying clients also need others to *be* with them and to *listen* to them in addition to *doing* something to them or for them (Pumphrey & Ramsden, 1979). Support and assistance at an emotional as well as a practical level help clients maintain self-sufficiency and dignity during the dying process. However, health professionals and kin often withdraw from dying persons behaviorally and symbolically, thereby denying that emotional support (Fox, 1981).

The Effect of Cancer on the Person: A Summary

Cancer and its treatment represent a multitude of shifting challenges and threats that require adaptation. These challenges and threats range from disruption of physiological integrity to loss of self-sufficiency and social isolation. Successful adaptation requires a broad array of problem-solving and coping skills. Because the demands of cancer and its treatment are numerous and outside clients' previous experience, and because reality sets limits on how actively clients can meet these demands, support, information, and assistance from family and health providers are integral resources in promoting adaptation. Anxiety, anger, and depression are common responses to cancer and its treatment. These reactions range from mild to severe, with no clear line between what is "normal" or "expected" and what might be considered "abnormal" or "morbid."

The availability of personal, social, and health care resources promotes successful adaptation by reducing clients' emotional and behavioral distress. These resources may also enhance outcome at a physiological level. By reducing stress, clients' immune and endocrine defenses against cancer may be mobilized or enhanced (Levy, 1983). Prognostic studies have found that clients who have few coping skills and little social support have a shorter survival time than individuals who have better coping resources (Sklar & Anisman, 1981). Some prognostic studies have not found this relationship (Miller & Spratt, 1979). Effective treatment of cancer at physical as well as psychosocial levels requires interventions to reduce stress and promote active coping strategies.

One important resource is social support. Survival time, recovery, and psychosocial adjustment are better for individuals who have good social support systems at the time of diagnosis (Lichtman & Taylor, 1986) and later in treatment (Carey, 1974). The effectiveness of social support depends on its nature and source (Wortman, 1984). Dunkel-Schetter (1984), for example, found that emotional forms of support from the family were perceived as most helpful and that informational and appraisal support from the family was perceived as less helpful. In a similar manner, emotional support from health providers was perceived as extremely helpful. But unlike family sources, informational support and advice from providers was also perceived as very helpful.

Specifically, health professionals can reduce client distress by minimizing the discontinuity in the client's life that results from cancer and its treatment. The type and scheduling of treatment should be planned in a manner that is medically effective yet also compatible with the client's work, familial, and social responsibilities. By providing accurate information, involvement in treatment planning, and preparation for specific procedures and likely outcomes, health providers can foster transactions that maximize clients' self-determination, control, and sense of predictability. There are four times during the course of intervention when clients are particularly vulnerable: diagnosis, primary treatment, relapse, and terminal illness. Health professionals can make a special effort to aid clients during these periods. Some clients are more vulnerable than others. Clients who have few personal coping skills and social supports or whose cancer and treatment seriously disrupt their lives are in particular need of assistance from health providers (Meyerowitz, 1980).

Adaptation is also influenced by the coping skills of persons with cancer. The first reports of associations between psychological and behavioral coping styles and cancer prognosis were published in the 1950s (e.g., Bacon, Renneker, & Cutler, 1952). Since then, studies have continued to find that persons with cancer who express negative affect, are assertive without alienating others, and who have a fighting spirit have a better prognosis than those who are passive, nonexpressive, polite, and cooperative (Temoshok & Fox, 1984). This has been found for persons with metastatic breast cancer, (Derogatis, Abeloff, & Milisaratos, 1979), malignant melanoma (Rogertine, Fox, VanKammen, Rosenblatt, Docherty, & Bunney, 1979), and testicular cancer (Edwards, DiClemente, & Samuels, 1985). Much of the coping done by cancer clients is palliative. It involves managing somatic and emotional distress caused by cancer and its treatment. However, direct forms of coping are also important. Clients can seek information, exercise an active role in treatment, actively cooperate and comply with medical procedures, and become actively involved in rehabilitative procedures. Successful adaptation requires the use of different coping modes to meet the changing threats and challenges posed during the course of the disease and its treatment (Lazarus, 1982).

SUMMARY

While cancer is an often life-threatening, serious, and debilitating disease, it is not totally mysterious and hopeless. Many environmental carcinogens have been identified, and contact with these carcinogens is strongly influenced by personal behavior and collective political and economic choices. Although cancer is influenced by the occurrence of random events over which we have minimum control, it is also influenced by events over which we have a good measure of control. We are also not without body defenses against cancer. The immune and endocrine systems play an important surveillance and protective role against cancer. We may weaken those defenses by creating a lot of stress in daily transactions with the environment.

The adjustment, recovery, and survival time (the prognosis) of persons with cancer are complexly determined. Prognosis depends on the biological characteristics of the person and the disease. It is influenced by the efficacy of surgery, chemotherapy, radiation therapy, and other forms of medical intervention. During the past twenty years, these medical interventions have significantly enhanced the prognosis in cancer (Silverberg, 1985). Forty percent of persons currently diagnosed as having cancer have successfully completed a disease-free five-year interval (American Cancer Society, 1985). Even when cure was not possible, technical advances have prolonged survival time in many cases.

However, these gains have not come without costs. Such interventions exact a heavy toll from clients. The transformation of cancer from a uniformly fatal disease to a condition characterized by chronicity and possible cure has led to the recognition of the importance of psychosocial and behavioral variables as pivotal facets of treatment. Social support, coping skills, ability to access and utilize health care services, and adherence to and cooperation with treatment are as relevant to prognosis as biological state and medical intervention (Derogatis, 1986). The client, from this perspective, is an active participant and collaborator in treatment.

REFERENCES

Alexander, P. (1977). Innate host resistance to malignant cells not involving specific immunity. In S. Day, W. Myers, P. Stansley, S. Garattini, & M. Lewis (Eds.), *Cancer invasion and metastases: Biologic mechanisms and therapy*, 259–276. New York: Raven Press.

American Cancer Society. (1985). *Cancer facts and figures, 1985*. New York: Author.

Bacon, C. L., Renneker, R., & Cutler, M. (1952). A psychosomatic survey of cancer of the breast. *Psychosomatic Medicine 41*, 453.

Baldanado, A., & Stahl, D. (1978). *Cancer nursing: A holistic, multidisciplinary approach*. Garden City, NY: Medical Examination.

Boyd, W. (1966). *The spontaneous regression of cancer*. Springfield, IL: Charles C. Thomas.

Bridbord, K., Decoufle, P., Fraumeni, J. F., Leary, M., Johnson, L., & McKay, R. (1978). *Estimates of the fraction of cancer in the United States related to occupational factors*. Bethesda, MD: National Cancer Institute.

Burish, T. G., & Carey, M. P. (1984). Conditioned responses to chemotherapy: Etiology and treatment. In B. Fox & B. Newberry (Eds.), *Impact of psycho-endocrine systems in cancer and immunity*, 311–320. Lewiston, NY: C. J. Hogrefe.

Carey, R. C. (1974). Emotional adjustment in terminal patients: A quantitative approach. *Journal of Counseling Psychology, 21*, 433–439.

Clark, R. L. (1976). Psychologic reactions of patients and health professionals to cancer. In J. W. Cullen, B. H. Fox, & R. N. Isom (Eds.), *Cancer: The behavioral dimensions*, 207–231. New York: Raven Press.

Derogatis, L. R. (1986). Psychology in cancer medicine: A perspective and overview. *Journal of Consulting and Clinical Psychology, 54*, 632–638.

Derogatis, L. R., Abeloff, M. D., & Milisaratos, N. (1979). Psychological coping mechanisms and survival time in metastatic breast cancer. *Journal of the American Medical Association, 242*, 1504–1508.

Doll, R., & Petro, R. (1981). *The causes of cancer*. New York: Oxford University Press.

Dunkel-Schetter, C. (1984). Social support and cancer: Findings based on patient interviews and their implication. *Journal of Social Issues, 40*, 77–98.

Edwards, J., DiClemente, C., & Samuels, M. L. (1985). Psychological characteristics: A pretreatment survival marker of patients with testicular cancer. *Journal of Psychosocial Oncology, 3*, 79–94.

Eisenberg, J. M. (1979). Economics of cancer and its treatment. In B. R. Cassileth (Ed.), *The cancer patient*, 45–58. Philadelphia: Lea & Febiger.

Fox, B. H. (1976). The psychosocial epidemiology of cancer. In J. W. Cullen, B. H. Fox, & R. N. Isom (Eds.), *Cancer: The behavioral dimensions*, 101–134. New York: Raven Press.

Fox, B. H. (1978). Premorbid psychological factors as related to cancer incidence. *Journal of Behavioral Medicine, 1*, 45–133.

Fox, B. H. (1981). Behavioral issues in cancer. In S. M. Weiss, J. A. Herd, & B. H. Fox (Eds.), *Perspectives on behavioral medicine*, 163–191. New York: Academic Press.

Henderson, B. E. (1981). Descriptive epidemiology and geographic pathology. In J. H. Burchenal & H. F. Oettgen (Eds.), *Cancer: Achievement, challenges and prospects for the 1980s*, 51–70. New York: Grune & Stratton.

Herberman, R. B., & Holden, H. T. (1984). Natural killer cells as antitumor effector cells. *Journal of the National Cancer Institute, 62*, 441–445.

Jemmott, J. B., & Locke, S. E. (1984). Psychosocial factors, immunological mediation, and human susceptibility to infectious diseases: How much do we know? *Psychological Bulletin, 95*, 78–108.

Lazarus, R. S. (1982). Stress and coping as factors in health and illness. In J. Cohen, J. W. Cullen, & L. R. Martin, (Eds.), *Psychosocial aspects of cancer*, 74–98. New York: Raven Press.

Leopold, R. L., & Ramsden, E. L. (1979). Rehabilitation services. In B. R. Cassileth (Ed.), *The cancer patient*, 119–132. Philadelphia: Lea & Febiger.

Levy, S. M. (1983). Host differences in neoplastic risk: Behavioral and social contributors to disease. *Health Psychology, 2*, 21–44.

Lichtman, R. R., & Taylor, S. E. (1986). Close relationships and the female cancer patient. In B. L. Andersen (Ed.), *Women with cancer: Psychological perspectives*, 106–121. New York: Springer-Verlag.

Mages, N. L., & Mendelsohn, G. A. (1979). Effects of cancer on patients' lives: A personological approach. In G. Stone, F. Cohen, & N. Adler (Eds.), *Health psychology: A handbook*, 255–284. San Francisco: Jossey-Bass.

McIntosh, J. (1974). Processes of communication, information seeking and control associated with cancer: A selective review. *Social Science and Behavioral Medicine, 8*, 167–187.

Meyerowitz, B. E. (1980). Psychosocial correlates of breast cancer and its treatments. *Psychological Bulletin, 87*, 108–131.

Miller, D. G. (1980). On the nature of susceptibility to cancer. *Cancer, 46*, 1307–1318.

Miller, T., & Spratt, J. S. (1979). A critical review of reported psychological correlates of cancer prognosis and growth. In B. A. Stoll (Ed.), *Mind and cancer prognosis*, 63–97. New York: John Wiley & Sons.

Morrison, T. R., & Paffenbarger, R. A. (1981). Epidemiological aspects of biobehavior in the etiology of cancer: A critical review. In S. M. Weiss, J. A. Herd, & B. H. Fox (Eds.), *Perspectives on behavioral medicine*, 135–162. New York: Academic Press.

Nerenz, D. R., Leventhal, H., & Love, R. R. (1982). Factors contributing to emotional distress during cancer chemotherapy. *Cancer, 50*, 1020–1027.

Newberry, B. H., Liebelt, A. G., & Boyle, D. A. (1984). Variables in behavioral oncology: Overview and assessment of current issues. In B. H. Fox & B. H. Newberry (Eds.), *Impact of psychoendocrine systems in cancer and immunity*, 3–29. Lewiston, NY: C. J. Hogrefe.

Peck, A., & Boland, J. (1977). Emotional reactions to radiation treatment. *Cancer, 40*, 180–184.

Poste, G. (1977). The cell surface and metastasis. In S. Day, W. Myers, P. Stansley, S. Garattini, & M. Lewis (Eds.), *Cancer invasion and metastasis: Biological mechanisms and therapy*, 19–48. New York: Raven Press.

Prehn, R. T. (1976). Tumor progression and homeostasis. In G. Klein & S. Weinhouse (Eds.), *Advances in cancer research* (Vol. 3), 207–219. New York: Academic Press.

Pumphrey, J. B., & Ramsden, E. L. (1979). Patient adaptation to terminal illness. In B. R. Cassileth (Ed.), *The cancer patient*, 219–232. Philadelphia: Lea & Febiger.

Redd, W. H., & Andrykowski, M. A. (1982). Behavioral intervention in cancer treatment: Controlling aversive reactions to chemotherapy. *Journal of Consulting and Clinical Psychology, 50*, 1018–1029.

Rogers, M. P., Dubey, D., & Reich, P. (1979). The influence of the psyche and the brain on immunity and disease susceptibility: A critical review. *Psychosomatic Medicine, 41*, 147–164.

Rogertine, G. N., Fox, B. H., VanKammen, D. P., Rosenblatt, J., Docherty, J. P., & Bunney, W. E. (1979). Psychological and biological factors in the short term prognosis of malignant melanoma. *Psychosomatic Medicine, 41*, 647–655.

Silverberg, E. (1985). Probabilities of eventually developing or dying of cancer. *Cancer Statistics, 35,* 36–56.
Sklar, L. S., & Anisman, H. (1981). Stress and cancer. *Psychological Bulletin, 89,* 369–406.
Stephenson, H., Adams, C., Hall, D., & Pennypacker, H. (1979). The effects of certain training parameters on detection of simulated breast cancer. *Journal of Behavioral Medicine, 2,* 23–25.
Temoshok, L., & Fox, B. H. (1984). Coping styles and other psychosocial factors related to medical status and prognosis in patients with cutaneous malignant melanoma. In B. Fox & R. Newberry (Eds.), *Impact of psychoendocrine systems in cancer and immunity,* 417–430. Toronto: C. J. Hogrefe.
Turk, D., & Rennert, K. (1981). Pain and the terminally ill cancer patient: A cognitive social learning perspective. In H. J. Sobel (Ed.), *Behavior therapy in terminal care: A humanistic approach,* 95–124. Cambridge, MA: Ballinger.
Ultman, J. E., & Golomb, H. M. (1977). Approach to diagnosis and management in oncology. In G. Thorn, R. Adams, E. Braunwald, K. Isselbacher, & R. Petersdorf (Eds.), *Harrison's principles of internal medicine.* New York: McGraw-Hill.
U. S. Department of Health and Human Services, Public Health Service, National Institute of Health. (1987). *Incidence and mortality trends among whites in the United States.* Washington, DC: U.S. Government Printing Office.
Wortman, C. B. (1984). Social support and cancer. *Cancer, 53,* 2339–2368.

9

Pain

INTRODUCTION

Pain is a frequent complaint. The incidence of acute and chronic pain is staggering. There are 20 to 50 million sufferers of arthritis, with 600,000 new cases each year (Arthritis Foundation, 1976), and 25 million people who suffer from migraine headaches (Paulley & Haskell, 1975). Low back pain has disabled 7 million Americans and accounts for 8 million physician office visits a year (Clark, Gosnell, & Shapiro, 1977). Up to 80% of physician visits involve pain-related complaints (Bresler, 1979). More than 900 million dollars are spent annually for aspirin and similar over-the-counter pain relievers, with each person in the United States consuming an average of 225 tablets of these substances per year (Koenig, 1973).

The understanding of pain and the development of procedures for its relief are central concerns in medicine. In this chapter, the nature and causes of pain will be explored. A model of pain will be developed using the systems paradigm, and the implications of the model for treatment will be discussed.

PAIN AS A MULTIDIMENSIONAL PROCESS

We have all experienced the attention-riveting, noxious quality of pain. Whether the pain is sharp and intense or a generalized throbbing, there is a subjective hurt that is experienced as a basic lack of well-being. Pain certainly involves the subjective experience of discomfort.

When you experience pain, you react in a reflexive manner to protect yourself. You reflexively verbalize discomfort. When you pick up a hot skillet with a bare hand, you drop it, shake your hand, and moan or scream. If the pain continues, you communicate this to others, try to find relief, and change your body posture to reduce it. Pain involves a complex set of reflexive and learned behaviors, often dramatically altering normal roles and actions.

When you verbally or nonverbally communicate pain, other people react with concern and provide aid. The expression of pain captures others' attention. If you see a child fall off of a bicycle, skin her hands and knees, and cry, you provide comfort and may exempt her from her usual roles, like putting the bicycle back in the garage. Pain is thus also a social and environmental event.

When you are in pain, you try to identify the noxious stimulus that caused the pain or to assess the damage to the body caused by that stimulus. If you feel a sharp pain when sliding your hand along a piece of wood, you look for a sliver. If you feel pain after accidentally bumping into a chair, you feel for a tender spot or look for a bruise. Pain can be defined on the basis of either the agent that caused the pain or the biological damage resulting from that agent.

Pain has multiple components. We tend to think of it as a thing or an entity, but it is really a kind of shorthand label applied to a complex set of interrelated phenomena: subjective, behavioral, social, environmental, and physiological. It is easy to forget it is a label and to treat pain as if it were a material thing. This reification (changing pain as a label into a thing) results in conceptual and practical confusion.

This discussion of the complexity of pain and the emphasis on pain as a label may seem unnecessary. Often, these various facets of pain are considered together such that consistency is observed in the various facets used to ascribe the label "pain." From this point of view, selecting and using one facet of pain is as good as selecting and using any other. However, this unidimensional simplification can severely limit our understanding of pain and the procedures used to treat it.

THE BIOMEDICAL PARADIGM OF PAIN

The traditional biomedical paradigm of pain and pain treatment is based on mechanistic and reductionistic tenets. It simplifies and reduces pain to biological or physical-chemical components. Consider a physician dealing with a patient who is complaining of pain in the lower back and left leg. The assumption is made that the patient's complaint is a reflection of some underlying pathology: A symptom has an underlying cause. A diagnostic search is made, using x-rays, a neurological exam, and a history of the patient's experience, to localize and identify the biological damage causing the pain. Let us assume that the x-rays show a compression of two disks in the lower spine. Treatment would involve fixing the damage, perhaps by surgically fusing the two vertebrae. However, if the x-rays and other diagnostic procedures failed to find a cause for the reported pain, the validity of the patient's complaint would be questioned. The presence of observable tissue damage is the *sine qua non* definition of pain. A strong relationship should exist between the severity of pain and the amount of biological damage. If there is an inconsistency, observable biological evidence is the acid test (Fordyce, 1978).

The Specificity Theory of Pain

The traditional biomedical approach to pain is closely tied to the specificity theory of pain (Melzack, 1973). The specificity theory proposes that specific neural pathways carry pain information from peripheral receptors to the sensory cortex of the brain. A schematic of this specific system is shown in Figure 9-1. These pathways are specialized to carry pain information. The theory assumes that the sensation of pain is directly related to stimulation of free nerve endings. There is a direct-line fixed communication system between the free nerve endings and the brain. This implies an invariant relationship between the amount of pain experienced and the intensity of the noxious stimulus (or the amount of tissue damage). If a person feels pain, there should be some identifiable cause. The intensity of the pain and the amount of damage should be proportional to each other.

The specificity theory suggests that other dimensions of pain (e.g., affective, behavioral, social, and motivational) are reactions to the sensation of pain. These dimensions do not affect the intensity, quality, or duration of pain. The affective, behavioral, social, and motivational aspects of pain are seen as secondary to the basic sensation of pain (Melzack & Casey, 1968).

Usually, when we experience pain, we can locate some type of injury. In most cases, persons' complaints and the amount of damage are roughly proportional; healing of the tissue brings about a reduction in pain. The specificity theory is often accepted as a fact. However, the specificity theory and its biomedical applications do not adequately account for experimental and clinical data that indicate that the relationship between tissue damage and pain is variable. There are many clinical cases in which clients complain of severe, persistent pain for which the health care provider can find no adequate biological cause.

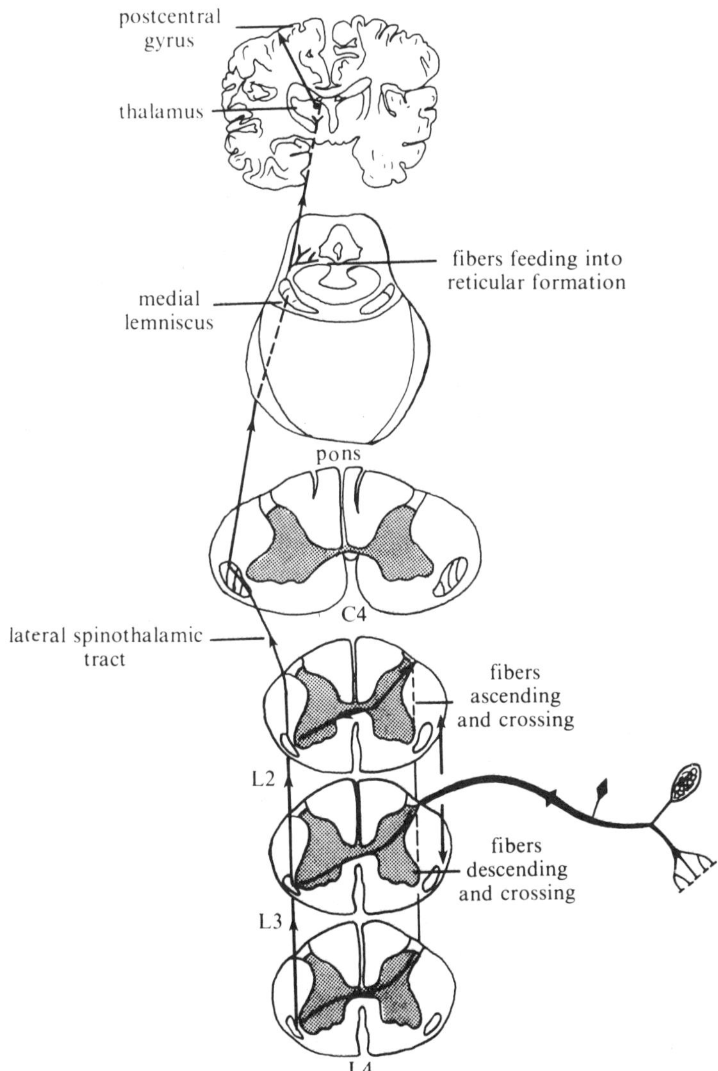

FIGURE 9-1 Spinal and Brain Mechanisms Involved in Pain: The Specificity Theory. (From *An Introduction to the Neurosciences* (p. 306) by B. A. Curtis, S. Jacobson, and E. M. Marcus, 1981, Philadelphia: W. B. Saunders. Copyright 1981 by W. B. Saunders. Reprinted by permission.

The other extreme, in which a person has massive tissue damage but makes few or no complaints, also occurs. Beecher (1959) observed that wounded soldiers returning from battle in World War II complained very little and requested minimal painkilling medication. These men were not in shock and were able to feel pain, for they complained vigorously at inept vein punctures. After the war, Beecher observed that civilians who had wounds similar to those incurred by the soldiers complained of severe pain and pleaded for painkillers. Beecher (1959) concluded:

> The common belief that wounds are inevitably associated with pain, and that the more extensive the wound the worse the pain, was not supported by observations made as carefully as possible in the combat zone. . . . The data state in numerical terms what is known to all thoughtful clinical observers: there is no simple direct relationship between the wound *per se* and the pain experienced. (p. 63)

In between these two extremes of pain without identifiable damage and damage without pain, there is much variation in how closely the various facets of pain are related.

If the specificity theory is valid, the surgical severing of pain pathways should stop the pain. Despite the many locations at which these surgical ablations occur, these ablations do not produce significant, lasting reductions in chronic pain (Melzack, 1973). An alternate theory that accounts for these phenomena is thus needed. The gate control theory presents such an alternative.

The Gate Control Theory of Pain

The gate control theory conceptualizes pain as a multidimensional phenomenon having sensory, motivational-affective, and cognitive-evaluative components. Pain involves multiple levels within the system. The theory hypothesizes a number of complex structures in the central nervous system that contribute to pain. The interplay among these structures determines the quality and degree of pain experienced and the relationship of that experience to noxious stimuli or tissue damage (Melzack & Wall, 1982). Specifically, the theory hypothesizes that there are a series of neurophysiological mechanisms located in the dorsal horn of each segment of the spinal cord. These mechanisms act as gates, controlling transmission cells that send information about pain to the brain. When these gates are open, information is transmitted that elicits brain activity mediating the experience of pain. When the gates are closed, no pain is experienced. The status of the gate depends upon several inputs.

One input is the pattern of sensory information from the external environment (e.g., temperature and touch) and from the body (e.g., stretch receptors in the muscles and distension of the stomach). Low intensity (i.e., normal, nonnoxious) sensory information, carried by large diameter nerve fibers, closes the gate and inhibits the transmission of pain information to the brain. The second input is high intensity (i.e., noxious) sensory information. This information, carried by small diameter nerve fibers, opens the gate and facilitates the transmission of pain information to the brain. This is shown in Figure 9-2.

The third input to the gates comes from the brain. Information about peripheral stimulation bypasses the gate, ascends in the dorsal columns of the spinal cord, and terminates in the cortex, where it activates brain processes related to attention, emotional state, past learning experiences, and expectations. The meaning given to the stimulation by this processing is then transmitted back to the gate via nerve fibers that descend from the brain to the spinal cord (see Figure 9-2). Depending on the meaning given to the stimulation, this descending information can also open or close the gate and consequently influences the transmission of pain information to the brain. There is a fourth powerful inhibitory input to the gate coming from the brain stem reticular formation. This input appears to exert a tonic or constant influence that tends to close the gate. We will discuss this input in more detail in the next section.

The gate is in a fluctuating state. It constantly "averages" the inputs from sensory stimulation and from cognitive-affective processing in the brain. When the gate is sufficiently open and its output exceeds a critical level, it activates neurophysiological systems in the brain that mediate pain perception, experience, and behavior. In other words, whether a person experiences pain and the intensity and quality of pain depend on noxious sensory input (tissue damage), nonnoxious sensory input, and the psychological and behavioral state of the person when the noxious stimulation occurs.

FIGURE 9-2 The Spinal Gating Mechanism and Ascending and Descending Influences in the Gate Control Theory. (From *The Challenge of Pain* (p. 235) by Ronald Melzack and Patrick D. Wall. Copyright © 1982 by Ronald Melzack and Patrick D. Wall. Reprinted by permission of Basic Books, Inc., Publishers.)

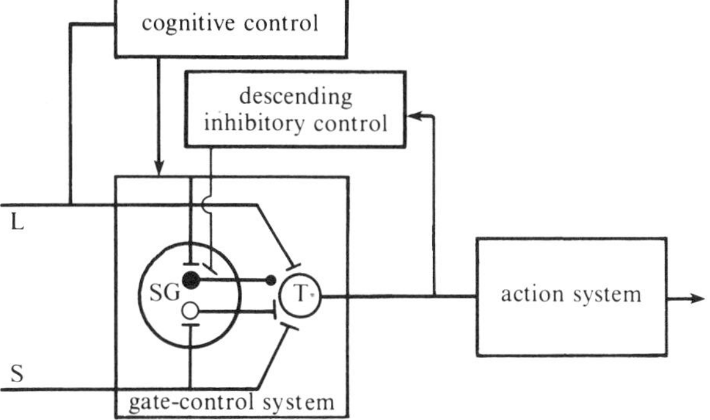

The influence of nonnoxious stimulation and the state of the organism on pain can be made clearer by a couple of examples. When you injure yourself by cutting your finger, gently squeezing your finger reduces the pain for a short period. In other cases, a gentle touch, with an intensity that would not normally cause pain, near a wound may elicit excruciating pain. In each of these cases, a nonnoxious sensory input modulates or alters the pain resulting from an injury. Or recall a pain that persisted for a period of time. If the pain was of moderate intensity, you could ignore it at first because you thought it would go away by itself. It hurt, but not a lot. Then the pain continued. You began to wonder about it more, perhaps became increasingly anxious because you were afraid it meant something was seriously wrong. It seemed to hurt more. In this case, your attentiveness to and anxiety about the pain may have increased its intensity.

The output of the gate ascends in several tracts in the spinal cord and is projected to two brain systems: (1) the thalamus and sensory cortex, and (2) the subcortical areas of the brain called the reticular formation and the limbic system (see Figure 9-3). These areas of the brain mediate the experiential correlates of pain. Information sent to the thalamus and cortex serve primarily a sensory-discriminative function. Processing of information in these areas permits the person to recognize and localize the noxious stimulation and perhaps to identify the nature of the noxious stimulation (Casey, 1979). Projections to the reticular formation and limbic system (including the thalamus, hypothalamus, hippocampus, amygdala, and limbic cortex) mediate the emotional and motivational facets of pain. Activation of these areas is responsible for the aversive quality of pain and the desire to avoid or escape the source of pain (Casey, 1979). These brain systems interact to provide the cognitive, perceptual, affective, and motivational facets of the experience of pain. This activity in turn activates motor mechanisms used to express and to reduce pain. These motor mechanisms mediate the complex ways in which pain is expressed, ranging from basic reflexes to verbal complaints.

In summary, the gate control theory postulates that the experience of pain depends on the pattern of information converging on the gate from multiple sources. Physiologically, it is not a one-way transmission system. There is information descending from the brain that influences transmission from the spinal cord about noxious and nonnoxious stimuli. Pain does not occur in an empty organism, but is influenced by the physiological, psychological, and behavioral status of the person. The brain mechanisms that mediate the experience of pain are activated when the gate is open. The pain is experientially the same regardless of the variables that open the gate.

Although the gate control theory is not a final or definitive model of pain, it is able to account for many experimental and clinical pain

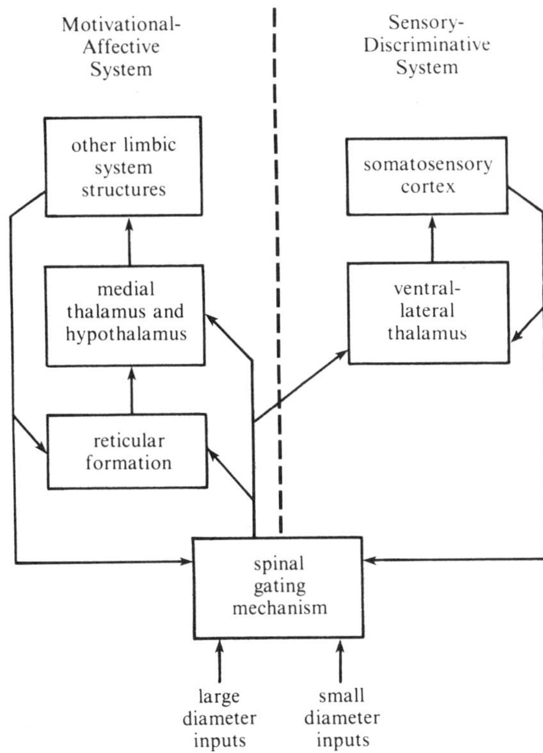

FIGURE 9–3 Spinal and Brain Mechanisms in Pain. (From "The Neurophysiological Basis of Pain" by K. L. Casey, 1973, *Postgraduate Medicine, 53*(6), p. 62. Copyright 1973 by McGraw-Hill. Reprinted by permission.)

phenomena better than the specificity theory. Rather than viewing pain as a simple, discrete sensation that is directly related to the intensity of a noxious stimulus, the gate control theory suggests that pain is a complex, multifaceted process. Pain is not only elicited by noxious stimulation. It is also influenced by other sensory inputs, the meaning given to the stimulation, the context in which it occurs, the emotional state of the person, and the behavior in which the person is engaged. A person is not an empty organism that passively receives noxious stimulation.

Natural Analgesic Mechanisms

According to the gate control theory, higher nervous system processes exert some control over pain. In fact, there are data suggesting that the nervous system may contain a natural, built-in pain suppression mechanism. Electrical stimulation of the part of the brain stem called the periaqueductal gray produces analgesia without disrupting consciousness and other behaviors. The activation of the periaqueductal gray inhibits pain by sending inhibitory messages to the spinal gating mechanisms (Melzack & Wall, 1982; Reynolds, 1969).

Recent research on the physiology of pain has also identified endogenous opiatelike substances in the central nervous system. Opiate substances (e.g., morphine and codeine) have a long history of clinical use in pain relief. These substances have their analgesic effects by acting on neural tissue in the central nervous system. Opiates bind with receptors of neurons in the periaqueductal gray of the reticular formation and limbic system (Snyder, 1977). These are the same areas at which stimulation-produced analgesia can be elicited.

Snyder and other researchers reasoned that if opiates have their analgesic effects by binding with receptors at specific brain sites, it was possible that the nervous system produces natural painkilling substances at these sites. Evidence suggests that these naturally occurring painkilling substances are endorphins and enkephalins. Endorphins and enkephalins act as neurotransmitters at opiate-active sites in the nervous system. Opiate-binding sites and endorphin-containing neurons are distributed in the same areas of the nervous system (Cannon, Liebeskind, & Frank, 1978). These neural sites integrate the sensory with motivational and affective aspects of pain. Morphine's effect at these sites does not obliterate a person's awareness of pain (the sensory component), but seems to reduce the aversiveness of the pain. Morphine is most effective for those individuals who are highly anxious about their pain (Ray, 1978).

The functional role of endorphins and enkephalins is not completely understood. The evidence suggests they play a role in modulating pain by affecting neural activity at reticular, limbic, and spinal sites in the nervous system. High levels of these substances are associated with reduced pain and low levels with enhanced pain. The injection of endorphins and enkephalins in these areas induce analgesia. Cerebrospinal fluid levels of these substances are lower than normal in persons experiencing chronic pain and higher than normal in persons congenitally insensitive to pain. Various treatments to reduce pain (e.g., acupuncture, transcutaneous electrical nerve stimulation, and analgesic central nervous system stimulation) are associated with increasing the levels of endorphins and enkephalins (Cannon et al., 1978). Other research suggests that placebo effects may be mediated by these substances (Levine, Gordon, & Field, 1978) and that stressful events may activate these substances (Akil, 1982).

The research on endorphins and enkephalins suggests that pain is not solely and directly tied to noxious stimuli, but that environmental, behavioral, and psychological factors influence the pain experience. Let us look at the behavioral and psychosocial facets of pain in more detail.

PSYCHOSOCIAL ASPECTS OF PAIN

Pain is a valuable biological signal that tissue damage is impending or has occurred. But pain involves more than tissue damage. There are a host of psychological, social, and behavioral factors that are involved in the pain experience. Pain happens to people. Noxious stimuli are embedded in an array of stimuli that make up the person's immediate environment. The person on whom the noxious stimuli impinge has a learning history of dealing with the noxious and nonnoxious stimuli. This history influences the meaning given to noxious stimuli. The person is actively engaged in purposeful behavior to accomplish selected goals. The person's behavioral expression and reaction to pain occurs in the context of this purposeful activity. In this section, we will explore how environmental, psychological, and behavioral factors influence the experience of pain.

Environmental Variables

We do not passively receive noxious stimuli. Rather, we actively evaluate the meaning, duration, and intensity of pain on the basis of the situation in which it occurs. To get a sense of this, try a quick experiment. Pinch a very small bit of skin on the inside of your arm just below the armpit. Even though this area is quite sensitive, you will find that you can pinch quite hard without feeling too much pain. Now imagine that a stranger sitting next to you suddenly pinched that skin area with the same intensity. You would probably experience more pain. Environmental or situational cues provide us with information about the expected intensity and duration of pain. They give us some idea of the degree to which pain is under our control or is predictable. When you pinched yourself, you knew that you were doing it to yourself, that you would not pinch too hard, and that you could stop when it hurt too much. There was a feeling of control and predictability. If a stranger did it, you would not know why he did it, how hard or long he would pinch, and whether you could get him to stop. The situation provides little control or predictability.

Situational variables play an important role in experimental and clinical pain. Craig and Weiss (1972) demonstrated how the social environment can influence experimentally induced pain. They administered a series of electric shocks to two groups of individuals. The shocks were all of equal intensity and not usually reported to be painful. Prior to receiving the shocks, one group was exposed to a model who made judgments about the shocks that ranged from undetectable to painful as the series progressed. The other group was not exposed to the model. Both groups then received an equal number of constant intensity shocks. The group exposed to the model reported nearly 80% of the shocks to be painful, while the nonmodel group reported only 2% of the shocks to be painful. Environmental cues that suggest that some stimulus is likely to be painful influence how those stimuli are experienced. The experience of pain is commonly influenced by environmental cues. Recall the last time you went to the dentist. As you sat in the chair before any procedure began, it is likely that you tensed your body and gripped the arms of the chair tightly. Because the dentist's office has been associated with pain, it provides cues such that you anticipate its occurrence.

Situational stimuli can also decrease the intensity of pain. Intense or important stimuli distract us from noxious stimuli and reduce the pain. For example, Kanfer and Goldfoot (1966) studied how long subjects could keep their arms immersed in ice water under differing environmental conditions. One group was asked to view and describe an interesting set of slides during the immersion, while another group was asked to watch a clock to time their tolerance. The distracted group showed significantly longer immersion time than the pain-focusing group. Common experiences validate this effect. Football players, for example, sustain severe blows with minimal pain. This may be the result of the focusing of attention on the game and the immediate task. It may also be influenced by the potential ridicule of opponents if pain is displayed. Situational cues may serve to reduce the experience of pain.

There are clinical examples analogous to these experimental and commonsensical examples. Beecher's (1959) observations of wounded soldiers in World War II is a good example. Recall that soldiers having massive battlefield wounds reported little pain even though they were capable of experiencing pain associated with medical procedures. In this situation, the injury was a "ticket home." It provided escape from an even more threatening situation, death on the battlefield. Wall (1979) suggests that the relative absence of pain in this situation occurred because the soldiers' attention focused on that escape.

The reduction of clinical pain as a function of situational cues is evident in placebo effects. A placebo is any therapy or component of therapy that is deliberately used for its nonspecific psychological or psychophysiological effect or for its presumed specific effect but is without specific, direct activity on the condition being treated. The placebo effect is the change in some condition (e.g., pain) produced by a placebo (Shapiro & Shapiro, 1984). Beecher (1972) has shown that approximately 35% of patients with pathological pain obtain relief from placebo medications. The placebo effect may depend on environmental cues that have been associated with changes in the symptoms. The cue may be a pill that in the past has been associated with pain relief. The cue may be the reassurance of a health provider. The occurrence and strength of a placebo effect are related to a client's perception of the provider as likable, attractive, caring, and competent (Shapiro & Shapiro, 1984). Insofar as these qualities have been associated with successful treatment, the presence and knowledgeable action of the health provider may result in pain reduction. Placebo effects have been demonstrated in many interventions used to relieve pain. This includes the use of opiates, audio analgesia, hypnosis, biofeedback, and imagery (Turk, Meichenbaum, & Genest, 1983).

Placebo effects may be negative as well as positive. Beecher (1959) has reported that placebos can elicit toxic and painful effects such as headaches, nausea, rashes, heart palpitations, abdominal cramps, constipation, and diarrhea. Placebos may even reverse the usual physiological effects of drugs. Wolf (1950) has shown that emetic (i.e., vomiting- or nausea-producing) drugs can reduce vomiting and nausea if the person believes the drug is effective for that purpose.

Placebo effects vary in their persistence. Klopfer (1957) reported a case history of a man dying of lymphoma. He had multiple tumors, was anemic, and his chest was filled with fluid. He was given a month to live. He begged for an experimental drug, Krebiozen, which was a widely touted cure for cancer. Within two days of his first injection, the tumors were half their original size and the fluid in his chest was gone. He was discharged in ten days and continued in good health for two months. He then read conflicting reports about the efficacy of the drug and relapsed to his original state. His physicians told him to ignore the reports and that his relapse was due to the deterioration of the drug. They offered him a "new double strength dose," which was actually water. There was a dramatic improvement until the client read an American Medical Association report that indicated the drug was worthless. His health quickly declined and he was dead in two days.

The exact mechanisms that mediate the placebo effects and, more generally, the effects of environmental cues on pain are not known. Psychologically, those cues that enhance expectations of relief, predictability, and control seem to reduce pain while those that reduce predictability and control and that focus attention on pain seem to enhance pain. These expectations, beliefs, and evaluations could potentially influence neural activity, which mediates pain in several ways. These cognitive processes may alter visceral activity (e.g., sympathetic nervous system activation) or muscle tension and thus affect the pattern of sensory input to the gate. Information resulting from these cognitive processes may also influence the status of the gate via the tracts that descend from the cortex to the gating mechanisms in the spinal cord. These effects could also be mediated by endorphins and enkephalins (Levine et al., 1978).

Situational or environmental cues, then, can have a powerful effect on pain. The power of cues to alter pain is the result of learning that these cues predict certain outcomes. Cues associated with a change in pain take on the power to actually effect that change. From the systems frame of reference, pain needs to be understood at many levels that reciprocally influence each other. In this case, the body not only affects the mind, but the mind also affects the body.

Personality Variables

Personality refers to a cross-situational and temporal stability in how an individual interprets and responds to the environment. Personality variables account for consistency in persons' actions in contrast to the situational influences just discussed. Many studies have attempted to associate personality characteristics with reactions to pain. One such characteristic is persons' coping style. Augmenters are persons who magnify sensory input, whereas reducers minimize stimulation. Augmenters tolerate less pain than reducers (Petrie, 1967); this difference may even influence neural firing in response to noxious stimulation (Mushin & Levy, 1974).

Differential responsiveness to pain is also found between persons described as sensitizers and repressors. Sensitizers react to stimulation by actively trying to cope with it. Repressors play down the importance of stimulation by denying or avoiding it. Repressors have more tolerance for pain than sensitizers when the pain initially occurs. As pain continues, sensitizers become more tolerant (Davidson & Bobey, 1970). Similarly, repressors show less anxiety than sensitizers a few days before surgery, but after surgery show more anxiety (DeLong, 1970). Denial works for a period of time, but with continued pain, it is a less effective strategy than active coping.

A number of other personality dimensions (e.g., field dependence-independence, extraversion-introversion, hysteria, and hypochondriasis) have been studied in relation to pain (see Weissenberg, 1977, for a review). While many of these personality variables have been shown to be related to the pain experience, most of the experimental and clinical data supporting the pain modulating effect of these personality variables are based on group comparisons and have not been consistently replicated across studies. Generalizing these data to specific individuals must be done with caution.

The central idea is that noxious stimuli do not impinge on an empty organism, but rather the organism actively interprets and responds to the stimuli on the basis of past experience. The response of a person to pain-producing stimuli is influenced by the characteristics of the person.

Mood States

The mood of the individual also plays a role in the perception of and reaction to pain. Anxiety has been found to be directly related to pain. Anxiety-prone individuals are more sensitive to experimentally induced pain in terms of both behavioral and physiological measures. Experimentally elicited anxiety enhances the perceived intensity of a noxious stimuli while a reduction in anxiety reduces the perceived intensity of a noxious stimulus (Sternbach, 1968).

The relationship between anxiety and pain is also seen in clinical pain. Persons who are highly anxious complain more frequently and intensely about pain than less anxious persons (Sternbach, 1974). Many interventions used to reduce pain may be effective in part because they provide the individual with a feeling of control or predictability. These interventions provide the client with information and teach coping skills such as relaxation or cognitive strategies (see Chapters 11 and 12) and are generally successful in increasing pain tolerance (Turk, 1982). Probably the best known example of this type of intervention is prepared childbirth. In this program, the mother is given information about the childbirth process and is taught breathing exercises and relaxation skills. The prepared childbirth program increases pain tolerance and reduces the use of analgesics and anesthetics (Genest, 1981). In a similar manner, depression is often correlated with clinical pain, especially when that pain is chronic (Sternbach, 1968). The use of antidepressant medication has also been reported to result in relief from pain (Sternbach, 1974).

The manner in which anxiety and depression influence pain perception is unknown. It may be that pain is worse when a person feels the pain is uncontrollable and poses a serious threat (anxiety) or when the pain is associated with a loss of normal roles and helplessness (depression). Experientially, pain and negative affective states may be elicited by similar types of stimuli. Pain is often associated with injury and punishment. Injury is a threat to well-being and thus elicits anxiety. Punishment often involves a loss of love and access to desired activities and is thus associated with depression. When one member of a class of responses (e.g., pain, anxiety, and depression) is elicited by some event, other members of that class may also be experienced (Fordyce, 1976; Leventhal & Nerenz, 1983). The physiological correlates of anxiety and depression, including increases in muscle tension, sympathetic arousal, and changes in brain neurotransmitters, may alter the neural mechanisms mediating the pain experience.

PAIN BEHAVIOR

Pain behavior refers to overt responses made by persons experiencing pain. There are several classes of pain behavior. It may involve a reflexive movement like withdrawing one's hand from a hot radiator. Pain behavior also entails verbalizations or complaints that indicate the presence of pain. These range from nonspecific moans and groans to elaborate descriptions of the location and quality of the pain. Pain is also expressed by the alteration of body posture or movement (e.g., limping after spraining an ankle or flexing the torso to one side to reduce back pain). Pain is also apparent in reduced role functioning. Activity level may be reduced (e.g., no heavy lifting during a backache), and normal activities (e.g., not going to work) and modes of social-sexual relating ("Not tonight dear, I have a headache") may be avoided. Pain can also be inferred from illness behaviors like taking aspirin or visiting a health provider (Turk et al., 1983).

The various classes of pain behavior are not necessarily correlated. A person may groan and complain a lot but still carry out normal vocational and social roles. It is not uncommon, in cases of chronic pain, to see inconsistencies in pain behavior. For example, a person may indicate that pain necessitates eating in bed rather than at the kitchen table yet be able to sit through a double feature movie without complaint.

The expression of pain varies from person to person and from situation to situation. It is influenced by past learning, environmental cues and consequences, and the extent and nature of the tissue damage. The expression of pain is subject to modeling and reinforcement influences. Developmentally, an infant's response to pain is diffuse and nonspecific. It involves crying and vigorous, gross body movement. Over time, the expression of pain becomes more specific and refined (Craig, 1980). Among the first words learned are those used to express pain. The child has many opportunities to observe the expression of pain by parents, peers, and siblings. These observations provide the child with modes of expressing pain and with information about which modes are acceptable (approved and reinforced) and unacceptable (disapproved and punished). Thus, by observing an older sibling, a child may learn that loud screaming quickly results in parental attention. The child is then likely to use that mode of expression when hurt. Through observation, the child may also learn that appropriate ways of expressing pain vary depending on the situation. Loud screaming may result in derision from peers in contrast to its usefulness in the home setting. Based on modeling, certain modes of expressing pain are facilitated and others are inhibited (Craig, 1978). These modeling influences may lead to pain expression styles ranging from stoic to histrionic.

Modeling influences are apparent in clinical pain. Apley (1975), for example, found that children who complained of recurrent abdominal pain were more likely to have parents or siblings who complained of similar problems. Modeling influences may also suppress pain complaints. Russian Cossack soldiers and Roman legionnaires were reported to place their arms in a fire without complaint to demonstrate their bravery and comradeship.

Pain behavior is also shaped by its immediate consequences. Pain behavior has a strong effect on others. It has a "pull" for empathic and care-taking responses. If you saw a four-year-old child fall off a swing and begin crying, you would likely try to comfort the child. Pain complaints by professional football players may lead to derision from opponents. These consequences shape the behavior that is used to express pain in various situations. Fordyce (1978) provides a detailed discussion of social reinforcers for pain behavior.

The frequency of pain behavior is also influenced by its effectiveness in reducing pain. Taking aspirin for a headache is common because it leads to quick relief. Behaviors that make pain worse, like walking on a sprained ankle, are suppressed because the pain acts as an immediate, intense punishment for the behavior.

Pain behavior is of course influenced by the intensity, quality, and duration of the pain. The expressions and actions made by a person who has had a splitting headache for three days are different from those made by a person who has just begun to notice a mild headache. Your reaction to having your finger mashed in a car door is different from your reaction to being pinched by a friend.

Pain behavior is the person's best possible solution to a noxious stimulus given the situation and available resources. It has as its goal the reduction or alleviation of pain. Some behaviors are more effective than others in this regard. In some cases, as we will see with chronic pain, the behaviors may make pain worse.

Pain behavior is not only a reaction to the experience of pain but also can serve as a means to modify it. The relationship is reciprocal. Going to a health provider to get a broken bone set leads to a reduction in pain. Taking high doses of analgesics and sedatives and limiting exercise, while initially adaptive in promoting healing, may also alter the pattern of sensory input to the gate and sustain pain after the tissue is healed (Fordyce, 1976; Turk et al., 1983).

A SYSTEMS CONCEPTUALIZATION OF PAIN

As described in Chapter 5, the systems paradigm views persons as active agents. Persons are sensitive to changes in the external environment and the body. Via physiological and behavioral self-regulation, persons attempt to adapt to change. Adaptation occurs at many interrelated levels, from biochemical to social. Pain is one of these adaptational processes. A person does not "have" pain. Rather, pain describes a set of responses made by the person physiologically, psychologically, and behaviorally to deal with tissue damage and noxious stimuli.

The level at which pain is observed and analyzed is arbitrary. Confining these observations and analyses to one level (as the specificity theory does in its focus on tissue damage) limits the understanding of pain and the scope and power of diagnostic and treatment procedures to alleviate it. Pain involves the integrated process made up of the interaction of biochemical (endorphins), physiological (spinal gating mechanisms), psychological (personality and mood), behavioral (pain behaviors), and social-environmental (situational influences and consequences) variables.

Observations about pain made at one level are variably related to observations made at another level for two reasons. First, there are many factors that make up pain. What is observed at any one level is influenced by processes at subordinate and supraordinate levels. For example, pain behavior is influenced by both the intensity and duration of the noxious stimulus (subordinate) and by the consequences of that behavior (superordinate). Second, pain is a process. There are constant changes in responses observed at different levels and in the relationship between those responses over time.

Imagine a forty-year-old male who prides himself on "never being sick." One Saturday while working in the yard, he feels a pain in his back when lifting a tree limb. He figures it is nothing and decides to "work out" the pain with exercise. He is not worried about the pain and goes about his daily routine, experiencing occasional pain. On waking Sunday morning, he experiences an intense, shooting pain when he tries to get out of bed. It is difficult to move much less put on his socks and shoes. He is now concerned and focuses on the pain. His wife suggests aspirin and a heating pad. Following those suggestions, he gets some relief. What happens at one level changes over time. Subjectively, the man experiences no pain, minor pain, severe pain, and then less pain. These changes are affected by and affect other levels. His lifting caused the initial damage, which was then exacerbated by his continued exercise. His anxiety increased with the pain and interference with his normal routine, but abated as rest and aspirin reduced the pain.

CLINICAL PAIN

Acute Pain

Clinical pain can be characterized as acute or chronic. Acute pain has a sudden onset and is tied directly to a noxious stimulus or tissue damage. Most pain we experience is acute. The pain is quickly and reflexively elicited by the noxious stimulus. Acute pain serves the important adaptive function of protecting a person from harm and motivating corrective behavior. The treatment of acute pain consists of an attempt to locate the cause for pain. If a person hobbles into a physician's office and describes a shooting pain in his knee, the physician would take x-rays and palpate the knee to identify the tissue damage causing the pain. One of two types of treatment is then initiated, definitive or symptomatic. Definitive treatment is directed at the removal or repair of the source of pain. Setting a broken bone or repairing a torn ligament are examples of definitive treatments. Definitive treatment depends on a health provider's ability to identify the underlying cause of pain and on the availability of a means to alter it. If the cause cannot be identified or if no effective treatment is available, symptomatic treatment is used. Symptomatic treatment is directed at reducing the client's experience of pain without altering its cause. Often, a combination of definitive and symptomatic strategies is used. Analgesic medication is a common symptomatic treatment of pain. In more extreme cases, it is possible to try to block neural transmission of pain by cutting pain pathways or by using electrical stimulation to alter the pattern of neural firing.

The treatment of acute pain using the specificity theory (biomedical paradigm) and the medical model of helping is adequate and effective in treating acute pain. However, the importance of a systems paradigm of pain and a compensatory model of helping is still evident. In acute pain, there is still variability in the manner in which a client describes the pain depending on the context in which it occurs, client mood and characteristics, and the outcomes for the pain behavior. Skilled clinical diagnosis and management of acute pain require the clinician to recognize the impact of these variables. Definitive and symptomatic treatment of acute pain require the active cooperation of the client. This may entail taking medication, engaging in rehabilitative tasks, or altering normal activities. The compensatory model provides the client with shared responsibility for treatment and consequently fosters cooperation and adherence to treatment recommendations.

Chronic Pain

Chronic pain is the continuation of pain despite treatment and personal coping efforts by the client. It usually begins as an acute episode. The continuation of pain for a long period has no protective or adaptive role, and frequently leads to serious physical, social, and emotional deterioration. By definition, definitive and symptomatic forms of treatment are ineffective in providing relief. Chronic pain may be associated with a stable or progressive but persistent type of tissue damage such as arthritis or cancer, or it may occur in the relative absence of any identifiable biological cause, such as phantom limb pain. In either case, clinical treatment is unsuccessful because the source of pain cannot be identified, is resistant to treatment, or both.

The experiences of acute and chronic pain are quite different. In acute pain, if it begins slowly, there may be an initial, barely perceptible awareness that something is wrong, which is then ignored. As the sensations become more intense and are experienced as painful, they become the focus of attention. This results in anxiety and in a search for a reason for the pain. If the pain persists or increases, anxiety also increases, and relief is sought via self- or professional care. Usually, the pain is thought to be of finite duration and intensity and amenable to treatment.

In chronic pain, the sufferer has difficulty finding a reason for the pain. He may "understand" its cause as explained by the health provider, but the pain makes no sense as a warning signal because it does not lead to successful avoidance, escape, or treatment. The person does not "deserve" the pain. In acute pain, the pain is due to a sprained ankle or cut finger for which the person is responsible. But in chronic pain, the suffering has a less specific source and purpose. It seems endless and may increase over time.

This lack of understanding, predictability, and control moves the person from initial anxiety to depression and anger (Sternbach, 1974). Pain becomes the primary focus of attention. Rest is difficult. The person is irritable with family and friends. The pain interferes with normal social, vocational, and recreational activities. The person becomes even more preoccupied with the pain and is often upset by the health professionals' inability to relieve the pain. The client will move from one provider to another to find relief. The person is often subjected to multiple surgeries, and may take heavy doses of tranquilizers, analgesics, muscle relaxants, and antidepressants. None of these interventions is successful for long. Searching for meaning, control, and effective treatment becomes more frantic. The pain, time spent in treatment, loss of normal roles, and alienation of others exhaust the person emotionally, physically, and financially.

Psychogenic Pain

Chronic pain for which health providers cannot find adequate biological cause is often called "psychogenic." There is a discrepancy between pain behavior and observable tissue damage to explain that behavior. While the term is often used descriptively, it also has explanatory implications. It suggests that if no adequate physical cause can be found to account for pain, it then has a psychological cause, usually some type of personality disturbance (Fordyce, 1976). It is a diagnosis (or explanation) made by exclusion. It reflects the dualism inherent in the biomedical paradigm.

The "psychogenic" explanation of pain has questionable validity. While personality problems are associated with chronic pain, it is not clear whether pain is the cause or result of personality problems. It is often *not* possible to differentiate persons who experience chronic pain with and without observable physical cause of the basis of personality tests (Sternbach, 1974). The application of the term "psychogenic" does not lead to effective treatment. In fact, it may interfere with treatment. The notion that the pain is psychologically caused suggests it is not real or as legitimate as pain that is organically caused. This leads to a destructive relationship between the client and the provider. The notion also suggests that treatment consists of altering the client's personality. This mode of conceptualizing and changing pain behavior does not lead to effective treatment (Fordyce, 1976). Psychogenic pain is explained on the basis of personality variables; this unidimensional view is as limiting as the sole focus on organic variables.

Operant and Respondent Pain

An alternate conceptualization of pain has been suggested by Fordyce (1976). He suggests the use of two terms, respondent and operant, to refer to pain. Respondent refers to pain experience and behavior that are elicited by an antecedent noxious stimulus. Respondent pain is comparable to acute pain. Operant pain refers to pain experience and behavior that are not associated with a recent, sufficient, antecedent noxious stimulus, but rather is maintained by the consequences of experience and behavior. There are, of course, mixtures of operant and respondent pain.

How does operant pain develop? Several conditions contribute to its development. Operant pain often begins as an acute, respondent episode. A broad set of behaviors are used to express that acute pain. The person engages in illness behaviors like reducing exercise, staying in bed, and not going to work. The person may display anxiety and concern and persistently communicate his pain to others. If there is sufficient opportunity for these behaviors to be powerfully reinforced and if there are few potent reinforcers for well behavior (e.g., exercising, getting out of bed, and going to work), operant pain may develop.

This process takes place slowly over time. Potent reinforcement for pain behavior is more likely if the acute or respondent pain is severe and of long duration. The person who is in severe pain will obtain more potent attention and assistance from others, will be excused from more duties, and will receive compensation for the disabling condition. The person is more likely to be not only exempted but actively discouraged (nonreinforcement) from engaging in well behavior as a part of the treatment. The longer these conditions are in effect, the more likely they are to have a lasting effect.

Initially, then, pain behavior is not only elicited by antecedent noxious stimuli but also strongly reinforced. After the noxious stimulus or tissue damage diminishes, the pain behavior persists because of potent, frequent reinforcement. This process is shown in Figure 9-4.

Not all individuals who experience severe, persistent respondent pain develop operant pain. The usual consequences for the illness and pain behaviors (e.g., staying in bed, avoiding work, and being waited on) may not be reinforcing, and the external and intrinsic reinforcers for well behavior (e.g., living with their pain) may remain strong (Sternbach, 1974).

The development of operant pain is also associated with a person's

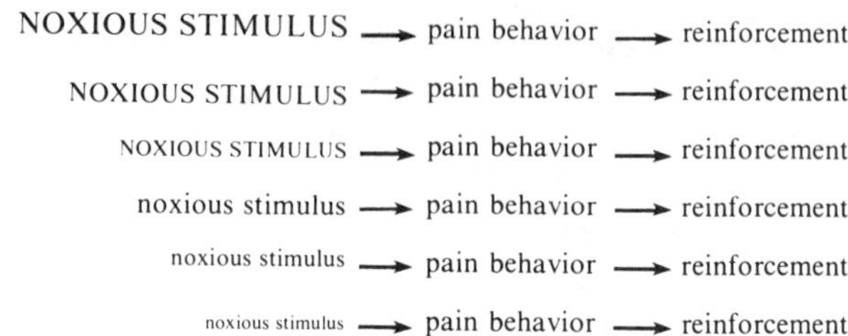

FIGURE 9-4 The Sequential Development of Operant Pain

learning history in dealing with pain. As suggested in the section on pain behavior, tolerance and expression of pain are influenced by observation and reinforcement during socialization. Those persons whose learning history fosters a low tolerance for pain and persistent, vociferous expression of pain are more likely to develop an operant pain syndrome. Persons displaying operant pain report that their parents' response to their pain, as children, was one of two extremes. Either a great deal of concern and support was elicited when illness or pain occurred, or both parents were reluctant to respond and did so only when the pain was severe. In both cases, parental nurturing and attention were pain contingent. Pain syndromes are also more likely in those individuals whose parents displayed operant pain, suggesting that modeling may also have an influence (Apley, 1975).

Various reinforcers are contingent on pain behavior. Many come in the form of social attention. Pain has a strong "pull" for caring and nurturing from family, friends, and health care providers. Fordyce (1976) reports the following illustrative case example of a forty-year-old male who was incapacitated by pain for twenty years. His wife worked to augment his disability income. After work she would return home to her husband, who spent much of the day in bed watching TV. She would prepare and bring dinner to the bedroom, where she would eat on a TV tray. She would express much concern about his pain at this and other times. On special occasions, he would try to get out of bed and eat at the kitchen table. She did not give him special attention on these occasions, but rather would wonder whether it was wise and chide him for taking risks. Her attention and nurturing were contingent on his pain behavior (staying in bed). He expressed appreciation and reported reduced pain when she was attentive and nurturing, thus reinforcing her just as she was reinforcing him. A host of idiosyncratic social reinforcers such as receiving back rubs and being excused from household chores were also operating. The case history also suggests that the amount and duration of monetary compensation are directly contingent on pain behavior.

In addition to the social attention from health providers, other pain-contingent reinforcers are available as a part of definitive and symptomatic treatment of pain. Medications for pain, especially when given PRN (as needed), may serve as a potent reinforcer. These medications are likely to provide some relief from pain and a sense of well-being (reduced anxiety). Some of these medications (e.g., opiates and minor tranquilizers) may also have positive (euphoric or pleasant) side effects. These consequences reinforce complaining about pain and taking medication. It is not uncommon for persons in chronic pain to take five or six analgesic, sedative-hypnotic, or other psychotropic medications simultaneously. The dosage is often high because of physiological tolerance to the drugs. It is common for these clients to use more than one physician as a source of medication. Because the client is persistent and demanding and because definitive treatment is unsuccessful, the physician's prescription of medication is reinforced by fewer demands and complaints and by avoidance of what could be seen as a treatment failure.

A second major source of reinforcement in the treatment of pain is reduced activity and prescribed rest. This is reinforcing because it reduces pain and legitimizes the avoidance of unpleasant activities and roles. For the person who hates work, dislikes socializing, and despises household chores, rest and inactivity provide a means to escape those activities.

The use of analgesic and other medications and the prescription of rest are part of effective definitive and symptomatic treatment for acute or respondent pain. At the same time, they may foster the development and maintenance of operant pain. Thus, the use of legitimate and effective modes of treatment may be iatrogenic (cause problems). This serves to emphasize the importance of a systems paradigm in treating acute pain. Actions that lead to a reduction in an aversive state of affairs (e.g., pain or unpleasant activities) are particularly resistant to extinction. Once developed, it is difficult to get rid of pain behaviors, especially if they are intermittently reinforced.

Operant pain has a broad negative impact on the person. The person's attention and activities are increasingly focused on pain. There are both anger and depression in response to the lack of effective treatment and to the inability to carry out normal roles and activities. There is an increased sensitivity to one's body to find meaning or to understand what is happening; this results in hypochondriacal concerns that further frustrate and confuse health providers. The impact and consequences of chronic pain and its treatment result in progressive social, emotional, and economic deterioration.

While Fordyce's (1976) analysis of operant pain is very useful, you might be thinking that these people are not "really" in pain and that what is being reinforced and maintained are pain behaviors, not the actual pain. Recall, however, that pain behavior, anxiety, depression, and attention to pain influence physiological processes. It is possible that those neurophysiological mechanisms that mediate acute or respondent pain are also activated in operant pain. There are several inputs to the gate that effect the transmission of pain information to the brain. These inputs are influenced by behavioral, situational, personality, and emotional variables. The anxiety, depression, attention to pain, and expectation that pain will continue and increase may open the gate via the input from the brain cortex. The use of analgesic and other medication may alter the pattern of input to the gate or other nervous system activity (e.g., reduction in endorphins and enkephalins in the limbic system) and activate those neural structures that mediate pain. The lack of activity and exercise may likewise alter normal sensory input to the gate.

Operant pain is not simply in the person's head (psychogenic), or in the person's transaction with the environment (operant), but involves an ongoing, mutual interaction of pain-related processes at various organizational levels. It is not different from acute pain in that the whole system is involved. Operant pain, compared to other types of pain, is less strongly associated with tissue damage and is more strongly influenced by situational, psychosocial, behavioral, and environmental facets of the system.

SUMMARY

In this chapter we have developed an integrated, multidimensional model of pain as an alternative to the traditional biomedical paradigm that confines pain to a unitary cause (organic or psychogenic). The multidimensional or systems paradigm suggests that pain, as one subset of the process of adaptation, consists of a set of neurophysiological, psychological, behavioral, and environmental processes that reciprocally influence each other. This conceptualization suggests that the diagnosis and treatment of pain can and often should occur at levels in addition to the physiological level. In treating pain, the active collaboration and cooperation of the client and the health professional are needed. This compensatory model of helping is useful in addressing acute or respondent, chronic, and operant pain.

REFERENCES

Akil, H. (1982). On the role of endorphins in pain modulation. In E. L. Beckman (Ed.), *The neural basis of behavior*, 71–89. New York: SP Medical & Scientific Books.

Apley, J. (1975). *The child with abdominal pains*. Oxford: Blackwell.

Arthritis Foundation. (1976). *Arthritis: The basic facts*. Atlanta: Author.

Beecher, H. K. (1959). *Measurement of subjective responses: Quantitative effect on drugs*. New York: Oxford Press.

Beecher, H. K. (1972). The placebo effect as a nonspecific force surrounding disease and the treatment of disease. In R. Janzen, W. D. Keidel, A. Herz, L. Steichele, J. P. Payne,

& R. A. Burt (Eds.), *Pain: Basic principles, pharmacology, therapy*, 296–314. Stuttgart, West Germany: Georg Thieme.

Bresler, D. E. (1979). *Free yourself from pain*. New York: Simon & Schuster.

Cannon, J. T., Liebeskind, J. C., & Frank, H. (1978). Neural and neurochemical mechanisms of pain inhibition. In R. A. Sternbach (Ed.), *The psychology of pain*, 27–48. New York: Raven Press.

Casey, K. L. (1979). Supra-spinal mechanisms in pain. In H. W. Kasterlitz & L. Y. Terenius (Eds.), *Pain and society*, 63–86. Deerfield Beach, FL: Verlag Chemie.

Clark, M., Gosnell, M., & Shapiro, D. (1977, April 25). The new war on pain. *Newsweek*, pp. 48–58.

Craig, K. D. (1978). Social modeling influences on pain. In R. A. Sternbach (Ed.), *The psychology of pain*, 73–110. New York: Raven Press.

Craig, K. D. (1980). Ontogenetic and cultural influences on the expression of pain in man. In S. Bernhard (Ed.), *Pain and culture*, 143–167. Deerfield Beach, FL: Basil.

Craig, K. D., & Weiss, S. N. (1972). Verbal reports of pain without noxious stimulation. *Perceptual Motor Skills, 34*, 943–948.

Davidson, P. O., & Bobey, M. J. (1970). Repressor sensitizer differences on repeated exposure to pain. *Perceptual Motor Skills, 31*, 711–714.

De Long, R. D. (1970). *Individual differences in patterns of anxiety, arousal, stress-relevant information and recovery from surgery*. Unpublished doctoral dissertation, University of California, at Los Angeles.

Fordyce, W. E. (1976). *Behavioral methods for chronic pain and illness*. St. Louis: C. V. Mosby.

Fordyce, W. E. (1978). Learning processes in pain. In R. A. Sternbach (Ed.) *The psychology of pain*. New York: Raven Press.

Genest, M. (1981). Preparation for childbirth: A selected review of evidence for efficiency. *Journal of Obstetric, Gynecologic and Neonatal Nursing, 10*, 82–85.

Kanfer, F. H., & Goldfoot, D. A. (1966). Self control and tolerance of noxious stimulation. *Psychological Reports, 18*, 79–85.

Klopfer, B. (1957). Psychological variables in human cancer. *Journal of Projective Techniques, 31*, 331–340.

Koenig, P. (1973, April). The placebo effect in patent medicine. *Psychology Today, 60*, 37–40.

Leventhal, H., & Nerenz, D. R. (1983). A model for stress research with some implications for the control of stress disorders. In D. Meichenbaum & M. E. Jaremko (Eds.), *Stress reduction and prevention*, 102–139. New York: Plenum.

Levine, J. D., Gordon, N. C., & Field, H. L. (1978, September 23). The mechanism of placebo analgesia. *Lancet*, 654–657.

Melzack, R., (1973). *The puzzle of pain*. New York: Basic Books.

Melzack, R., & Casey, K. L. (1968). Sensory, motivational and central control determinants of pain: A new conceptual model. In D. Kenshalo (Ed.), *The skin senses*, 423–443. Springfield, IL: Charles C. Thomas.

Melzack, R., & Wall, P. D. (1982). *The challenge of pain*. New York: Basic Books.

Mushin, J., & Levy, R. (1974). Average evoked response in patients with psychogenic pain. *Psychological Medicine, 4*, 19–27.

Paulley, J. W., & Haskell, D. J. (1975). Treatment of migraine without drugs. *Journal of Psychosomatic Research, 19*, 367–374.

Petrie, A. (1967). *Individuality in pain and suffering*. Chicago: University of Chicago Press.

Ray, O. (1978). *Drugs, society and human behavior*. St. Louis: C. V. Mosby.

Reynolds, D. V. (1969). Surgery in the rat during electrical analgesia induced by focal brain stimulation. *Science, 164*, 444–445.

Shapiro, A. K., & Shapiro, E. (1984). Patient-provider relationships and the placebo effect. In J. D. Matarazzo, S. M. Weiss, J. A. Herd, N. E. Miller, & S. M. Weiss (Eds.), *Behavioral health: A handbook of health enhancement and disease prevention*, 371–383. New York: John Wiley & Sons.

Snyder, S. H. (1977). Opiate receptors and internal opiates. *Scientific American, 236*, 44–56.

Sternbach, R. A. (1968). *Pain: A psychophysiological analysis*. New York: Academic Press.

Sternbach, R. A. (1974). *Pain patients: Traits and treatments*. New York: Academic Press.

Turk, D. C. (1982). Cognitive-learning approaches in health care. In D. M. Doleys, R. L. Meredity, & A. R. Ciminero (Eds.), *Behavioral medicine: Assessment and treatment*, 387–414. New York: Plenum.

Turk, D. C., Meichenbaum, D., & Genest, M. (1983). *Pain and behavioral medicine: A cognitive-behavioral perspective*. New York: Guilford Press.

Wall, P. D. (1979). On the relation of injury to pain. *Pain, 6*, 253–264.

Weissenberg, M. (1977). Pain and pain control. *Psychological Bulletin, 84*, 1008–1044.

Wolf, S. (1950). Effects of suggestion and conditioning on the action of chemical agents in human subjects: The pharmacology of placebos. *Journal of Clinical Investigation, 29*, 100–109.

10

Basic Behavioral Interventions: Operant, Respondent, and Observational Learning

In Chapters 10 through 13, basic behavior change principles relevant to health education, disease prevention, and clinical treatment and rehabilitation will be detailed. The theory, clinical application, and relevance of several methods are considered: contingency management, respondent conditioning, observational learning, self-control, cognitive therapy, biofeedback, and relaxation. Specific strategies used to implement these methods are provided. Examples of preventative and clinical applications to specific health problems are described.

INTRODUCTION

The systems model emphasized in the preceding chapters asserts that persons are not self-contained organisms. They are in constant interaction with their larger bioecological environment. Such transactions are important determinants of health and illness and are highly relevant to preventative and clinical medicine. Person-environment interactions involve psychological and behavioral processes: attention, perception, affect, memory, learning, thinking, and motor actions.

Traditional clinical medicine alters clients' health status primarily by manipulating elements within the organism (e.g., by surgery and drugs). These interventions are powerful and effective but limited in focus. The beneficial effects of such biological interventions can be complemented and amplified by interventions that focus on psychological and behavioral processes. Preventative medicine and epidemiology have long recognized the importance of behavioral and environmental factors in understanding health and altering health actions. However, because health providers in these fields have been trained from a biological perspective, there is a need for more emphasis and a clearer involvement of psychological and behavioral processes in their work.

In this and the two subsequent chapters, we will examine intervention principles whose application has been shown to alter psychological and behavioral processes relevant to health and illness effectively. The application of such principles in clinical and preventative health settings is commonly called behavioral health and medicine (Matarazzo, 1980; Pomerleau & Brady, 1979; Schwartz & Weiss, 1977).

In this chapter, we will review behavior change principles based on classic modes of learning: operant and respondent conditioning and observational learning. Using these principles, behavior change strategies relevant to health and illness along with examples of their application will be described in detail. The behavior change strategies described in this and the following two chapters will serve as the basis for a description of the interventions applied to specific health and illness problems in Chapters 13 through 16.

OPERANT CONDITIONING

The principles of operant conditioning describe the relationship between behavior and consequent environmental events that influence the occurrence of that behavior. More specifically, operant theory states that the performance of behavior is influenced by the consequences it produces. We work for a salary, study to get good grades, and interact with people who are pleasant. We desist from actions that lead to pain or that have no payoff. This may sound very simplistic, but much of our behavior is influenced by its consequences. As discussed in Chapters 2 and 3, health-promoting and health-impairing behaviors, and illness-related decisions and actions are strongly influenced by their consequences. Thus operant principles are relevant to the direct effects of behavior on health and illness. Coping responses to stress are also operants. In Chapter 4, we learned that the availability of effective coping responses in an individual's repertoire influences the impact of stress on health status, and that the short- and long-term consequences of coping responses in reducing or exacerbating stress influence the kinds of responses made to stress. Thus, operant principles are relevant to understanding both the direct and indirect effects of the environment and behavior on health and illness.

Several types of contingent relationships between behavior and consequences are possible. The major operant principles refer to these relationships: reinforcement, punishment, and extinction.

Reinforcement

Reinforcement refers to an increase in the frequency of a behavior when it is contingently followed by a "desirable" event. Any event that is contingent on a behavior and that increases the frequency of that behavior is defined as a reinforcer. A reinforcer may be positive or negative. Positive reinforcers are events that are presented after a response occurs that increase the frequency of that response. Negative reinforcers are events that are removed after a response occurs that increase the frequency of that response.

Positive reinforcement, then, refers to an increase in the frequency of a response that is followed by a favorable event or positive reinforcer (Kazdin, 1984). In everyday life, positive reinforcers are called rewards. There are two categories of positive reinforcers: primary and secondary. Primary reinforcers are events that are innately reinforcing, such as food, water, and sex. Most reinforcers that control behavior are events that acquire their reinforcement value through learning; such secondary reinforcers are money, praise, and grades. When identifying reinforcers, two considerations are important. First, an event may serve as a reinforcer for one person but not another. Second, an event may be a reinforcer for a given person in one situation but not in another.

There is no a priori guarantee that an event will serve as a reinforcer. Status as a reinforcer must be established empirically. Only when an event is actually made contingent on a behavior and increases the frequency of the behavior can the event said to be reinforcing. The proof is in the pudding. Access to activities can also serve as a positive reinforcer. This is called the Premack principle (Premack, 1965): Of any pair of responses in which a person engages, the more frequent one will serve as a reinforcer for the less frequent one. Parents often use the Premack principle on their children: "No TV until your homework is finished," or "No dessert until you clean your plate."

Negative reinforcement refers to an increase in the frequency of a response by the removal of an aversive event after the response is performed. There are many common examples of negative reinforcement. Taking an aspirin when experiencing a headache is negatively reinforced by a reduction in headache pain. Turning up the thermostat when feeling cold is negatively reinforced by a reduction in discomfort. Like positive reinforcement, negative reinforcement results in an *increase* in the frequency of a behavior; the operations effecting the increase are simply different (see Figure 10-1).

Punishment

Punishment refers to the presentation of an aversive event or the removal of a positive event contingent on some response that results in a decrease in the frequency of that response. Note that there are two types of punishment (see Figure 10-1). In the type referred to as punishment, an aversive event is presented after the response is performed. For example, attempting to walk on a sprained ankle results in pain and thus discourages such attempts. Receiving failing grades in anatomy and physiology discourages enrollment in biology courses.

The second type of punishment, response cost, entails the removal of a positive reinforcer after a response is performed. Paying a traffic ticket for illegal parking is an effective response cost if it reduces illegal parking in the future. Being grounded for misbehavior is another common example of a response cost, in this case involving the loss of activity reinforcers.

Punishment does not necessarily entail pain or physical force. It is defined empirically by its effect on behavior. Only if the frequency of a behavior is reduced by the contingent application or removal of some event can punishment be said to occur. Punishment suppresses behavior; it only teaches a person what *not* to do.

Extinction

Extinction refers to the reduction in the frequency of a behavior when it is no longer reinforced. Unlike punishment, which also leads to a reduction in response frequency, extinction provides no consequence for a response; no event is taken away or presented. You stop putting money in vending machines if they do not work.

FIGURE 10-1 Principles of Operant Conditioning: Reinforcement and Punishment. (From *Behavior Modification in Applied Settings*, 3rd edition (p. 35) by A. E. Kazdin, 1984, Homewood, IL: The Dorsey Press. Copyright 1984 by The Dorsey Press. Reprinted by permission.)

Type of Event Used

Operation performed after a response		Positive	Aversive
	Present	Positive Reinforcement	Punishment
	Remove	Punishment (Response Cost)	Negative Reinforcement

Antecedent Stimulus Control

Thus far, we have focused on the relationship between behavior and consequent stimulus events. Stimulus control refers to the influence of antecedent events on behavior, because they provide information about the consequences that are likely to follow a specific behavior. Antecedent stimuli that indicate that a reinforcer or punisher will follow a response are called discriminative stimuli. For example, opening a door for someone (behavior) may result in a "thank you" (positive reinforcer). But we do not stand there and repeatedly open the door when no one is present. We only do so when someone is close by (discriminative stimulus), because that presents the occasion for reinforcement. Discriminative stimuli also operate in predicting punishment. Traffic fines for speeding may not lead to a reduction in speeding at all times, but only when police are sighted or on certain stretches of road. We learn to respond in a different manner depending on antecedent stimuli as a result of differential reinforcement: A response is reinforced (or punished) in the presence of one stimulus but not another.

The notion of antecedent stimulus control is very important. Most behaviors are situation specific. In some cases, we may want to enhance stimulus discrimination (i.e., to increase the power of certain discriminative stimuli and to decrease others). For example, we learned in Chapter 2 that "hypochondriacs" may be overly responsive to physiological stimuli and interpret any such stimuli as illness. We could attempt to teach such persons to distinguish normal physiological stimuli from those that are indicative of illness using operant principles.

Stimulus generalization refers to the transfer of a response to situations or stimuli other than those in which the reinforcement or punishment was experienced. This works in the opposite direction from stimulus discrimination. Generalization may be problematic. An individual who avoids being immunized because of a painful injection by one health provider at one time in one situation is displaying problematic stimulus generalization. There are instances when we may wish to promote such generalization. The police want people to obey the speed limit even when the police are not present. Dental hygienists want people to floss their teeth at home on a daily basis after demonstrating the technique in the office.

Stimulus control is important for another reason. Quite often, the behavior we wish to reinforce either does not occur or occurs so infrequently that we have difficulty encouraging it. We can use prompts (events functioning as discriminative stimuli) to initiate the behavior we wish to reinforce. Prompts may include verbal instructions, physical guidance, or modeling (see below). For example, teaching children how to floss their teeth via reinforcement would be extremely inefficient if we simply handed them a piece of dental floss and waited to reinforce them for the correct response. Health providers use prompts to elicit the behavior: They describe how to do it, model the procedure, and then physically guide the children in flossing their teeth. Prompts have wide application in teaching any new skill (e.g., self-injection of insulin), in retraining a skill that has been lost (e.g., physical rehabilitation), or in eliciting a behavior that is in the person's repertoire but infrequently displayed (e.g., your biannual dental checkup).

Once a behavior is reliably performed, we may want it to occur independently of such prompts. Fading refers to the gradual removal of prompts once the behavior occurs reliably. Fading may also be used to reduce stimulus-controlled undesirable behavior. Suppose, for example, that a child on a pediatric ward screams each time his mother leaves the room. Mother absence is a powerful discriminative stimulus for screaming. Fading would entail having the mother leave for a very brief period of time and return before the screaming begins. The length of the mother's absence would be slowly increased until the child could tolerate her absence without upset.

Developing and Implementing Operant Programs

Implementing a behavior change program using operant principles requires the careful attention to a number of practical matters: (1) identifying, selecting, and measuring the target behavior to be changed; (2) deciding how and when to reinforce, punish, or extinguish and how and when to prompt; and (3) assessing the effectiveness of the program. Let us look at each of these matters in more detail.

Defining Target Behaviors. Most problems can be defined as behavioral excesses (undesirable behaviors that occur frequently or behaviors that are inappropriate to a setting) or deficits (desirable behaviors that fail to occur or fail to occur at the right time or place). In either case, the target behavior to be decreased (if excessive) or increased (if deficit) must be specified objectively, clearly, and completely. Objective refers to a definition of the problem in terms of overt, observable behavior. A clear definition is one that can be repeated and paraphrased by others. In a complete definition, the boundary conditions are specified such that responses to be included and excluded as targets are specified (Kazdin, 1980).

Assessing Target Behaviors. Once clearly specified, it is necessary to assess the extent to which the target behavior is performed prior to treatment. The target behavior may be assessed via observation in terms of its frequency, strength, or duration (see Reese, 1978, for a more thorough discussion). This provides the base line or comparison point needed to assess the effectiveness of the treatment program once it has been initiated. Thus, observational assessment of the target behavior begins prior to treatment and continues until treatment has been completed.

During the initial base line assessment, it is also useful to identify antecedent and consequent events that serve as discriminative stimuli and reinforcers (or punishers) for the target behavior in the natural environment. It is these events that need to be systematically altered in order to implement an effective treatment program.

Developing and Implementing Operant Programs: Positive Reinforcement. After defining, operationalizing, and measuring the behavior to be altered, consequences are then systematically manipulated in order to bring about the desired effect. This may also require the use of prompting, shaping, and fading. Whether addressing behavioral excesses or deficits, it is critical to use positive reinforcement. For deficits, the object is to increase the frequency of the desired behavior. For excesses, where the primary intent is to eliminate an undesirable behavior via extinction or punishment, it is still critical to reinforce a desired behavior to take the place of the excessive behavior. Punishment only teaches what *not* to do; it does not teach the person what to do.

After selecting an event as a consequence and empirically demonstrating that it serves as a reinforcer for the client, several guidelines need to be followed to maximize the effectiveness of the reinforcer. There should be minimal delay between the performance of the target response and the delivery of the reinforcer. The amount or strength of the reinforcer should be sufficient to motivate the person but not so great that the person is satiated or loses interest in the reinforcer. When initially reinforcing a behavior, each occurrence of the behavior should be reinforced. This is referred to as a continuous schedule of reinforcement. Once the behavior is well established via continuous reinforcement, it should then be reinforced on an intermittent schedule, usually on a variable ratio (on the average, every 5th, 7th, or *n*th response is reinforced) or on a variable interval (on the average, the first time the behavior occurs after 5 minutes, 10 minutes, *n* minutes, reinforcement occurs). The shift from continuous to intermittent schedules should occur gradually. The shift is made because intermittently reinforced responses are harder to extinguish, because the client is less likely to lose interest in the reinforcer, and because an intermittent schedule is less time-consuming for the clinician.

As described earlier, several types of reinforcers can be used. Selection is based primarily on client preference; that is, use what works. However, as shown in Table 10-1, other considerations may influence reinforcer selection.

A slightly different but very useful application of reinforcement principles entails the development of behavioral contracts between in-

TABLE 10-1 Advantages and Disadvantages of Various Positive Reinforcers

TYPE	EXAMPLE	ADVANTAGES	DISADVANTAGES
Consumables	Food, gum, soda	Strong if gauged to individual preference	Consumption interferes with ongoing behavior, cumbersome and difficult to dispense
Social behaviors	Verbal praise, attention, physical contact	Easily administered, not disruptive of ongoing behavior, generalizes to the natural environment	Not necesarily reinforcing
High probability behaviors	Any kind of preferred activity (e.g., TV and rest)	Readily available	Often delayed access after the response; often all or none, i.e., cannot be parceled out in small units; ethical constraints against deprivation
Tokens	Chips, stars, points that can be used to purchase backup reinforcers	Potent and flexible, bridge delay between response and reinforcement; backed up by a variety of reinforcers, less satiation, do not disrupt ongoing behavior, can be parceled out in small units	Transfer poorly to the natural environment, have to establish token value

dividuals. Contracts are written statements that specify the relationship between behaviors and consequences. Such contracts are negotiated by two parties, each specifying the target behavior desired of the other person and the consequences to be provided contingent on that behavior. Good contracts have five characteristics (Stuart, 1977): (1) contracts should detail the reinforcers each party will gain after engaging in the specified behavior; (2) contracts should concretely specify the behavior to be reinforced in terms of its timing and frequency (the behavior must be observable); (3) the contract should specify sanctions (punishers) for failure to meet the contract terms; (4) the contract should include bonus reinforcers for consistent compliance; and (5) the contract should specify the means of keeping track of the target behaviors and the reinforcers given and received. Generally, it is better to specify the targets as behaviors to be increased rather than as problems to be decreased. Contracts are highly flexible and involve the client in the behavior change process. Contracts can be renegotiated or adjusted. They are particularly useful in structuring relationships between individuals who have ongoing and frequent contact with each other (e.g., parents and children, marital partners, health provider and client). A case example using contracting will be presented later in this chapter.

Developing and Implementing Operant Programs: Punishment and Extinction. Undesirable or excessive behaviors can be suppressed using contingent punishment. However, the use of punishment requires careful consideration for several reasons. First, it does not teach the person what to do, only what *not* to do. It should thus only be used in conjunction with reinforcement of the desired response. Second, it is difficult to effectively implement punishment in the natural environment; very careful control of that environment is required. Third, punishment may result in negative side effects. However, punishment does have its place. It may be useful when the undesirable behavior is life threatening and requires immediate suppression (e.g., the head banging of an autistic child). Punishment may also be required to suppress undesirable behaviors that occur with such frequency that the desired behavior does not occur and therefore cannot be reinforced (e.g., self-stimulation in a retarded individual). Punishment may also be used to suppress an undesirable behavior temporarily while reinforcing the desired behavior that will take its place. The therapeutic use of punishment is controversial and should only be used when necessary, with consent of the client, and by clinicians who are skilled in its use.

There are many popular misconceptions about punishment. Not all punishment entails physical pain. In fact, in only very extreme cases is painful physical punishment used and justified. Recall that a punisher is defined by its effects; many events that function as punishers are not painful and are not physical. Verbal statements, including reprimands, warnings, and disapprovals may function as punishers. Because they are easily administered, cause no physical discomfort, and occur frequently in the natural environment, maintenance of behavior change is likely. However, negative verbal statements have inconsistent effects.

They sometimes suppress behavior, sometimes have no effect, and sometimes even serve as reinforcers.

Time-out from reinforcement is a type of punishment that entails the withdrawal or removal of access to reinforcement for a specified period. In time-out, the person is physically isolated from reinforcing stimuli and activities. When a parent sits a child in the corner after misbehavior, time-out is being used. Time-out is quite effective and requires only brief isolation (5 to 10 minutes) from reinforcement. Removal of the person from opportunities for reinforcement may be difficult if the person physically resists. Time-out also precludes the opportunity for reinforcement of desired responses during the time-out period.

Response cost refers to the loss of a positive reinforcer already in the person's possession or to a penalty entailing work or effort. It may involve the loss of a material reinforcer (e.g., paying a fine for a traffic ticket) or of an activity reinforcer (e.g., being grounded, or having no TV privileges) contingent on the undesired behavior. Response cost is easily implemented, but cannot be used too frequently because, as the person "goes into debt" (e.g., being grounded for 7 months), motivation is lost. A clear benefit of response cost is that it does not remove the person from the learning environment.

Another type of punishment that involves a penalty but is usually distinguished from response cost is called overcorrection. In overcorrection, the penalty for engaging in the undesirable response is performing some behavior that corrects the environmental effects of that behavior. This is like restitution. Quite often, overcorrection also entails practicing the appropriate response, or positive practice. Suppose a child has the bad habit of throwing his coat on the floor when he comes in the front door. Overcorrection would entail the child picking up the coat and putting it in the closet, and perhaps straightening the rest of the living room as well. Positive practice would involve having the child repeatedly come in the door with his coat on and hanging it in the closet. One nice feature of overcorrection is that it focuses on teaching the desired response. However, the client must be guided through the corrective actions and positive practice. This requires time and effort from the clinician and is difficult to implement when the client is physically resistive.

Each of the punishment procedures discussed has been found to be effective. The procedure selected is determined by its ease of implementation, the training required of the person who will administer the program, and the degree to which the treatment is acceptable to the client. To be maximally effective, the punishment should be delivered immediately after every occurrence of the undesirable behavior (a continuous schedule). The punishing event should have an intensity that is the minimum required to suppress the behavior. In most cases, undesirable behaviors occur because they are reinforced in the natural environment. Naturally occurring reinforcers need to be identified and removed for punishment to be effective. It is also important to reinforce the desired alternate response.

As mentioned, punishment may result in negative side effects. It may elicit an emotional reaction like anger. It may lead to escape or avoidance from the punishing situation or agent. It may lead to counter-aggression, for it models the use of aversive control techniques for the person to whom it is applied. Most of these side effects can be minimized by using the mild forms of punishment described above and by reinforcing incompatible desired behaviors.

Extinction refers to systematically withholding reinforcement from a previously reinforced response. This leads to a gradual reduction in the frequency of the target behavior. Extinction is implicitly used in almost all operant treatment programs but may be used as a specific means of reducing undesirable behaviors. To be effective, *all* reinforcement of the behavior must be withheld. This requires a very careful and thorough analysis of naturally occurring contingencies. If only some or even most but not all reinforcement is withheld, the target undesired behavior is on an intermittent reinforcement schedule that may unwittingly actually foster the continued performance of the undesirable behavior. Consequently, the use of extinction as a sole mode of treatment is usually impractical. Usually, it is necessary to reinforce the desired behavior as well.

The process of extinction is gradual. When extinction is first initiated, the frequency of the targeted behavior may increase. This extinction burst may be difficult to tolerate, but such behaviors must not be reinforced. Even after extinction has led to a reduction in the targeted response, that response may again temporarily reappear in the absence of reinforcement. This spontaneous recovery again must be met with the systematic nonreinforcement of the response.

Developing and Implementing Operant Programs: Response Maintenance and Transfer. After the implementation of reinforcement, punishment, or extinction procedures has resulted in observable changes in the target behavior, it is necessary to alter the operant program to insure that these changes transfer to new settings and that they are maintained over time.

There are a number of strategies that may be utilized to promote the transfer and maintenance (often called the generalization) of behavior change. First, the behavior can be brought under the control of contingencies in the natural environment. This entails selecting target behaviors that have a high likelihood of being reinforced in the natural environment. It may also require working with the individual in the client's natural environment to encourage continued reinforcement of the behavior change.

The second strategy is to gradually remove or fade the contingencies in the operant program. This entails shifting to more highly intermittent schedules of reinforcement over time to further increase resistance to extinction. The delay between the performance of the response and the delivery of the reinforcement may also be increased; in the natural environment, most responses do not lead to immediate reinforcement. In a sense, this strategy involves slowly altering the reinforcement program so that it operates in a manner similar to contingencies in the natural environment. Self-control procedures can also be used to promote generalization. These procedures are described in detail in the next chapter.

Developing and Implementing Operant Programs: A Summary. While operant principles appear to be relatively simple, implementing these principles to change behavior requires skill and patience. A number of steps have been discussed, and a summary is presented in Figure 10-2. Each step requires the successful completion of the previous steps. Although difficult and complicated, operant procedures are widely applicable and very powerful means of changing health- and illness-related behaviors. Let us now turn to an example of the application of these procedures. The utilization of operant proce-

FIGURE 10-2 General Procedure for Implementing an Operant Program

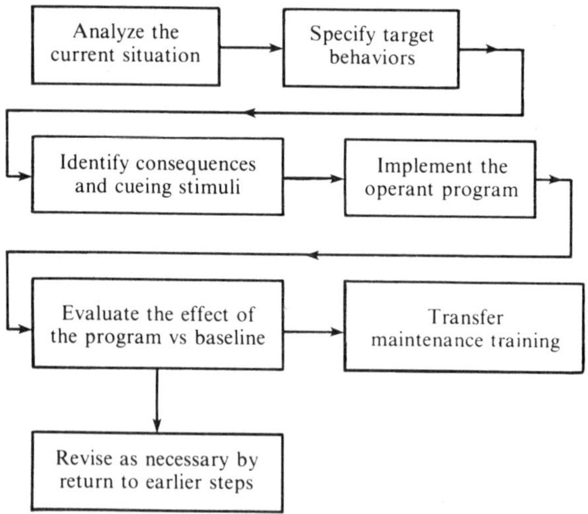

dures for other behavioral health and illness targets will be discussed in Chapters 13 to 16.

Operant Procedures: A Clinical Example

The following example is an abbreviated description of a study that utilizes operant procedures to deal with a serious medical problem (Snyder, 1987). A male adolescent was referred for treatment because of his unwillingness to engage in appropriate self-care for diabetes. The client had Type 1, insulin-dependent diabetes since age six. Although he was quite knowledgeable and capable of caring for his diabetes by self-administering insulin, doing urine glucose tests, and eating appropriate foods as scheduled, his self-care had become increasingly erratic during the nine months previous to referral such that he had been frequently hospitalized for both hypoglycemia (low blood sugar resulting from the failure to eat sufficient calories or the use of too much insulin) and hyperglycemia (high blood sugar resulting from the ingestion of too much sugar or the failure to take enough insulin).

Four target behaviors were clearly defined and systematically assessed: (1) the child's diabetes self-care practices; (2) the child's aggressive, noncompliant behavior; (3) the child's school attendance; and (4) the verbal conflict between mother and child. A functional analysis of these target behaviors indicated that the child and his mother were engaged in a temporal cycle of aversive control. At the beginning of a cycle, the child would engage in relatively good self-care but frequent aggression and noncompliance. In response to his aggression and noncompliance, the mother would increase her nagging and threats. Her nagging and threats reduced his aggression and noncompliance, thus negatively reinforcing her behavior. However, he also deliberately reduced his self-care in an attempt to turn off her nagging and threats. Poor self-care would continue until a diabetic crisis occurred, resulting in a termination of the nagging and threats (negative reinforcement of his poor self-care) and in maternal expressions of caring and concern (positive reinforcement). After his diabetes restabilized, the cycle would begin anew.

Three biobehavioral mechanisms appeared to be operating in which disregulation at one level interfered with regulation at other levels. The primary mechanism was an aversive behavior exchange between the client and his mother. The mother's nagging and threats were evoked (discriminative stimulus) by her son's aggression and noncompliance, and negatively reinforced by his short-term reduction in that behavior after her nagging and threats. The son's poor self-care was in turn elicited by nagging and maintained by a reduction in nagging and threats when a diabetic episode ensued (negative reinforcement) and by the attention engendered by his medical condition (positive reinforcement). The son used poor self-care to thwart his mother's disciplinary actions. Two secondary mechanisms may also have been operating. The short-term decrease in aggression and noncompliance resulting from maternal nagging and threats may have been mediated by the son's poor self-care rather than by the effectiveness of her actions. That is, poor self-care in response to nagging and threats may have disrupted the biobehavioral homeostasis requisite to aggression and noncompliance. The son's deteriorating self-care, as well as being deliberate, may have been the result of an indirect, stress-induced glucose metabolism lability that complicated the self-care.

Treatment entailed the development of a behavioral contract. As

TABLE 10-2 Behavioral Contract for Diabetic Self-Care and General Behavior

RESPONSIBILITIES OF SON	CONSEQUENCES FROM MOTHER
1. Will eat specified foods for morning meal (by 8 A.M.), morning snack (by 10 A.M.), noon meal (by noon), afternoon snack (by 4 P.M.), evening meal (by 6 P.M), and evening snack (by 10 P.M.)	1. Will make appropriate foods of son's choice available, will remind son only once for each meal or snack, will pay 25 cents per each episode of eating proper amount and type on time
2. Will take insulin twice daily, at 7 A.M. and 5 P.M.	2. Will make insulin available, will remind only once, will pay 50 cents per each on-time injection
3. Will be in bed by midnight with lights and TV off on Sunday through Thursday nights	3. Will remind only once at 11:55 P.M., son will be able to keep his own TV in his room the following day
4. Will be at school at 9 A.M. each weekday morning, will stay in school until 3:30 P.M.	4. For each day, will earn 1 chip; chips are exchangeable for backup rewards (e.g., dirt bike or time at video arcade)
5. Will engage in no aggression or noncompliance	5. Will earn 1 chip for each day; chips are exchangeable as in number 4

Bonus: Perfect week on numbers 1 and 2 will result in a $2.50 bonus

Penalty: If son fails to maintain eating and insulin injection such that a hyperglycemic or hypoglycemic episode occurs resulting in the loss of consciousness, he will be taken to the hospital and admitted for 2 days with no TV, visitors, magazines, etc.

If son fails to attend school regularly (less than 4 days per week), juvenile authorities will be contacted and adjudication proceedings will be initiated

If son engages in any antisocial behavior (e.g., aggression or stealing), he will work at a task defined by his mother as commensurate with his action's seriousness shown in Table 10-2, this contract specified both desirable self-care actions and general behavior for the adolescent that were exchangeable for material and activity reinforcers. Failure to meet the terms of the contract led to punishment. This contract was developed in close consultation with the client's physician, hospital staff, and juvenile authorities. Its contents were negotiated by both the mother and the son.

The contract was implemented and led to a reduction in hyperglycemic and hypoglycemic episodes, improved self-care, improved school attendance, and a reduction in aggression and noncompliance. At the termination of treatment, the client was engaging in an average of ten proper self-care behaviors daily (out of a possible total of 11), mother-son conflict had been reduced to one-third of its pretreatment level, aggression and noncompliance were reduced to one-quarter of their pretreatment levels, the son was attending school daily, and a diabetic episode did not occur for over three months (compared to a monthly occurrence prior to treatment). These gains were maintained for at least two months after treatment had ended.

This example demonstrates the complexity involved in assessing health- and illness-related problems and in implementing operant programs to correct those problems. Other examples of the use of operant techniques in behavioral health and medicine are described in Pinkerton, Hughs, and Weinrich (1982).

RESPONDENT CONDITIONING

The second type of stimulus-response learning is referred to as respondent, or classical, conditioning. Certain stimuli reflexively elicit a response. Food elicits salivation, light elicits pupil constriction, pain elicits flexion of the body. These stimuli are called unconditioned stimuli (US). The connection between an unconditioned stimulus and a response is automatic or unlearned. In respondent conditioning, a stimulus that does not automatically elicit a response (called a conditioned stimulus, or CS) is made to elicit the response. To do this, the CS is repeatedly paired with the US such that the CS alone will eventually elicit the response. In contrast to operant conditioning, respondent conditioning entails the manipulation of events preceding the response. Unlike operant conditioning, in respondent conditioning the organism does not freely emit the response. Rather, the response is elicited.

The classic example of respondent conditioning, of course, is Pavlov's demonstration of salivation in dogs. Food is the US and salivation the response. After pairing a tone (CS) with the presentation of food (US) for several trials, Pavlov found that the tone alone elicited salivation. There have been many demonstrations of respondent conditioning in humans. Persons experiencing an asthmatic attack often use inhalators (CS) that contain a medication (US) that results in respiratory relief (the reflexively elicited response). After repeatedly obtaining relief via the use of inhalated medication, the inhalator alone (CS), even if it no longer contains any medication (in the absence of the US), brings relief (the response).

Once established, a classically conditioned response can be extinguished by presenting the CS repeatedly in the absence of the US. If the asthmatic continues to use an inhalator that contains no medication, the use of the inhalator will cease to be effective. There is also stimulus generalization and stimulus discrimination. In stimulus generalization, stimuli similar to the original CS will also elicit the response, even though they were never paired with the US. If Pavlov had used a 700 Hz tone as the CS, a 900 Hz tone would also elicit the response. However, it is also possible to teach discrimination. If the 700 Hz tone was consistently paired with the US and the 900 Hz tone was repeatedly presented but never paired with the food, the dog would learn to salivate in response to the 700 Hz tone but not to the 900 Hz tone. Finally, higher order conditioning has also been demonstrated. In this case, a CS, once it effectively elicits a response by repeated pairing with a US, can then be used to establish a different CS (Kalish, 1981).

A large number of visceral responses, such as heart rate, galvanic skin response, immune response, brain activity, respiration, and stomach contractions, can be classically conditioned. Respondent conditioning is particularly relevant to behavioral medicine because of its role in conditioned emotional responses, including fear, anger, anxiety, and guilt. Painful stimuli reflexively produce "emotional" behavior (e.g., withdrawal or avoidance), physiological responses (e.g., increases in heart rate, blood pressure, and sweating), and subjective feelings of distress. Through classical conditioning (perhaps in combination with operant conditioning), subjective, behavioral, and physiological aspects of emotional responses may be elicited by innocuous, formerly neutral stimuli even though no real threat exists. For example, let us suppose that a child experiences a painful dental procedure. The procedure is the US that elicits physiological arousal and the experience of pain. Other stimuli associated with the procedure, such as the dentist and the office (the CS), may elicit physiological arousal, anxiety, and behavioral avoidance. As discussed in Chapter 8, classical conditioning is also thought to be responsible for the anticipatory nausea and vomiting experienced by persons receiving chemotherapy for cancer.

Fear and anxiety associated with health care procedures may interfere with timely health care actions, accurate symptom recognition, adjustment to hospitalization, cooperation with surgical and rehabilitative procedures, and adherence to treatment regimens. These direct effects of behavior on health were described in Chapter 2. Conditioned emotional responses may serve as a cue for health-impairing habits such as smoking and drinking, as described in Chapter 3. Finally, conditioned emotional responses may also have an indirect effect on health. The psychophysiological arousal accompanying frequent and prolonged elicitation of conditioned emotional responses may contribute to psychosomatic illnesses such as ulcers, high blood pressure, and colitis (Lachman, 1972). Respondent conditioning may play a mediating role in the association of stress and illness.

Clinical Procedures Derived from Respondent Conditioning

Two clinical procedures for extinguishing conditioned emotional responses have been derived from respondent conditioning: flooding and systematic desensitization. Extinction is a process in which a conditioned emotional response is eliminated by repeatedly presenting the conditioned stimulus in the absence of the unconditioned stimulus. Flooding entails extended exposure to the most threatening situation without escape until behavioral and physiological arousal are no longer evident. Systematic desensitization is often preferable because it is less stressful for the client and less likely to result in premature termination of treatment (Pinkerton et al., 1982).

In systematic desensitization (Wolpe, 1969), a response alternate to emotional arousal is substituted in the emotion provoking situation. In this case, a hierarchy of feared situations is developed. Such a hierarchy varies according to the client and is developed with the assistance of the client. The hierarchy should consist of ten to fifteen concrete situations, ranging from those that provoke very little anxiety to those that provoke severe anxiety. These are rank ordered according to the client's subjective evaluation. Suppose, for example, that a child is highly anxious about going to the dentist. When taken to the office, the child cries, resists, and is physiologically and behaviorally aroused. Systematic desensitization would entail exposing the child to the office, dental personnel, and nonaversive dental procedures. This could be done gradually over a period of days. On subsequent days, the child may visit the waiting room and the hygienist's office, sit in the chair, and undergo mild procedures like a checkup, x-rays, teeth cleaning, and so forth. The exposure is gradual and hierarchical, beginning with the least threatening situation and proceeding to more threatening situations as the less threatening ones are mastered. A hierarchy of a client with a fear of dental procedures is presented in Table 10-3. The client is also taught a response that is incompatible with emotional arousal, usually some form of relaxation (see Chapter 12).

Systematic desensitization, or counterconditioning, is then implemented. The client self-induces relaxation. When relaxed, the client is briefly exposed to the situation in the hierarchy that elicits minimal anxiety (or the client can be asked to imagine this situation). This exposure is repeated until the individual can experience (or imagine) the situation without experiencing any arousal. The client is

TABLE 10-3 Hierarchy of Dental Fear

1. Thinking about going to the dentist
2. Calling to make an appointment to go to the dentist
3. Traveling to the dentist's office
4. Sitting in the waiting room
5. Hearing your name called
6. Getting into the dental chair
7. Being reclined in the chair
8. Seeing the hygienist lay out the instruments
9. Having a probe put in your mouth
10. Feeling the probe scrape against your teeth
11. Having the probe touch a cavity
12. Seeing the dentist reach for a drill
13. Hearing the noise of the drill
14. Feeling the drill on your teeth

then exposed to the next situation in the hierarchy using the same procedure. Progression through the hierarchy is gradual and depends on the complete extinction of the emotional response to prior hierarchy situations. Thus, via a series of gradual steps, the client is exposed to all of the emotion-provoking stimuli with minimal subjective distress. Not only is the client's conditioned emotional response extinguished, but the client is also provided an adaptive coping skill (relaxation) relevant to the situation.

Flooding and systematic desensitization have been used effectively to treat a variety of conditioned emotional responses (for reviews see Emmelkamp, 1982; Kazdin & Wilcoxon, 1976). For example, Hallsten (1965) treated a twelve-year-old anorectic female by systematic desensitization. Several years prior to treatment, the client had been teased for being overweight and then went on a diet, losing an excessive amount of weight. She was fearful of being fat and periodically self-induced vomiting. After training in self-relaxation, a hierarchy of situations related to her fear of being fat and being teased about her weight was constructed. These situations included being called to the dinner table, eating high calorie foods, and looking at herself in the mirror. Desensitization was conducted over twelve sessions during which she began to eat complete meals. There was an increase in her weight such that five months after treatment, she was within the normative weight range for her height and age.

The effectiveness of systematic desensitization and flooding is well established. The application of these and other classical conditioning procedures to other health and treatment problems will be further detailed in Chapters 13 to 16.

Operant and Respondent Treatment Procedures: A Summary

Preventative and clinical procedures based on operant and respondent principles are basic and important tools in addressing problems in behavioral health and medicine. The distinction between operant and respondent conditioning is often obscured in real life. It was originally postulated that respondent conditioning was restricted to involuntary (visceral or smooth muscle) responses and operant conditioning to voluntary (striated muscle) responses. This may not be the case (see Chapter 12). In the natural environment, a response may be both elicited (respondent) and controlled by the consequences that follow it (operant); an excellent example is the mixed operant-respondent pain syndromes described in Chapter 9.

OBSERVATIONAL LEARNING

Observational learning (also referred to as modeling and vicarious learning) refers to a process by which an individual's behavior changes as a function of observing, hearing, or reading about the behavior of another person. Via observation, the person extracts information about how to engage in certain behaviors, when it is appropriate to behave in certain ways, and which consequences are likely to result from certain behaviors. In this manner, it is possible to acquire new behaviors rapidly without having to perform them or to shape them in a trial-and-error fashion. Via observation, the frequency and situational performance of behaviors already in a person's repertoire can be altered without actual reinforcement, punishment, or extinction of those behaviors (Bandura, 1969).

Observational learning is ubiquitous. Teenagers imitate rock stars and fashion models in terms of dress, hair styles, and vocabulary. Young children readily imitate the behavior of parents and cartoon characters. Adults imitate the behaviors and styles of persons who are deemed successful or esteemed.

In contrast to operant and respondent conditioning, a person can learn via observation without engaging in an overt response or directly experiencing environmental stimuli. A response is acquired or its performance altered through cognitive coding of the observed events. Bandura (1977) suggests that four basic processes are involved in observational learning: (1) attention—not everything observed is learned; to learn, the observer must attend to and comprehend the information provided by the model; (2) retention—once attention to and comprehension of the modeled behavior occurs, the observer must remember the material by actively processing the information; (3) motoric reproduction—the person must practice the behaviors to become skilled and proficient; and (4) motivation—the actual performance of the behavior depends on anticipated and actual consequences of that behavior.

In understanding observational learning, it is helpful to make a distinction between acquisition and performance. A person can acquire a new response via observation without ever performing that response. Most of us know how to fire a pistol as the result of watching cowboys and detectives on TV, even though most of us have never really fired a pistol. Whether the acquired response is performed depends on the expected contingencies for the response. Observation can influence the frequency with which we perform responses already in our repertoires. If we consistently observe that others drive over the speed limit without getting caught, we may also drive over the speed limit more frequently.

Types of Observational Learning

Observation can result in increases or decreases in the frequency or strength of responses. Increases will be discussed under three rubrics: acquisition effects, disinhibitory effects, and facilitation effects. Acquisition effects refer to a new behavior that is learned by observing a model. A diabetic, for example, may be taught how to self-administer insulin by observing a health provider demonstrate the technique. Disinhibitory effects occur when the observer's inhibited behavior becomes more frequent after viewing a model perform the behavior without suffering any adverse consequences. A person who fears dental procedures and thus avoids dental treatment (inhibited) may be more likely to seek treatment after hearing that treatment was not painful and observing the model's improved appearance. Facilitation effects refer to an increase in the performance frequency of a behavior already in the observer's repertoire as the result of observing a model engage in or be reinforced for that behavior. Children, for example, may brush their teeth more frequently after watching "Sesame Street"'s Grover model such behavior. Relative to acquisition effects, disinhibitory and facilitation effects refer to changes in the frequency of behaviors already in the person's repertoire.

Decreases in the frequency or strength of behavior as a result of observation come under two rubrics: inhibitory effects and incompatible behavior effects. Inhibitory effects occur when a person observes a model being punished or nonreinforced for a behavior and consequently engages in the behavior less frequently. The use of TV advertisements in which a fashion model, rock star, or movie personality denigrates drug use would hopefully have inhibitory effects on the drug use of the viewers. Incompatible behavior effects result from the observation of a model who performs a response that is incompatible with some behavior. To continue with the previous TV advertisement example, the fashion model or rock star may be shown asking for a nonalcoholic beverage at a party or refusing an offer of marijuana. Quite often, it is possible to promote increases in desired behaviors and decreases in undesirable behaviors in one modeling sequence, as in a combination of the two TV ad scenarios.

Generally, observational learning is most effective when the action targeted for change is actually performed by the observer. Participant modeling entails the actual shaping and the verbal and physical guidance of a behavior of the client after the client has observed a model engage in the behavior. In participant modeling, a model displays the behavior, the client performs the behavior, and corrective feedback is provided about the client's performance, with repetitions of the sequence until the behavior is performed adeptly. Such a procedure is probably more powerful than observation alone (as in the TV ads) because it entails all four of the elements that promote observational learning (as detailed above). Participant modeling is applicable to increasing or decreasing the frequency of behaviors already in the person's repertoire as well as to acquiring new responses. Participant modeling is frequently used to teach motor skills like swimming strokes, tennis serves, and dance steps.

Observational Learning: Clinical Examples

An excellent example of the use of observational learning in a medical setting focuses on reducing children's fear of hospitalization and surgery (Melamed & Siegel, 1975). Children who were to be hospitalized for surgery were shown a film called *Ethan Has an Operation* prior to admission. The film depicted a seven-year-old boy being hospitalized for a hernia operation. The children viewed Ethan's progress through admission, ward orientation, physical examination, preoperative procedures, postoperative recovery, reunion with his parents, and discharge from the hospital. Throughout this sequence, Ethan described his feelings and fears at each stage and his manner of resolving them. Melamed and Siegel found that children who observed the film prior to hospitalization and surgery showed less behavioral and physiological arousal and reported less subjective distress throughout hospitalization and surgery than children who observed a control film about a boy's trip into the country.

Melamed and Siegel's study exemplifies the use of modeling to extinguish anxiety. Observational learning can also be used to facilitate the performance of infrequent behaviors. Maccoby and Farquhar (1975), for example, used mass media procedures to inform the public about how personal health habits (e.g., diet, exercise, smoking) affect the risk of heart disease and how to alter this risk-related behavior. Multiple media were used to create interest in the program, and instructional manuals and personal influence relying on modeling, guided practice, and feedback were used to encourage health-promoting habits. Persons in the communities targeted by this media and educational campaign significantly increased their health-promoting behaviors.

Modeling is a very powerful and efficient treatment procedure. Research has documented its effectiveness in promoting behavior change, either to increase desirable behaviors or to decrease undesirable behaviors. A review of the applications and efficacy of observational learning can be found in Rosenthal and Bandura (1978). Additional applications of modeling will be presented in Chapters 13 to 16.

SUMMARY

In the first nine chapters, we repeatedly learned the multiple and intimate roles of behavioral and environmental factors in health, illness, and treatment. Efficient, effective, and powerful intervention necessitates the development of means to change behavior. In this chapter, the principles of three basic types of learning were described. Interventions derived from the principles of operant and respondent conditioning and of observational learning were outlined. These interventions have a strong record of effectiveness and are relevant to a broad range of behaviors associated with health and illness. These interventions complement more traditional biological and pharmacological interventions and can be used to promote health and to prevent and treat illness. They supply health providers with powerful means of altering cognitive, emotional, and behavioral processes.

REFERENCES

Bandura, A. (1969). *Principles of behavior modification*. New York: Holt, Rinehart and Winston.

Bandura, A. (1977). *Social learning theory*. Englewood Cliffs, NJ: Prentice-Hall.

Emmelkamp, P. M. (1982). Anxiety and fear. In A. S. Bellack, M. Hersen, & A. E. Kazdin (Eds.), *International handbook of behavior modification and therapy*. New York: Plenum Press.

Hallsten, A. E. (1965). Adolescent anorexia nervosa treated by desensitization. *Behavior Research and Therapy, 3*, 87–91.

Kalish, H. I. (1981). *From behavioral science to behavior modification*. New York: McGraw-Hill.

Kazdin, A. E. (1984). *Behavior modification in applied settings*. 3rd Edition. Homewood, IL: The Dorsey Press.

Kazdin, A. E., & Wilcoxon, L. A. (1976). Systematic desensitization and nonspecific treatment effects: A methodological evaluation. *Psychological Bulletin, 83*, 729–758.

Lachman, S. (1972). *Psychosomatic disorders: A behavioristic interpretation*. New York: John Wiley & Sons.

Maccoby, N., & Farquhar, J. W. (1975). Communication for health: Unselling heart disease. *Journal of Communications, 25*, 114–126.

Matarazzo, J. D. (1980). Behavioral health and behavioral medicine: Frontiers for a new health psychology. *American Psychologist, 35,* 807–817.

Melamed, B. G., & Siegel, L. J. (1975). Reduction of anxiety in children facing hospitalization and surgery by use of filmed modeling. *Journal of Consulting and Clinical Psychology, 43,* 511–521.

Pinkerton, S. S., Hughs, H., & Weinrich, W. W. (1982). *Behavioral medicine: Clinical applications.* New York: John Wiley & Sons.

Pomerleau, O. F., & Brady, J. P. (1979). Introduction: The scope and promise of behavioral medicine. In O. F. Pomerleau & J. P. Brady (Eds.), *Behavioral medicine: Theory and practice,* xi–xxvi. Baltimore: Williams & Wilkins.

Premack, D. (1965). Reinforcement theory. In D. Levine (Ed.), *Nebraska symposium on motivation,* 123–179. Lincoln: University of Nebraska Press.

Reese, E. P. (1978). *Human behavior: Analysis and application.* Dubuque, IA: W. C. Brown.

Rosenthal, T. L., & Bandura, A. (1978). Psychological modeling: Theory and practice. In S. L. Garfield & A. E. Bergin (Eds.), *Handbook of psychotherapy and behavior change: An empirical analysis* (2nd ed.), 621–658. New York: John Wiley & Sons.

Schwartz, G., & Weiss, S. (1977). What is behavioral medicine? *Psychosomatic Medicine, 36,* 377–381.

Snyder, J. J. (1987). Behavioral analysis and treatment of poor diabetic self-care and antisocial behavior: A single subject experimental study. *Behavior Therapy, 18,* 251–263.

Stuart, R. B. (1977). *Client-therapist treatment contracts.* Champaign, IL: Research Press.

Wolpe, J. (1969). *The practice of behavior therapy.* Elmsford, NY: Pergamon Press.

11

Self-Control and Cognitive Therapy

INTRODUCTION

The behavior change procedures outlined in the previous chapter based on operant and respondent conditioning and observational learning emphasize alteration of behavior by an external agent. The client is a relatively passive participant in the change process. Such external control is contrary to the perspective detailed in earlier chapters. Operant and respondent procedures also treat persons as if they are "black boxes." There is little attention paid to the psychological processes occurring within the individual that mediate learning: thinking, planning, and evaluating. Evidence supports the notion that persons exert control over their own behavior and are not just robots who react passively to environmental stimuli. Human behavior cannot be adequately explained without focusing on internal psychological processes.

In this chapter, we will consider two behavior change strategies, self-control and cognitive therapy, that emphasize that individuals' behavior is often self-determined and that recognize the importance of psychological processes—the workings within the "black box." Self-control interventions recognize that persons create and control their own environment as well as being influenced by it (Bandura, 1969). Cognitive interventions recognize that human learning entails cognitive processes that are causally interactive with the environment and behavior (Mahoney, 1977). Let us begin with self-control.

SELF-CONTROL

Definition

In operant procedures, one person manipulates environmental stimuli and response contingencies to alter the behavior of another. In contrast, self-control refers to actions taken by individuals to alter their own behavior to achieve a self-selected outcome. Self-control entails engaging in one response (a controlling response) to change another response (the controlled response). In self-control, persons are their own behavior modifiers.

Self-control occurs frequently in our day-to-day behavior. We write appointments in a calendar so that we will be in the right place at the right time. We set the alarm clock to wake at a certain time. Thus, we engage in antecedent stimulus control. We also set up reinforcement contingencies for our own behavior. We denigrate (punish) ourselves for poor test performance. We praise (reinforce) ourselves for success. We put off watching TV (an activity reinforcer) until we are finished studying. We buy new clothes after losing weight. We also engage in responses to control our own emotions. We may have a drink when feeling anxious, try to recall pleasant experiences when feeling sad, or "whistle in the dark" when feeling afraid.

Generally, individuals are said to engage in self-control when they regulate a response that has conflicting short- and long-term consequences. Self-control may entail forgoing the performance of a behavior that is immediately reinforcing to avoid long-term aversive consequences. Behaviors in this category include limiting food consumption, not smoking, and moderately using alcohol. Self-control may also entail engaging in a behavior that has aversive short-term but positive long-term consequences. Behaviors in this category include exercising, studying, and getting medical and dental checkups. In other words, acts of self-control are characterized by forgoing immediate rewards to obtain future rewards (Kanfer & Phillips, 1970).

Self-control is learned. Developmentally, the behavior of young children is controlled by external agents like parents or teachers. They set standards for children's behavior and provide consequences to encourage appropriate and to discourage inappropriate behavior. As children become socialized, these standards and consequences become internalized such that children begin to control their own behavior. Achievement of standards then becomes reinforcing because of its past association with external reinforcement. Failure to achieve standards is punishing because of its prior association with external punishment.

Self-control is learned via operant and observational processes (Kazdin, 1980).

Self-control, as described here, is different from "willpower." Willpower is a trait that someone has. As such, it is hard to define and to change. It is tautological: Persons engage in self-control because they have willpower, and willpower is inferred from the self-controlling act. Self-control is better considered as something a person does rather than has. Self-control is learned and it is situational. A person may display self-control in one context but not in another (Mahoney & Arnkoff, 1978).

Applications and Advantages

Self-control training has been utilized to alter many behaviors relevant to health and illness. It has been used to enhance adherence to treatment recommendations (e.g., taking prescribed medication), to alter health-impairing and health-promoting habits (e.g., eating, exercising, smoking, and displaying Type A behavior), to alter conditioned emotional arousal (e.g., anxiety and guilt), and to alter the behavioral components of pain syndromes.

Self-control interventions have a number of advantages over operant strategies. First, self-control procedures can be applied to behaviors that are not easily observed by external agents because they are infrequent (panic attacks), covert (hallucinations), or private (sexual activity). Second, self-control procedures do not require the clinician to have strong control over the client's environment, as is necessitated by operant procedures. Such control is not typically available to the health provider or relinquished by the client. Third, self-control procedures involve the client in the change process, which is congruent with the compensatory model of helping. Fourth, behavior change resulting from self-control may be more likely to persist because the change is shaped in the natural environment. Fifth, self-control training is cost effective. It requires less therapist time, can be applied in groups, and provides the client with generalized skills that can subsequently be applied to other problems.

Procedures

Several techniques have been used to teach individuals to control their own behavior more adeptly. These include goal specification, self-observation, stimulus control, self-reinforcement and punishment, and alternate response training. Each of these techniques will be detailed. However, successful self-control interventions also entail client-relational and client-educational issues that provide the conditions for change. Our discussion will initially focus on establishing the therapeutic conditions that maximize the likelihood of success.

Establishing Therapeutic Conditions for Success. Recall that behaviors targeted for self-control are under conflicting contingencies. These behaviors have strong payoffs and costs. Therefore, clients are often ambivalent about changing a problem behavior. In a self-control program, the client has to make a genuine commitment to change. How can the client be motivated to make such a commitment? Clients often have tried to change their problematic behavior without success. Consequently, clients may harbor feelings that change is hopeless. How can positive expectations be engendered?

Kanfer (1975) suggests several strategies to enhance client commitment and motivation. First, when possible, the clinician should reduce external reinforcement for the problematic behavior. Second, the clinician should provide strong emotional support (referent power) and hope for change (expert power), and make change appear desirable. Third, while providing support and hope, the clinician should make clear the aversive consequences of the problem behavior. These consequences are often ignored by the client ("It won't happen to me," or "I'll stop smoking after Christmas"). Fourth, the client should be asked to sign a contract with the clinician, spouse, friend, or children that indicates commitment to change. Fifth, it is important to empathize with the client's ambivalence and hopelessness about change but then to develop a shared conceptualization of the problem, goals for change, and the means to effect that change. This provides a sense of hope and control that the client may not have previously experienced.

Client responsibility is inherently communicated in the initial procedures used in self-control: target specification and self-observation. Let us turn to these procedures.

Target Specification and Self-Observation. As in operant programs, in self-control procedures it is first necessary to specify clearly and carefully the target behavior to be changed. This can be a problem behavior to be decreased or a desired behavior to be increased. The client is then given the task of self-observing the target behavior. Self-observation serves several functions. It parallels the continuous observation in operant programs and as such provides a base line against which the effectiveness of a self-control intervention can be assessed. It communicates, very early in treatment, that the client is required to take an active role in the behavior change process. Incidental to self-observation, clients may also come to feel that change is possible. Systematic self-observation often results in behavior change, although change due solely to self-observation is usually short-lived. It also provides clients with a better understanding of their problem than one based on previous haphazard analyses. Self-observation provides the data needed to establish realistic short- and long-term goals. In self-observation, clients are also asked to observe and record the temporal, situational, emotional, and cognitive stimuli that precede and follow the target behavior. These data are needed to formulate effective self-control strategies.

When implementing self-observation, the following steps are recommended: (1) discuss the purpose and importance of self-observation and self-recording, and give examples of how the data collected will be used; (2) specify, with the client, the behavior to be observed, and discuss examples to illustrate that behavior; (3) select unobtrusive and convenient means of recording the behavior, and make materials necessary for recording available to the client; (4) role play and rehearse the entire sequence of observing and recording the target behavior; (5) begin modestly by selecting one or two simple behaviors to be observed (more complex observation of antecedent and consequent stimuli can be added as the client becomes adept at simpler assignments); (6) select the time or setting in which the behavior is to be observed and recorded; (7) call during the initial week of self-observation to remind the client to do so and to troubleshoot any problems; and (8) thoroughly discuss the data collected each week in terms of identifying stimuli that evoke and maintain the behavior.

As an illustration, let us suppose we are working with a nineteen-year-old college student who weighs 180 pounds. She wishes to lose weight. We might select two target behaviors for initial self-observation and self-recording: eating and exercising. The self-observation might be introduced in the following manner:

> It seems that you're really motivated to lose some weight, but your attempts to do so in the past have not worked well. What I think we need, before we try to change your eating and exercising habits, is some idea of your current eating and exercising patterns. This will give us a better handle on the specifics of the problem, what our goals ought to be, and how to go about changing your behavior. Let's begin by figuring out what you need to observe and record.

Let us suppose that after four weeks of self-observation and self-recording, the client delivers the information shown in Figure 11-1. Of course, we would have to work up to the complexity reflected in this sample slowly. What specific information is included for self-observation and self-recording depends on the target behavior and the individual client. Self-monitoring continues throughout treatment. It provides information concerning the effectiveness of the various self-control interventions, and any adjustments that may be required.

The next step is to set short- and long-term goals for behavior change. Short-term goals indicate how much change is expected on a daily or weekly basis. Long-term goals refer to the ultimate product to be achieved by the end of treatment (over months). Goal attainment is facilitated by having the client publicly state these goals to spouse or

Day: Thursday Date: 7/16

Weight: 183

Calories eaten: 3828
Calories exercise: 100
Total "meals": 7

Time	Place	Activity	People	Mood	Amt. Food	Calories	
7:30	dorm	breakfast	?	bitchy	1 o.j. 1 HB egg 2 toast, butter 1 coffee, cream & sugar	120 48 210 40	448
10:30	College Inn	class break	Debbie, Alice, Tom	bored	1 danish 1 coffee, c & s	125 40	165
12:00	dorm	lunch	Barb, John	ok	1 milk 1 spaghetti 2 p. cake	160 not eat 500	660
4:30	snack bar	after bio lab	Tom, Denise	hungry	1 cheeseburger 1 fries	470 250	720
6:30	dorm	dinner	Barb, Alice, Jean	good	1 meat (lamb) 1 peas 2 sm potato 1 choc. ice cream	470 115 120 100	805
10:30	snack bar	break frm study	Tom, Jean	tired	2 beers 1 pot chip	300 230	530
11–12	room	studying	no one	tired	10 choc. chip cookies	500?	500

Exercise:	Moderate		Vigorous		Strenuous
Walk:	15 min.	Walk fast:	10 min.	Sports:	
Bicycle:		Horse ride:		Dance:	
Housework:		Swim:		Jog:	
Total time:	15		10		
Calories:	50		50		

FIGURE 11-1 Sample of Self-Observation and Self-Recording for Weight Control

friends, specify the goals in terms of behavior change (e.g., eating frequency or amount rather than weight), and set graduated performance demands (more modest at first to insure success experiences). The frame of mind with which the client approaches behavior change is important. A coping model in which the client anticipates that effort, discomfort, doubt, and distress will be encountered in achieving these goals is useful. Dichotomous thinking and moralistic evaluations of one's performance as success versus failure or good versus bad are less helpful.

For the overweight client, the following goals might be jointly specified by the client and the therapist. Over the next two weeks, one evening and one daytime snack will be eliminated. Exercise will be increased to 30 minutes of moderate activity and 15 minutes of vigorous exercise per week. In the long run, eating will be limited to three meals per day for a total of 1,500 to 1,700 calories. Other snacks will be calorie free. Exercise will be increased to 30 minutes of vigorous exercise per day.

Once sufficient information has been obtained from self-observation and short- and long-term goals have been set, the treatment program is implemented. The client and the therapist develop a behavior change program that usually entails a combination of stimulus control, self-reinforcement, and alternate response training. Let us consider each of these in turn.

Stimulus Control. As discussed in the last chapter, behavior is controlled in part by antecedent or discriminative stimuli. Manipulation of these stimuli will alter the frequency of the behavior that they evoke. Stimulus control is a commonsensical remedy for problems. The use of chastity belts in the Middle Ages, mothers' use of mittens for children who suck their thumbs, and the use of cash rather than charge cards when shopping are obvious examples.

In self-control, clients engage in stimulus control by reducing or eliminating contact with stimuli that evoke problematic behavior, or by increasing contact with stimuli that evoke desired behavior. The stimuli that are manipulated may be physical and social aspects of the external environment or the client's own cognitions, feelings, and physiology. Most problematic behaviors are the end products of a chain of stimuli and responses. Stimulus control is most easily effected early in the chain, when elements in the chain are relatively weak and serve as discriminative stimuli for many behaviors in addition to the problematic one. For example, it is much easier to say "no" to a door-to-door salesman when he first knocks on the door than when he is in the house.

Stimulus narrowing is used to decrease the frequency of problematic behavior. The client arranges the environment so that the range of stimuli that evokes the undesirable behavior decreases. In self-control programs for smoking, stimulus narrowing may involve progressively restricting the environment in which the person can smoke. First, there can be no smoking in the living room at home, then while driving, then around children, and so on. Some individuals smoke when they have a cup of coffee. Reduction in coffee consumption may lead to reduced smoking. Stimulus narrowing may be combined with response cost. In addition to restricting the behavior to certain times and places, other demands may be made that make the execution of the behavior cumbersome and time-consuming. A smoker, for example, may be required to put cigarettes in one place and matches in another, chew a stick of gum for ten minutes before lighting up, and sit in a specially designated smoking chair. The manipulation of physiological cues as a part of stimulus control is often more difficult because such cues are often ambiguous. However, it is possible to help clients find ways to reduce the frequency or strength of physiological cues that evoke problematic behavior. A smoker, for example, may chew nicotine gum to reduce craving.

A desired behavior can be encouraged by establishing stimuli that evoke that behavior or by increasing exposure to stimuli that already evoke the behavior. Insomnia, for example, has been treated by establishing stronger discriminative stimuli for sleep: Lie down intending to go to sleep only when you are sleepy; do not use your bed for anything other than sleeping (except sex); if once in bed you cannot go to sleep within ten minutes, get up and go to another room until you are sleepy (Bootzin, 1977).

Stimulus control is established slowly. Only a few elements should be introduced at one time, and no new element should be added until those already introduced are mastered. Stimulus control is generally used in combination with self-reinforcement and other methods described below. Effective stimulus control strategies can only be designed after an adequate behavioral analysis of the problem has been accomplished using data from self-observation.

To continue with our clinical example, the self-observational data suggest that snacking is associated with class and study breaks, is a social event, and may be evoked by a number of emotional and physiological cues other than hunger. When she eats, the client selects high calorie foods. The short-term goal is to reduce snacking. An attempt to eliminate the morning snack by using stimulus control could be made by suggesting that immediately after class (early in the chain) the client should go to a vending machine and purchase a diet soda (a competing behavior) that will hopefully produce body cues of fullness without calories. A similar strategy could be used for evening snacking. As treatment progressed, a number of other stimulus control strategies could be used. At meals, she could first eat high bulk, low calorie foods such as salads, raw vegetables, and fresh fruit. She could progressively narrow the setting (e.g., only in the dorm cafeteria) and activity (e.g., not while studying or watching TV) cues associated with eating. She could eliminate the presence of food in her dorm room, not carry money to buy food during the day, and tell her friends of her attempts to lose weight and elicit their support. It would also be useful to develop stimuli that would promote exercise. One or more of her friends who exercise regularly might be asked to invite her to exercise with them at a specific time ("Let's go swimming before dinner. I'll pick you up in your room at 4:30"). Thus exercise is tied to social cues and a specific time of day, and may even be used as a competing behavior for eating.

Self-Reinforcement. Self-reinforcement involves teaching clients to self-reinforce or punish themselves when a designated target behavior has been performed. Self-reinforcement operations parallel those of operant procedures that were detailed in the last chapter. Self-reinforcement may entail positive self-reinforcement, negative self-reinforcement, self-punishment, and self-imposed response cost. These operations may involve the manipulation of material, activity, or verbal-symbolic events.

Persons engage in positive self-reinforcement when they contingently provide themselves with a desired material object (e.g., clothes, jewelry, records, or concert tickets), access to a desired activity (e.g., TV, a movie, or a night on the town), or self-praise (e.g., "Good job!" or "I did that well"). This may involve the presentation of a new or usually unavailable reinforcer (e.g., a luxury item) or the initial denial of an everyday positive reinforcer (e.g., TV, a cup of coffee, or time to socialize) and the later administration of that reinforcer contingent on performance of the desired behavior. Positive self-reinforcement is an integral part of nearly every self-control program and is as effective in changing behavior as external positive reinforcement (see, e.g., Bolstad & Johnson, 1972).

The other forms of self-reinforcement have been less frequently used in self-control programs. Self-punishment entails applying an aversive event (e.g., snapping your wrist with a rubber band), an aversive activity (e.g., doing disliked work like cleaning the toilet), or an aversive verbal-symbolic phrase (e.g., saying "What a screw up," or "You really blew that one!") contingent on the performance of an undesirable behavior. Self-imposed response cost involves the loss of positive materials (e.g., giving money to a disliked organization like the Ku Klux Klan) or access to a high probability activity (e.g., watching TV). Negative self-reinforcement is exemplified by not going out on a date until a study assignment is completed. Although there are data that support the effectiveness of self-punishment, self-imposed response cost, and negative self-reinforcement, more research is needed to establish their utility clearly. The problem with the use of self-administered aversive events is that events that are sufficiently aversive to be effective also jeopardize their self-administration; their successful use is somewhat masochistic (Mahoney & Arnkoff, 1978).

To be effective, self-reinforcement must be carefully implemented. Kanfer (1975) suggests the following steps. First, select appropriate reinforcers. Identify those events and activities that are reinforcing for the client. This may include luxury items, but it is often more effective to use everyday events and activities that the person normally self-administers noncontingently. Some novel reinforcers may be used as special incentives. Material, activity, and verbal-symbolic reinforcers must be selected on the basis of the client's history and preference; what is reinforcing depends on the client. Several reinforcers should be identified and may include both "small" and "large" reinforcers. Second, clearly and concisely define response-reinforcement contingencies. Variations in the target response should be listed, and the concise conditions and methods for the delivery of the self-reinforcement should be discussed. The type of reinforcement should be compatible with the target behavior. Eating a large meal as a reinforcer for losing weight would be counterproductive. Third, practice the self-reinforcement procedure. Rehearse with the client several instances of the target behavior and the contingent application of the reinforcer. This insures that the client understands and is able to implement the procedure. Fourth, continue self-observation and revise the self-reinforcement procedures as warranted by the data. It is also useful to incorporate self-observation and self-recording of self-administered reinforcement to assess the client's correct use of these procedures.

Let us apply these principles to our clinical example. A number of positive verbal-symbolic self-reinforcers could be identified: "Good, I didn't snack this morning"; "When I exercise, I really care about myself"; "I'm looking good and feeling better"; "Terrific, I ate more salad and didn't have any dessert." These would be contingently applied each time the client drank a diet soda rather than snacked, selected low rather than high calorie foods, ate only in the dorm cafeteria, and went swimming with her friend. A daily tally of successes and failures could be kept, with backup activity and material reinforcers then exchanged for these successes and failures. Thus, for a specified number of successes, she could purchase jewelry, makeup, and clothing; make phone calls; or go to sporting events or the movies. Sometimes idiosyncratic reinforcers also work well. For example, this client might draw a silhouette of her body and, contingent on her successes, snip off small portions of that silhouette. Failures could be punished by giving money to a "right to life" organization that she dislikes.

Alternate Response Training. In alternate response training, a client is taught a response that is incompatible with the response to be controlled or eliminated. To replace the problematic behavior successfully, the alternate response must be in the client's repertoire and be at least somewhat reinforcing.

The most common form of alternate response training in self-control interventions focuses on the reduction of anxiety or stress. Relaxation (see Chapter 12) has been widely used as an alternate response to negative emotions and stress. After the person learns how to relax deeply and quickly, relaxation can be used in a self-controlling manner in those situations that evoke anxiety or stress.

In the clinical example, the client appears to eat in response to negative affect (e.g., feeling bitchy, tired, or bored) as well as to hunger. We would help her to differentiate negative emotions from hunger and teach her to engage in relaxation (or perhaps exercise) when she experiences negative affect.

Evaluation of Self-Control Interventions

Behavior change procedures can be viewed on a continuum in terms of the degree to which clients play an active role in altering their own behavior. In self-control programs, clients are obviously involved in the behavior change process but are still subject to influences from the external environment. Operant programs represent the other end of the continuum. In operant conditioning, external agents alter clients' environment to effect behavior change. But even then, clients exert control over what transpires. To the extent that clients have the ability and inclination to be involved in their own behavior change, they should be encouraged to do so. Such involvement is consistent with the compensatory model of helping, is congruent with the amount of control that individuals normally exert over their own environment and behavior, and enhances the likelihood that the behavior change will be maintained over time.

However, self-control programs are futile if clients do not accept a treatment goal or are not motivated to change a target behavior. Even when these conditions are met, self-control programs require that clients adhere to the recommended self-controlling actions. Such adherence is often difficult to attain. Natural contingencies discourage adherence to self-reinforcement. For example, if our client decided to have a high calorie snack (a big piece of cake) in the late evening, she could choose not to engage in the response cost and to purchase a backup reinforcer anyway. She thus has the pleasure of eating the snack at no cost (having your cake and eating it too?). In other words, it is often immediately reinforcing to cheat on the self-control program.

Motivating people to change behaviors that are reinforcing and maintaining positive treatment effects are critical issues. Recent reviews of the application of self-control procedures to two major health problems, smoking and obesity, reflect these concerns. Self-control training does lead to a reduction or a cessation of smoking in those clients who complete the training, but about 50 percent of clients who begin training drop out. Of those who do complete training, only 25 to 40 percent have maintained these gains a year later (Leventhal & Cleary, 1980). A similar although somewhat brighter picture can be painted for the self-control of weight. The average weight reduction resulting from self-control programs is 10 to 15 pounds. But approximately 15 to 20 percent of clients drop out before training is completed. Those who do complete self-control training maintain the 10- to 15-pound weight loss during the year after program completion (Brownell, 1982). This suggests that we need to focus on strategies to keep people in treatment (i.e., enhance the motivation to change) and to maintain self-controlling behaviors over a long period. Let us look at how we can accomplish this.

Dropout and Relapse Prevention. Many individuals who drop out of treatment feel that they simply cannot change. Their numerous past attempts to alter the problem have resulted in failure. They often are unable to avoid temptation completely, even when in a self-control program, and view their failure as proof of their lack of willpower. As a consequence, they give up. The goal of relapse prevention programs is to prevent dropout and to enhance the maintenance of behavior change (Marlatt & Parks, 1982).

Relapse is the failure to abstain from or to modulate habitual behavior appropriately. Our client, for example, may "slip" one evening by drinking two beers and eating half a pizza. She may construe this failure as proof that she cannot change (i.e., will always be fat) and consequently terminate her efforts to change. Such failure experiences are common. Clients must be taught the skills needed to anticipate and cope with potential failure. High-risk situations for relapse need to be identified. These typically entail experiences of negative emotion, interpersonal conflict, or direct and indirect social pressure to engage in the problematic behavior. For our client, feeling boredom and other negative affect and going to the snack bar with friends after class are high risk situations. Without the specific skills to deal with these situations, she may fail and give up trying.

Self-observation can be used to help clients identify high-risk situations. These situations are characterized by multiple, strong cues for engaging in the problematic behavior. The client can then develop strategies to avoid such situations if possible. If they cannot be avoided, other coping skills need to be learned and practiced to deal with temptation. Our client might simply decide not to go to the snack bar. She may assertively tell her friends that she would like to spend time with them, but would prefer not to go to the snack bar. If she does go or finds herself in other situations that are strong occasions for eating, she could select low calorie foods and learn to refuse offers to split a pizza or to share a pitcher of beer.

Despite our best efforts, most persons will succumb to temptation and engage in the undesired behavior (e.g., eat candy, have just one beer, or bum a cigarette). Clients often interpret this one failure as a complete or total failure and therefore as "justification" for giving up further efforts. An individual who has successfully dieted for five days eats a forbidden cookie and then goes on to finish all the cookies. An individual with an alcohol problem has one glass of wine at a wedding after abstaining for three months. He feels he has "fallen off the wagon" and might just as well drink all he wants. The list could be extended for other behaviors. It is thus important to teach clients to anticipate possible failure and to engage in cognitive and behavioral responses to modulate and control that behavior despite the failure (e.g., to get right back on the wagon). In fact, failure may be purposefully programmed into treatment to provide the client with opportunities to experience and then to cope with failure.

COGNITIVE THERAPY

The term cognitive refers to the private or internal representation and manipulation of external events and experiences: evaluation, thinking, imagery, problem solving, and memory. It refers to the processing that occurs between our experience of environmental stimuli and our production of some overt response to those stimuli (see Figure 11-2). We have already referred to cognitive mediation in discussing observational learning, systematic desensitization, and self-control. Cognitive processes are involved in all forms of human learning, including operant and respondent conditioning. In operant conditioning, for example,

FIGURE 11-2 Steps in Cognitive Processing

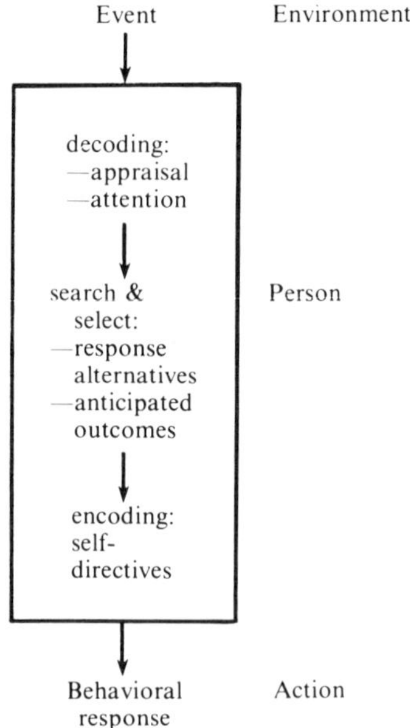

learning from response consequences is attributable to the informational and incentive functions of rewards and punishers. That is, we learn to anticipate that certain behaviors will lead to predictable outcomes: If we study hard, we will get good grades; if we do not wear seat belts, we are more likely to be seriously injured. Respondent conditioning requires that an individual realizes that conditioned and unconditioned stimuli are correlated. Conditioned stimuli do not automatically elicit a response but do so because they enable a person to predict the occurrence of unconditioned stimuli. Thus, operant and respondent conditioning are not automatic "stamping in" processes but depend on a cognitive representation of environmental stimuli and contingencies (Wilson & O'Leary, 1980).

Cognitive intervention consists of a diverse set of principles and procedures that share certain basic assumptions: (1) individuals learn adaptive and maladaptive behavior and affect through cognitive processes like selective attention, symbolic coding, problem solving, and self-instruction; (2) these cognitive processes can be activated and altered via basic learning principles; and (3) the therapeutic task is the assessment of maladaptive cognitive processes and the subsequent arrangement of learning experiences to alter these processes and the behavior with which they are correlated (Mahoney, 1977). The focus of cognitive therapy is to identify those attributions, thoughts, images, and self-verbalizations that contribute to problematic emotions, actions, and physiological responses, and then to modify those cognitive processes to promote better functioning. Let us survey in detail the procedures used in cognitive therapy.

Cognitive Intervention Procedures: Assessment and Conceptualization Training

The first objective in cognitive intervention is to assess thoroughly the behavioral, affective, and physiological components of the presenting problem and to identify those cognitive responses that contribute to the problem. The overt presenting problem must be identified and clearly defined as in operant or self-control procedures. The specification may be behavioral (e.g., smoking, failure to take medication, or avoidance of a health care procedure), affective (e.g., anxiety, depression, or anger), physiological (e.g., headaches, nausea, or heart palpitations), or some combination of the three.

The next step is to specify maladaptive cognitive responses that contribute to this problem. Initial specification is often accomplished in an interview. The client is asked to recall recent occurrences of the target problem and the context in which it occurred. The therapist probes for appraisals, thoughts, images, and self-talk that accompany the target problem. This interview assessment can be elaborated by simulating the recalled event via role playing or imagery. Client self-observation and self-recording are then utilized to assess the frequency and function of maladaptive cognitions systematically as they covary with the target problem in the natural environment. This also provides information about the range of environmental events that evoke the maladaptive cognitions and the target problem.

Several types of maladaptive cognitions may be assessed. Although oversimplified, the cognitive processing that occurs between experiencing an environmental event and making some response to that event entails three steps. The event must first be decoded, appraised, and interpreted. Then, of all the responses available to the person, one must be selected that is congruent with the goals of the person and the anticipated consequences of that response. Finally, once a response is selected, the execution of the response needs to be encoded and directed (McFall, 1982). This three-part process is shown in Figure 11-2. An example will clarify this processing. Suppose you are playing tennis. Your opponent's volley must be decoded in terms of its location and speed. You then need to search your repertoire of possible returns given the characteristics of the volley, your own capabilities, and the anticipated consequences of various kinds of returns. Finally, you must remind yourself how to execute the return you selected.

Two points are apparent from this example. First, a problematic outcome (an unsuccessful return) can result from incorrectly processing any of the three steps. You may misperceive an event (misjudge the location or speed of the volley), incorrectly scan your repertoire, and/or select a response in a way that is likely to produce a desired outcome (deciding to use a cross-court backhand when that is your weakness or when your opponent is likely to anticipate that return), or you may not carefully encode the response (not keeping your feet uncrossed and extending your arm). In other words, the problem may occur during decoding (see, e.g., Beck, 1976), response selecting and evaluating (see, e.g., D'Zurilla & Goldfried, 1971), or encoding (Meichenbaum & Goodman, 1969). The nature of the maladaptive cognitive processing varies from client to client.

The second obvious point from the example is that this cognitive processing seems more lengthy and elaborate than what we typically experience. In our daily experience, cognitive processing is abbreviated and often automatic. The seemingly automatic response we make to events is adaptive in many ways. Elaborate processing of stimuli in order to respond would often interfere with adaptation (you would never be able to return the volley if you had to do all of this thinking explicitly). In fact, most well-learned behaviors *are* automatic, for the processing is highly telescoped. However, the automatic and abbreviated nature of the day-to-day processing associated with overlearned responses may also be problematic. If some part of that processing is in error, we continue to experience bad outcomes while being relatively unaware of the causative processing error.

Consequently, cognitive assessment plays a second role in that it helps clients become more aware of automatic but problematic cognitive processing. It helps clients to conceptualize the target problem as a function of erroneous decoding, searching and selecting, and encoding processes. From the interview and self-observational procedures, clients inductively learn that their behavioral, affective, and physiological problems may result in part from "stinking thinking." This shared conceptualization is explicitly elaborated in client-therapist interaction and sets the stage for cognitive therapy. In addition to enhancing clients' awareness of maladaptive processing, the goals of cognitive intervention are to develop more adaptive modes of processing via rehearsal and practice and to use this adaptive processing to ameliorate the problem (Meichenbaum, 1977).

For a more concrete appreciation of cognitive intervention, let us again use a clinical example. Let us assume that we are working with a client who is scheduled for an endoscopic examination. In this procedure, the client is required to swallow a long tube that is used to assess gastric problems. This is a relatively distressing task for most clients, because the reflexive response to swallowing such an object is to gag. When clients respond with tension and a lack of cooperation, the discomfort and distress are increased. We have been informed that the client's general response to previous diagnostic procedures (like a GI series) has been characterized by extreme anxiety, vociferous complaints, and a lack of cooperation. A previous attempt at an endoscopic examination was a disaster.

We might begin by explaining to the client that our goal is to reduce the discomfort and anxiety he experiences when participating in diagnostic and treatment procedures by helping him find more effective ways to cope. Because we do not have the time or opportunity to have the client self-observe and self-record in this particular case, we will have to rely on assessment information based on an interview and imaginal recall. The client will be asked to describe diagnostic and treatment procedures he has previously experienced that resulted in distress. He will then be asked to recall them, one at a time, as vividly and completely as possible, just as if he were experiencing them right now, starting with his experiences before the procedure and continuing until the procedure was over. We want him to do a "slow motion replay" and to describe thoroughly the setting (e.g., where it took place, who was there, and what the equipment looked like), what was said by himself and others, what he was sensing (e.g., odors, tactile stimuli, and his own physiology), what he was doing, thinking and feeling, and how others responded. It might be useful to model such a recall for him and to ask him to do a "replay" of a salient but unrelated experience prior to engaging in the recall of the distressing medical procedures.

As he recalls several experiences, we are interested in assessing the manner in which he appraises the procedures (encoding), how he thinks about handling his distress (searching and selecting), how he tries to self-direct his response (encoding), and how this processing might exacerbate his anxiety, distress, and lack of cooperation. An abbreviated version of his cognitive processing of the previous endoscopic exam might be:

> [prior to the procedure] Oh, my God, I wonder what this is going to be like. I've heard it's really awful. My brother-in-law told me it was one of the worst things he's ever experienced. I want to get out of here. Jeez, I'm shaking like a leaf. Now they're putting on rubber gloves—this must be messy. Look at that hose, I'll never be able to get that down. Oh, this is going to be awful. I can't do it. [during the procedure] The tube makes me want to throw up. I can't help it. There's no way of letting them know. I'm choking, I want to scream. I have to stop them. They're forcing it anyway. Tears are running down my face, don't they notice? This is even worse than I thought. What if something gets torn down there? I can feel them pulling out the tube. [after the procedure] I feel weak. I might faint. I simply will not put up with this again. They can take their hose and shove it.

The client's processing clearly amplifies the discomfort associated with the medical procedure. He focuses on its most noxious aspects. He lacks basic information about what is going to happen, and he fantasizes about unrealistic dangers and outcomes. He lacks any coping strategies and feels helpless. He focuses on his own discomfort and negative affective and physiological reactions. He sees himself as a failure. This manner of thinking simply creates additional discomfort and distress; makes the procedure more difficult, painful, and lengthy; and sensitizes him to any medical procedures in the future.

In developing a shared conceptualization with our client, we might acknowledge that endoscopy and other procedures are often unpleasant and that it is natural to tense up and fight them. But it seems that his thoughts and actions are counterproductive, and that they make things even worse than they are. This is like tensing when you are trying to float in the water. The more you tense, the more difficult it is to float, so the more you tense, and thus a vicious circle develops. What we need to do is to work on ways to think about the procedure and on things to do during the procedure to minimize the discomfort rather than making it worse.

After an assessment and development of a shared conceptualization, we would work with the client to develop a set of cognitive and behavioral skills to correct the target problem.

Cognitive and Behavioral Skills Training. The primary goal of cognitive training is to teach the client to engage in more adaptive appraisal, problem solving, and self-instruction. This may be complemented by helping the client acquire effective behavioral coping skills. The first task is to generate a number of adaptive self-statements appropriate to the problem at hand. The relative utility of these statements is thoroughly discussed with the client. Some generalized examples of adaptive self-statements are shown in Table 11-1. These general statements can be elaborated and made more specific to the client, the presenting problem, and the nature of the maladaptive cognitions.

Modeling, rehearsing, and shaping are then used to enable the client to acquire and practice adaptive self-talk and imagery. First, the therapist models the process by verbally recalling and describing the problematic situations in slow motion and by engaging in adaptive self-

TABLE 11-1 Examples of Adaptive Self-Statements

Forming General Strategies
Be ready for maladaptive thinking.
Fear and tension are signals to cope.
Use problem- and coping-oriented thoughts.

Getting Ready for the Stressor
I'm prepared for this task.
Make plans. What can I do?
Worry is O.K.; it doesn't have to interfere.
I'm feeling tense—just need to relax.
What's happening now? How can I respond?
I'm feeling panicked. I can handle my feelings by describing them.

Confronting the Stressor
Remember my strategies; use as many as needed.
O.K., here it comes, just take it one step at a time.
Relax, breathe deeply and slowly.
Distract myself, think of the 1964 Yankees baseball line-up.
I can manage.
Keep it in proportion. What are the facts?

Dealing with Critical Periods
I knew this would happen. I can deal with it.
Focus on a strategy. What can I do?
I can't wipe this out but I can manage it.
Just a little longer; this will end.
Relax, focus attention.

Making Self-Evaluative Statements
I'm doing O.K. so far.
I've got a number of coping strategies going.
This is going well. What else can I try?
Good job. I'm staying with my plan.
It's working.

talk aloud. The client is then asked to do the same, and the therapist reinforces approximations of the desired cognitive coping responses and provides suggestions and feedback about possible improvements. Behavioral coping responses relevant to the problem are also modeled, rehearsed, and integrated with the cognitive coping training. This process continues until the client can adeptly engage in adaptive self-talk and behavior across multiple problem situations. A role-playing simulation of problem situations can also be used. Once the client becomes skilled at using overt coping verbalizations during these training trials, the client practices using covert verbalization during imaginal recall or role playing of the problem situations.

We could individualize the examples of self-talk listed in Table 11-1 for the client facing the endoscopic examination. More specific examples focusing on the sensations associated with the procedure (e.g., feeling the tube in his mouth and experiencing the gag reflex) could be developed. Self-directives and behavioral coping skills relevant to the procedure could also be developed. The self-directives might include, "I can feel myself gagging; I just need to relax as much as possible"; "Don't fight it; that only makes it worse"; and "This is time limited; only a few more minutes to go." Useful coping skills might include relaxation training.

Skills Transfer Training. The purpose of transfer training is to insure that the cognitive skills established in the therapeutic setting generalize to the client's natural environment. Thus, the focus of treatment is shifted to home practice and in vivo use of the newly acquired cognitive and behavioral skills. Initially, transfer training entails requesting the client to engage in daily practice of the skills at home. This practice is carefully structured. A list of problem situations, typical maladaptive cognitions, and adaptive self-statements and actions are provided. The client imagines the problem situations and practices replacing maladaptive cognitive and behavioral responses with more adaptive ones. The goal is overlearning. Ideally, the new skills should become "second nature" to the client.

When home practice appears to have resulted in overlearning, the second phase of transfer training begins. The client is now instructed to use the cognitive and behavioral skills in problem situations as they occur in day-to-day experiences. The client continues to self-observe problem situations as well as the cognitive and behavioral responses to those situations. The adequacy of the client's performance in the natural environment is monitored in therapy, and further practice and refinement of the skills occur as needed. Intervention continues until the client is capable of successfully coping with a wide range of problem situations and the target presenting problem improves.

In our clinical example, we would ask the client to practice self-statements and relaxation prior to the endoscopy. Insofar as the client appears to experience a generalized problem in coping with medical procedures that cause discomfort, it would be useful to extend the training and transfer practice to other medical procedures that he is likely to experience in the future. We could enhance the transfer to actual situations by exposing him to a series of graded experimental tasks (e.g., a cold pressor test and a rectal exam) that would provide him with the opportunity for practice "under fire."

Cognitive Intervention: A Summary

Cognitive intervention focuses on the systematic alteration of private thought processes to address overt affective, behavioral, and physiological problems. Cognitive intervention is an extension of the traditional learning approaches to covert responses. It differs from more traditional forms of psychotherapy in that covert, cognitive processes are carefully defined in observable terms and traditional learning processes (modeling, instructions, rehearsal, and reinforcement) are explicitly and systematically used to alter cognitions.

Cognitive intervention is clearly related to self-control. Clients learn to alter their own behavior by changing their thought processes. They are responsible for gathering the data and for practicing and utilizing the newly acquired skills. Cognitive and more purely behavioral methods can be integrated to provide a comprehensive multielement intervention that simultaneously addresses cognitive, behavioral, and physiological processes.

Cognitive-behavioral interventions have a broad range of applications in behavioral health and medicine. They have been used to modify both health-impairing and health-promoting behaviors in clinical and preventative contexts (e.g., smoking, overeating, and Type A behavior), to alter health-related decisions and actions (e.g., hypertension screening, genetic screening, and timely recognition of symptoms and utilization of services), and to alleviate distress related to illness, injury, and aversive diagnostic and treatment procedures (e.g., headache and operant pain, cardiac catheterization, and dental procedures). They have been used to enhance the adjustment and satisfaction of individuals with chronic medical problems and, in preventative programs, to enhance persons' general ability to cope with stress. Some of these applications will be described in Chapters 13 to 16.

HEALTH ENHANCEMENT AND EDUCATION

In providing examples of behavioral, cognitive, and self-control interventions, the primary focus has been on one-to-one or small-group interventions in clinical settings. However, these change technologies are also applicable to prevention and education in school, work, and community settings. Such large-group interventions have several advantages. First, they reach more people. This is an important consideration given the number of persons who could benefit and the economic costs involved in a wide-scale program. Second, intervention in the natural setting may actually enhance change. The behavior change process occurs in the natural environment, where it ultimately must be maintained. Community-based interventions can also take advantage of existing social support for behavior change. Third, effective education and prevention, by definition, must address a very broad audience. It would simply not be feasible to do this using small-scale approaches.

Research on risk reduction, health promotion, and health education on the community level is still in its infancy. The results of such programs are modest but promising (Matarazzo, Weiss, Herd, Miller, & Weiss, 1984). We will review several examples of these programs and provide a more explicit evaluation of their efficacy in Chapters 13 to 16.

SUMMARY

As detailed in Chapters 2 and 3, health status is strongly influenced by individuals' cognitions and behaviors. Traditional medical practitioners have failed to address these responses adequately due to a lack of an effective technology to engender change. In most cases, health providers cannot directly alter clients' environment and have not successfully altered clients' thinking. Self-control and cognitive interventions provide the means by which health practitioners can teach clients to alter their own covert and overt responses. Both types of intervention entail the use of basic learning principles detailed in the previous chapter. But in this case, clients act as their own change agents. This promotes clients' responsibility and involvement in their own health care. Outcome research suggests that self-control and cognitive interventions are potentially effective methods to alter a wide variety of health- and illness-related behaviors in clinical and preventative settings. The full potential of these methods has not been realized. The behavior change that results from self-control and cognitive interventions is often modest and relatively short-lived. These methods require additional elaboration and evaluation to attain their full potential. This may entail their combination with more traditional medical interventions (e.g., changing eating behavior and dieting, or changing smoking behavior and using nicotine gum). In any case, self-control and cognitive interventions provide a powerful tool to promote health and reduce risk for disease.

REFERENCES

Bandura, A. (1969). *Principles of behavior modification*. New York: Holt, Rinehart & Winston.

Beck, A. T. (1976). *Cognitive therapy and the emotional disorders*. New York: International Universities Press.

Bolstad, O. D., & Johnson, S. M. (1972). Self-regulation in the modification of disruptive behavior. *Journal of Applied Behavior Analysis, 5,* 443–454.

Bootzin, R. R. (1977). Effects of self-control procedures on insomnia. In R. B. Stuart (Ed.), *Behavioral self-management: Strategies, techniques and outcome*, 176–195. New York: Brunner/Mazel.

Brownell, K. D. (1982). Obesity: Understanding and treating a serious, prevalent and refractory disorder. *Journal of Consulting and Clinical Psychology, 50,* 820–840.

D'Zurilla, T. J., & Goldfried, M. R. (1971). Problem solving and behavior modification. *Journal of Abnormal Psychology, 78,* 107–126.

Kanfer, F. H. (1975). Self-management methods. In F. H. Kanfer & A.P. Goldstein (Eds.), *Helping people change*, 283–345. New York: Pergamon Press.

Kanfer, F. H. & Phillips, J. S. (1970). *Learning foundations of behavior therapy*. New York: John Wiley & Sons.

Kazdin, A. E. (1980). *Behavior modification*. Homewood, IL: The Dorsey Press.

Leventhal, H., & Cleary, P. D. (1980). The smoking problem: A review of the research and theory in behavioral risk modification. *Psychological Bulletin, 88,* 370–405.

Mahoney, M. J. (1977). Reflections on the cognitive trend in psychotherapy. *American Psychologist, 32,* 5–13.

Mahoney, M. J., & Arnkoff, D. B. (1978). Cognitive and self-control therapies. In S. L. Garfield & A. E. Bergin (Eds.), *Handbook of psychotherapy and behavior change* (2nd ed.), 689–722. New York: John Wiley & Sons.

Marlatt, G. A., & Parks, G.A. (1982). Self-management of addictive disorders. In P. Karoly & F. H. Kanfer (Eds.), *Self-management: From theory to practice*, 443–488. New York: Pergamon Press.

Matarazzo, J. D., Weiss, S. M., Herd, J. A., Miller, N. E., & Weiss, S. M. (1984). *Behavioral health: A handbook of health enhancement and disease prevention*. New York: John Wiley & Sons.

McFall, R. M. (1982) A review and reformulation of the concept of social skills. *Behavioral Assessment, 4,* 1–33.

Meichenbaum, D. (1977). *Cognitive-behavior modification*. New York: Plenum Press.

Meichenbaum, D., & Goodman, J. (1969). The development of operant motor responding by verbal operants. *Journal of Experimental Child Psychology, 7,* 553–565.

Wilson, G. T., & O'Leary, K. D. (1980). *Principles of behavior therapy*. Englewood Cliffs, NJ: Prentice-Hall.

12

Biofeedback and Relaxation Training

INTRODUCTION

> Before Harry Houdini performed one of his famous escapes, a skeptical committee would search his clothes and body. When the members of the committee were satisfied that the Great Houdini was concealing no keys, they would put chains, padlocks and handcuffs on him. . . . Of course, not even Houdini could open a padlock without a key, and when he was safely behind the curtain he would cough one up. He could hold a key suspended in his throat and regurgitate it when he was unobserved. . . . The trick behind many of Houdini's escapes was in some ways just as amazing as the escape itself. Ordinarily, when an object is stuck in a person's throat he will start to gag. He can't help it—it's an unlearned automatic reflex. But Houdini had learned to control his gag reflex by practicing for hours with a small piece of potato tied to a string (Lang, 1970, p. 39).

Many other seemingly unusual degrees of control over physiological processes have been reported. Anand (1961) reported that an Indian yogi confined in a sealed metal box was able to reduce his oxygen consumption and metabolism dramatically. Lindsley and Sassomon (1983) reported that a man had the ability to control the erection of hairs over his whole body. Such acts of control have previously been viewed as extraordinary; only a few individuals could accomplish such feats.

Recent work suggests that most people can exert control over what are usually considered "involuntary" physiological responses, such as blood pressure, heart rate, and brain activity. This control can be learned by using training procedures called biofeedback and relaxation training. Often, these procedures have been offered as effective treatments of illnesses not addressed by current medical intervention (Freeman, 1973) or as modes that allow you to control the state of your health, happiness, and well-being solely through the powers of your mind (Birk, 1973). These claims are grossly exaggerated. However, these procedures may offer an effective treatment modality different than that of traditional medicine.

In this chapter, the procedures described as biofeedback and relaxation training will be defined and described. The applications and effectiveness of these procedures will be assessed, and a conceptualization of how these procedures work will be made using the systems model of medicine and the compensatory model of helping.

BIOFEEDBACK

Biofeedback refers to a set of procedures used to teach a person to control visceral, somatic, and central nervous system activities by electronically recording and processing information about those activities and displaying it to the person. It makes available information about body processes that is usually unavailable. On the basis of this information, the person can learn to control physiological processes.

Feedback is integral to biological homeostasis. Feedback also provides the basis for learning. Consider a person learning to serve a ball in tennis. If the ball hits the net (discrepancy from the reference value), she may hit the ball harder or change the arc of her swing (corrective output). Reinforcement as described in the last two chapters is a form of informational feedback.

Viewed in this light, biofeedback is not new or startling. We have engaged in it since the first days of our lives, when we stuck our hands in front of our faces and watched where they went or what they did. At a descriptive level, biofeedback is not different than what continuously occurs within our bodies and in the process of learning. What is unique about biofeedback is its application to control body functions previously thought to be involuntary. Biofeedback simply involves the addition of special monitoring equipment to pick up and feed back information about these body functions. This information is then used by the individual to alter those body functions systematically and in a manner consistent with the instructions given (see Figure 12-1).

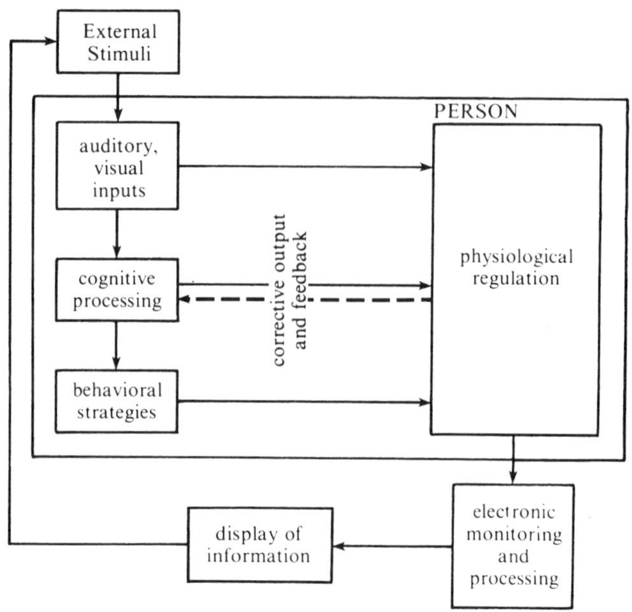

FIGURE 12-1 Biofeedback in the Feedback-Homeostasis Paradigm

Control over "Involuntary" Responses

Traditionally, visceral responses were thought to be altered only by classical conditioning procedures, whereas somatomotor (skeletal muscle) responses were thought to be altered via operant conditioning (see Chapter 10). For example, you could easily train someone to raise his arm by giving him a dollar each time he did so. But it would be difficult to get someone to raise his blood pressure via the same means. The person does not receive sufficient information about his blood pressure to know how it changes. However, during the 1960s several researchers demonstrated that, with biofeedback, persons could learn to control "involuntary" responses. For example, Kamiya (1969) showed that people could control the alpha rhythm activity of the brain, and Shapiro, Crider, and Tursky (1964) demonstrated that electrodermal activity could be operantly conditioned.

While the foundations for biofeedback were laid in these and similar studies, the "voluntary" control of visceral and central nervous system responses was not universally accepted. Many researchers suggested that subjects brought about these changes by altering skeletal-muscular activity or respiration. Thus, visceral control was really only a by-product of altering voluntary processes. A series of studies of visceral learning in animals (reviewed in Miller, 1969) established that the operant conditioning of visceral responses was not necessarily dependent on skeletal-muscular activity, and stimulated subsequent research on biofeedback. Miller and his colleagues used curare to block all skeletal-muscular activity in the subject animals, and then examined the degree to which the animals could control visceral activity using shock avoidance or brain stimulation as reinforcement. They found that the animals could vary heart rate and blood pressure independently, alter intestinal motility, and increase blood flow to one ear while decreasing it to the other.

The use of skeletal-muscular paralysis does not rule out other indirect means of influencing "involuntary" physiological responses, but how control is effected is not critical in many applications of biofeedback. Current research suggests there is some independence of skeletal-muscular and visceral activity and that the alteration of skeletal-muscular activity is not a necessary requirement for learned visceral control (Shapiro & Surwit, 1979). However, visceral and skeletal-muscular activity often vary together according to the situation (Obrist, 1976). From a clinical standpoint, how the person goes about controlling a visceral response is less important than being able to do so, as long as no destructive effects result from the mediating process.

The remarkable feature about biofeedback is the potential use of the selective control of specific physiological responses or patterns in treating various physical disorders.

Equipment

To understand the clinical use of biofeedback, it is necessary to know what types of physiological processes can be monitored, what the biofeedback apparatus does with that information, and how the information is displayed to the person. This describes what is going on in the monitoring half of the loop in Figure 12-1.

Although many different physiological processes may be monitored in biofeedback, the equipment has to carry out five basic functions: (1) detecting some electrical or mechanical signal of the body; (2) amplifying it; (3) filtering it; (4) converting it; and (5) displaying the signal to the individual. This is shown in Figure 12-2. To describe this process more specifically, let us use the feedback of skeletal-muscular activity (electromyographic, or EMG, biofeedback) as an example. (For the specifics of other physiological signals, see Olton & Noonberg, 1980.)

Muscle contraction is accompanied by electrical current from both neural and muscle activity. This activity can be measured by electrodes that are placed on the skin over the muscle of interest or by needlelike electrodes that are inserted into the muscle. The signal picked up at this point looks like a series of spikes that vary in frequency and amplitude with the firing (tension) of the muscle. The size of the current is very

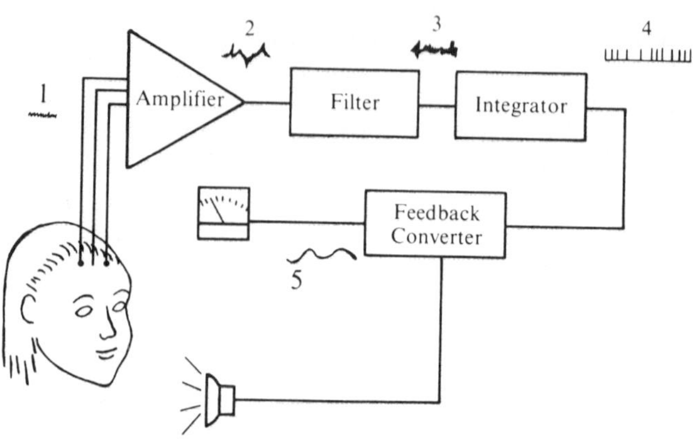

FIGURE 12-2 The Operation of Biofeedback Equipment

small (see Figure 12-1, step 1) and thus needs to be amplified (step 2). In addition to muscle activity, other electrical activity from the body (like heart beat) and from the external environment (e.g., the lights) is picked up, so that this unwanted information is filtered out (step 3). If the information was fed back to the person at this point, it would sound like static from a radio or look like a very complex series of spikes. In this complex form, it is not very useful. The equipment then integrates the information (sums the amount of muscle activity over a set period of time, e.g. every 30 seconds; see step 4) and converts it in a way to drive a speaker or meter that indicates the relative tension in the muscle being monitored. Thus, for example, a speaker's tone will increase in pitch as the muscle tenses and decrease in pitch as the muscle relaxes.

Two important aspects of biofeedback should be noted. First, the information is fed back quickly and precisely. Delayed feedback (e.g., seeing where a tennis ball lands hours after hitting it) is not useful. Precision is important so that the person can use changes in the desired direction to persist in the strategy that brought about that change. Second, the biofeedback apparatus does not do anything to the person. It does *not* cause a change in the person's physiology. The person must do that himself (the corrective output in Figure 12-1). The biofeedback equipment only provides the person with quick, accurate information about the physiological process being monitored.

In addition to EMG biofeedback, many other types of feedback are used. These include blood pressure, heart rate (electrocardiogram, or EKG), brain activity (electroencephalogram, or EEG), skin temperature, skin conductance (galvanic skin response, or GSR), and blood flow through body tissues. A detailed account of the physiology and biofeedback procedures associated with these responses can be found in Hassett (1978) and Gatchel and Price (1979).

Clinical Applications

Biofeedback can be used as a primary treatment in many disorders thought to be responsive only to medical treatment. Biofeedback cannot restore damaged tissue, but it can help persons to become more aware of physiological processes and to gain control over those processes. A list of some of the disorders to which biofeedback has been applied is presented in Table 12-1.

Several characteristics of these disorders should be noted. Some disorders, such as cardiac arrhythmias (irregular heartbeat) and postural hypotension (fainting when trying to stand up), are termed primarily organic because of the minimal involvement of psychosocial and behavioral variables. Other disorders, such as migraine headaches and essential hypertension, are termed functional because of the etiological involvement of psychosocial and behavioral variables. Even though biofeedback is mediated by learning, it is applicable to primarily organic as well as more functional disorders (Miller & Dworkin, 1977). In fact, Miller and Dworkin suggest that biofeedback alone may be less effective in more functional disorders because the symptoms are often strongly

TABLE 12-1 Clinical Applications of Biofeedback

DISORDER	TYPE OF FEEDBACK
Cardiovascular disorders	
Essential hypertension	Blood pressure GSR EMG
Postural Hypotension	Blood Pressure
Cardiac arrhythmias	EKG
Raynaud's disease	Skin temperature
Migraine headaches	Skin temperature EMG
Muscular disorders	
Muscle tension headaches	EMG
Neuromuscular disorder	EMG
Myofacial pain	EMG
Central nervous system disorders	
Epilepsy	EEG
Stress and anxiety	
Anxiety-related disorders	EMG EEG GSR
Stress management	EMG GSR EEG

reinforced by social attention or by avoidance of unpleasant activities or events (very similar to operant pain syndromes; see Chapter 9), and consequently the person is not motivated to use biofeedback to learn to control the symptom. In such cases, other cognitive-behavioral measures to teach more adaptive responses to aversive situations or to obtain positive reinforcement are needed. For example, if the assessment of a person who has migraine headaches indicates that the headaches occur primarily when the person is working with a supervisor and allow escape from the stressful situation, assertiveness training to teach the person more effective interpersonal skills may be used.

In primarily organic disorders, biofeedback may be used along with more traditional medical interventions. For example, blood pressure biofeedback may be used in conjunction with medication to treat essential hypertension. The point is that, although widely applicable, biofeedback is not the sole or primary treatment strategy for all disorders and all clients. Depending on the nature of the problem, biofeedback may be used as either an ancillary or a primary treatment.

Biofeedback has been applied to both tonic and phasic disorders. Tonic disorders are those in which the symptom is continuously present with only minimal variation in intensity. Cardiac arrhythmias and essential hypertension are examples of tonic disorders. Phasic disorders are those in which the symptom comes and goes, and varies in intensity depending on the situation. Migraine headaches and postural hypertension are examples of phasic disorders. Biofeedback strategies and goals are different for tonic and phasic disorders. In tonic disorders, the goal is to aid the person in developing continuous control over some physiological process. In hypertension, for example, the goal is a persistent reduction in blood pressure. In phasic disorders, biofeedback is used to teach a person to control a physiological process in those situations in which it becomes aberrant. With migraine headaches, the person needs to warm skin temperature when prodromal (warning) symptoms of a headache are first noticed.

Thus, biofeedback is useful for disorders that vary along the functional-organic and tonic-phasic dimensions. It will be used in different ways and in different combinations with other types of treatment depending on the characteristics of the disorder. An overview of the treatment of the four disorders is presented in Table 12-2. This, of course, oversimplifies matters because disorders can be tonic-phasic and functional-organic in many combinations and gradations.

The physiological information used as feedback for clinical disorders may be directly related to the clinical problem, as in blood pressure feedback for hypertension or EMG feedback for spastic muscles (see Table 12-1). However, the physiological information used as feedback is often related indirectly and perhaps in an unknown fashion to the physiological process causing clinical symptoms, as in EMG biofeedback

TABLE 12-2 Biofeedback Treatment Programs for Functional-Organic and Tonic-Phasic Disorder Combinations

DISORDER	EXAMPLE	TREATMENT
Functional-tonic	Essential hypertension	Feedback aimed at continuous control; use of cognitive-behavioral strategies and medical treatment
Functional-phasic	Muscle tension headache	Feedback aimed at situational control; use of cognitive-behavioral strategies and medical treatment
Organic-tonic	Cardiac arrhythmias	Feedback aimed at continuous control; medical treatment
Organic-phasic	Postural hypotension	Feedback aimed at situational control; medical treatment

for hypertension or skin temperature biofeedback for migraines. Indirect feedback is most often used when the physiological mechanism of the disorder being treated is unknown or when the biofeedback technology is not available to monitor a known physiological correlate of the disorder. Even when direct feedback is available, it is not necessarily more effective than indirect modes of feedback (see Patel, 1975, for an example).

Biofeedback has also been used for complaints that have predominantly behavioral or psychological rather than organic manifestations. This is particularly true for those problems associated with anxiety (and concomitant physiological arousal). Biofeedback can also be used as a facet of preventative interventions such as stress management (see Table 12-1).

Clinical Procedures

There is no standardized set of procedures used in the clinical application of biofeedback. To provide a general idea of its clinical use, a description of commonly used assessment and treatment strategies and a case study will be outlined. Remember, however, that the exact procedures used in any one case vary depending upon the nature of the disorder and the person being treated.

Assessment. As with any clinical problem, a thorough assessment of the presenting complaint is made from medical, behavioral, and environmental perspectives. In addition to the verbal description of the problem elicited in an interview, several other data sources and modes of collecting information are used. Consultation with the client's physician is needed. This consultative information includes the nature of the disorder, the types of interventions tried and currently in use, and the indications and contraindications for biofeedback. If the tonic-phasic and functional-organic natures of the disorder are unclear, self-monitoring of the problem by the client is initiated (and often continued throughout treatment). In self-monitoring, which was described in Chapter 11, the client observes and keeps a record of the frequency and intensity of the problem, the environmental antecedents and consequences associated with the problem, and a description of the cognitive-affective correlates of the problem. It is also common to obtain resting (nonstress) and stress-induced levels of physiological activity in several modalities (e.g., blood pressure, heart rate, and muscle tension).

Let us assume that a twenty-seven-year-old female client seeks biofeedback treatment because of recurring migraine headaches. These headaches occur three to four times per month and usually last from 12 to 18 hours. She describes them as beginning on one side of her head, around the eye, and slowly building in intensity over time. The pain is pulsating and intense, and is often accompanied by nausea and vomiting. Prior to a headache's onset, she is very sensitive to bright light and sees jagged lines in her visual field. A medical consultation confirms the diagnosis of migraine headaches. In the past, several drugs have been prescribed to control the headaches but have been ineffective.

The client works as a legal secretary and attends college classes in the evening. She describes herself as a perfectionist who likes to get her work done on time. She worries a great deal about her performance at both work and school. At this point, we would ask her to self monitor the frequency and intensity of her headaches and their environmental, cognitive, affective, and behavioral correlates. A record of one day of her recording is shown in Table 12-3.

These data are then analyzed to determine the nature of her disorder. Based on this analysis, the type of feedback to be used, if any, and the inclusion of other medical and/or cognitive-behavioral interventions are planned.

To continue with our clinical example, the disorder appears to be phasic and to have a functional component. The client's headaches occur in situations in which she feels pressured to perform with speed and accuracy. Typical thoughts in such situations focus on worry and self-criticism about her performance and on her inability to cope with others' (unreasonable) expectations. Feelings of anxiety and anger are often associated with these situations, and she may frequently receive attention from others contingent on her headache complaints. In this case, both biofeedback and cognitive-behavioral strategies would appear to be useful in helping her cope more effectively with pressure situations. Skin temperature biofeedback would be selected given the putative vascular involvement in migraine headaches. Assertiveness training (teaching

TABLE 12-3 Sample of Self–Monitoring Record of Events Associated with Onset of Headache

TIME	SITUATION	PHYSICAL SENSATIONS	THOUGHTS	FEELING (0–100)	BEHAVIOR
8 A.M.	Breakfast; husband says I look tired	—	Worry about getting to work on time, test at school tonight	Anxious (25) Hurt (30)	Rush through breakfast; forget my notebook
10 A.M.	At work; given a long report to type by noon	Upset stomach, tense neck	This is stupid; he could have given me this yesterday afternoon; now I won't have time to study at noon	Angry (60) Anxious (50)	Rush the typing; don't take time to talk to others
12 P.M.	At work; still typing	Tingling sensation, nausea	I'm making too many mistakes; how am I going to pass the test?	Angry (60) Anxious (70)	Eat and type at the same time; more coffee
2 P.M.	Given a 10-page report typed yesterday to be redone	Headache, left eye	Screw him; he should have edited the report before I typed it	Angry (80) Anxious (30)	Type frantically; make lot of mistakes; complain to a coworker
4 P.M.	Reports completed; cleaning up my desk	Headache worse, nausea worse	What a shot day! I feel crappy and there's nothing I could do about it.	Angry (50) Anxious (20)	Turn in reports; tell boss I'm ill and leave early

effective interpersonal skills) would be useful in teaching her to be more effective with her boss. Cognitive self-instruction (teaching her different modes of thinking and evaluating) may be used to alter her perfectionist demands and subsequent self-criticism of her own performance. Thus, the focus would be on physiological, behavioral, and cognitive facets of the problem.

Treatment. Treatment using biofeedback and other, ancillary procedures can be broken into several phases: control with feedback, transfer to self-control, and application.

Control with Feedback. Initially, treatment focuses on teaching new skills. Using biofeedback, the client is trained via shaping to control the physiological process being monitored. The client is given a series of trials with feedback and asked to alter the physiological process based on the feedback. Very small changes in the desired direction are reinforced via success and verbal praise. Over time, as the client can reliably demonstrate these small changes, larger changes in the desired direction are used as the criteria for reinforcement until the client can consistently bring about the desired amount of change. Specific strategies like relaxation, pleasant imagery, and the like (discussed later in this chapter) may be used to assist the client, or the client may be asked to experiment with her own strategies to see what works.

In the clinical example, hand temperature is fed back to our client using an auditory tone, with the increasing pitch of that tone indicating increasing hand temperature. The client is given a series of five-minute trials during a treatment session and is asked to try to increase her hand temperature by making the pitch of the tone increase using whatever strategies seem to work for her. The client's ability to raise her hand temperature during initial trials may be quite modest and variable. After each trial, verbal encouragement and reinforcement are given for small successes. The client may bring about a change in a direction opposite to that desired. This is often associated with thinking about some stressor (e.g., a task at work or an upcoming test) or simply trying too hard (perfectionism). This can be used to assist the client in becoming aware of the correlation between such events and decreasing hand temperature (and possibly headaches), and to use that awareness as a cue, after skills have been developed, to engage in more effective coping strategies. Over several sessions, the client learns to warm her hands via a continuation of the shaping process.

Following each biofeedback session, the clinician also helps the client learn cognitive and behavioral skills to cope more effectively with stress-producing situations. In the clinical example, this may involve role playing, modeling, and rehearsing more assertive ways to interact with her boss and alternative ways to evaluate her own performance.

Transfer to Self-Control. When the client has learned to increase skin temperature with feedback reliably, the next step is to teach her to generate that response without feedback so that it can be used in the natural environment. This is facilitated by trying to control the response on some trials when there is no feedback. When the client can reliably control the response without feedback, additional steps may be taken to insure that she can exert this control in actual stressful situations. This can be done by having her apply her recently acquired physiological, behavioral, and cognitive skills while imagining or role playing stress-evoking situations from the natural environment.

In our clinical example, we would ask our client to warm her hands on trials both with and without feedback. Once she could consistently warm her hands without feedback, we would ask her to imagine taking a difficult test while maintaining warm hands. Or we could role play an interaction in which her boss makes an unreasonable demand and ask her to respond in an assertive fashion while maintaining warm skin temperature. Thus, as a client acquires the various skills with assistance, that assistance fades away, and the various skills are practiced and integrated in an analog rehearsal of problematic situations from real life.

Application. As the client is able to engage in reliably effective physiological, cognitive, and behavioral responses in these analog situations, she would be asked to try them out in her natural environment. If effective, a reduction in the frequency and intensity of the symptoms would be expected. Further training, practice, and reinforcement would be carried out in subsequent sessions.

In the clinical example, the client would be asked to use her skills at work and school. Via continued self-monitoring, we would assess whether this resulted in a reduction of the frequency and intensity of her headaches, and provide her with additional practice or skills as needed.

Summary. The clinical application of biofeedback is a complex process. Biofeedback is not given to the client in mechanical manner. Throughout assessment and training, many strategies in addition to biofeedback are used. In all of these, the client is an active participant. The health provider and the client work together to understand and assess the problem and to develop and implement treatment to address it. The active involvement of the client is seen in self-monitoring during assessment, in learning control during biofeedback, and in practicing and using what is learned during generalization and application.

Biofeedback is usually only one part of a multifaceted program. Biofeedback focuses on learning to control some physiological process. Simultaneously, intervention may also focus on the cognitive-behavioral

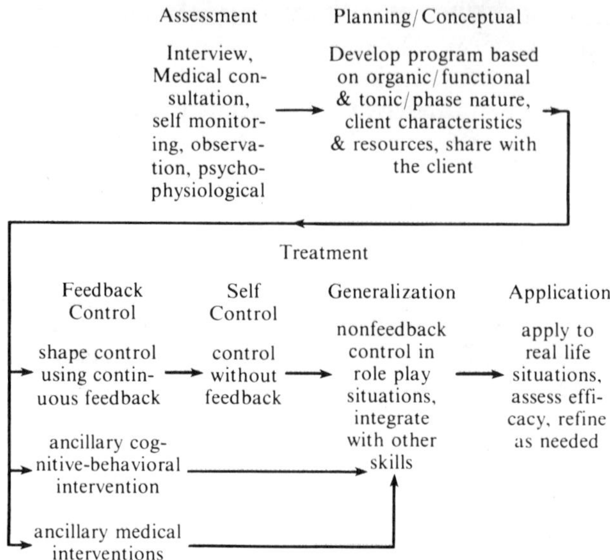

FIGURE 12-3 Flow Chart of Clinical Biofeedback

levels or on the physiological level via medical treatment. This is reflective of the systems approach to the assessment and treatment of clinical disorders. The exact combinations of treatments depend on the nature of the disorder and the characteristics and resources of the individual. A flow chart describing the clinical application of biofeedback is presented in Figure 12-3.

THE EFFECTIVENESS OF BIOFEEDBACK

Assessing the effectiveness of any treatment is a complex and lengthy process. Blanchard (1979) suggested six criteria for evaluating the effectiveness of biofeedback:

1. To what extent does treatment result in clinically significant change? To be effective, a change in the target symptom must be sufficiently large enough to be clinically meaningful. Small changes that are reliable may not be clinically significant.
2. To what extent do clinically significant changes persist over time? To be clinically useful, an effect must last a long time.
3. Do clinically significant effects transfer from the treatment to the natural environment? To be clinically effective, a client must be able to transfer reliably changes made in the treatment setting to the natural environment.
4. How many clients can exert a clinically significant change, make it persist, and demonstrate it in their natural environment? To be effective, the

treatment should be applicable to a broad range of individuals who have a given disorder.

5. To what degree are the changes observed due to the specific effects of biofeedback rather than placebo effects or the natural remission of the symptoms? Clients who receive biofeedback should show more improvement in target symptoms than those who receive either an equally believable but inert (placebo) treatment or no treatment.
6. To what extent are the results of biofeedback training replicated by several clinicians in different settings? Biofeedback effects should be robust enough to withstand small differences in procedures and characteristics of clinicians implementing treatment.

Other researchers have suggested the following additional criteria (American Psychiatric Association, 1979; Miller & Dworkin, 1977):

7. In terms of time, cost, and effectiveness, how does biofeedback compare with traditional medical and rehabilitative therapies and other cognitive-behavioral interventions? Biofeedback is time-consuming and costly. There may be alternate methods of treatment that are equally effective, less expensive, and more easily administered than biofeedback.
8. Are there any negative effects of biofeedback training? In clinical application, attention must be paid to unwanted or destructive effects of biofeedback.

A thorough, exhaustive review of data relevant to these questions would require a book in itself. A general view of current research on the effectiveness of biofeedback can be obtained from Table 12-4. This table is a compilation of several reviews of research on the common applications of biofeedback (Basmajian, 1979; Blanchard & Epstein, 1978; Gatchel & Price, 1979; Olton & Noonberg, 1980; Pepper, Ancoli, & Quinn, 1979; White & Tursky, 1982). Most of the criteria concerning the clinical effectiveness of biofeedback can be addressed from this summary table. The question of whether changes resulting from biofeedback training result in clinically significant changes can be assessed by looking at the column labeled "Results." For the disorders listed, biofeedback appears to result in significant clinical improvement in 50 to 70 percent of the clients treated (question 1 in the list above). The transfer and persistence of these effects (questions 2–4) can be assessed by looking at the column labeled "Maintenance." The long-term maintenance of the effects of biofeedback has not been convincingly demonstrated for many clinical applications. Thus, biofeedback seems to result in a clinically significant improvement for many disorders, but the duration of this effect may be short-lived.

The column labeled "Relative to Placebo or Relaxation" addresses whether the clinical improvement is due to nonspecific placebo effects or the specific effects of biofeedback. In many applications, biofeedback is not superior to less expensive relaxation procedures (question 7), and

TABLE 12-4 Summary of the Effectiveness of Biofeedback

DISORDER	RESULTS	RELATIVE TO PLACEBO OR RELAXATION	COMMENTS	MAINTENANCE
Hypertension	Positive but variable effects	Relaxation is equally effective	BP feedback has specific vascular effects	Transfer and maintenance not adequately demonstrated
Cardiac arrhythmias	Positive effects for tachycardia, maybe for PVCs		Has specific direct effects on HR	Transfer and maintenance not adequately demonstrated
Migraine headaches	Positive effects with temperature feedback	Relaxation is also effective; may be a placebo effect	Temperature feedback leads to general SNS effects	Transfer and maintenance adequately demonstrated
Tension headaches	Positive effects with EMG feedback	Relaxation is also effective; may be a placebo effect	EMG is not specific to tension headaches	Transfer and maintenance adequately demonstrated
Raynaud's disease	Positive effects with temperature feedback	Relaxation is also somewhat effective	Better than medical treatment	Transfer and maintenance not adequately demonstrated
Neuromuscular reeducation	Positive effects with integrated EMG in 60% of the cases		Integrated EMG has direct, specific effects	Transfer and maintenance adequately demonstrated
Epilepsy	EEG feedback effective in 60% of the cases	Better than placebo	Specific, direct effects	Transfer and maintenance not adequately demonstrated
Anxiety	EMG feedback decreases anxiety	No more effective than relaxation or behavioral exposure	Anxiety disorders are more than physiological arousal	

the demonstrated effects of biofeedback are not different from placebo effects. In addition, biofeedback is frequently not the only treatment used. Consequently, it is impossible to know whether the improvement was the result of biofeedback, other treatment, or both. These results come from a number of investigators, suggesting that the clinical effects of biofeedback are replicable by different clinicians in various settings (question 6). As suggested by the "Comments" column, biofeedback may be the most effective treatment available for Raynaud's disease, neuromuscular reeducation, and some drug-resistant types of epilepsy. Those types of biofeedback that address the specific physiological mechanism mediating a disorder (e.g., hypertension, cardiac arrhythmias, epilepsy, and neuromuscular reeducation) appear to have the most potential for success. Few negative effects have been reported in the clinical use of biofeedback (question 8). The exception is that some individuals report feelings of panic or loss of control during the procedures.

In summary, the clinical effectiveness of biofeedback for all disorders to which it has been commonly applied has not been clearly demonstrated. Although clinical improvement occurs, the persistence of that improvement has not been demonstrated and the manner in which biofeedback results in that effect is often unclear. Biofeedback may not be more effective than less expensive procedures for many disorders. Biofeedback is not a "cure-all" technique. But it is also not totally ineffective. At the current time, there are not enough data to make strong statements about its clinical effectiveness. Additional research is required to develop procedures that maximize the persistence of treatment effects and that demonstrate that those effects are specific and worth the time and effort required to bring them about. Biofeedback has clinical potential, but that potential has not been fully realized at this time. Biofeedback is most effectively used as one part of a treatment package. It provides clients with access to information about their physiology, but it is not a magic box that changes that physiology. Clients must effect that change themselves (Shellenberger & Green, 1986).

Mechanisms of Change in Biofeedback

Although the clinical effectiveness of biofeedback has not been clearly demonstrated, it is obvious that people can reliably alter several physiological processes and that biofeedback results in at least short-term clinical improvement. How does this occur? There are many specific theories of biofeedback (Schwartz & Beatty, 1977). These theories hypothesize that either a direct or an indirect mechanism brings about the observed changes. Biofeedback may have its effects in a direct manner when the client learns to control a specific physiological function that results in a concomitant reduction in the symptoms. This direct mechanism is apparent in some applications of biofeedback. In the case of the muscle rehabilitation of clients who have had strokes, EMG feedback focuses on increasing the activity of the muscles in areas of the body whose function were lost due to the stroke. Increased use of these muscles (symptomatic change) is directly related to the increased contraction of these muscle fibers (Basmajian, 1979). In this manner, biofeedback provides a behavioral strategy useful in modifying physiological processes underlying the symptoms of a clinical disorder.

However, biofeedback may also indirectly result in symptom change. Rather than influencing symptoms by altering an underlying physiological process, biofeedback may enhance the client's awareness of those situations that are stressful and of the maladaptive nature of her cognitive, affective, and behavioral responses to those situations. The client then alters these responses or learns new responses that are more effective in dealing with those situations (Schwartz, 1978). This indirect mode of effecting change is often just as powerful and useful as the more direct mode. In this way, improvement in symptoms may occur without the client ever learning to control substantially the physiological functions being monitored (Rugh, 1979).

It is possible that both direct and indirect mediation are responsible for change in some applications of biofeedback. In either case, biofeedback emphasizes that monitoring the problem and implementing treatment are the responsibility of the client as well as the health provider. Feedback, whether physiological or environmental-behavioral, provides the means by which a client can learn to recognize and correct clinical problems. Treatment is not done *to* the client but rather consists of the client learning a set of skills to recognize that the system is out of homeostasis as well as the means to return the body to homeostasis via physiological, cognitive, affective, or behavioral change.

RELAXATION TRAINING

Physiological processes can also be altered without electronically monitoring and feeding back information concerning a specific physiological function. Clients can learn to alter physiological activity when given specific instructions to do so and cognitive or somatic strategies to produce the desired changes. In this section, two commonly used procedures to teach relaxation will be described: progressive muscle relaxation and meditation. These procedures have the common goal of reducing physiological, cognitive, and behavioral arousal. The effectiveness of their clinical applications and the manner in which they reduce arousal will be discussed.

Progressive Muscle Relaxation

Progressive muscle relaxation training consists of a series of instructions that direct a client to relax his voluntary musculature. After a thorough assessment to determine the potential usefulness of relaxation, the client is provided with a conceptualization of the problem as one of excess tension or arousal. Relaxation training is suggested as an effective mode of reducing that arousal, thus having a beneficial impact on the presenting problem. A brief description of the procedure is then provided (Bernstein & Borkovec, 1973).

The client is seated comfortably in a quiet room. He is directed first to tense and then to relax sixteen muscle groups, one at a time, in the sequence given in Table 12-5. The client's attention is focused on the target muscle group, and at the predetermined signal from the clinician, the client tenses the muscle group for 5 to 7 seconds and then relaxes the muscle group for 20 to 30 seconds. During the relaxation phase, the clinician makes statements to keep the client's focus on the feelings of relaxation in that muscle group. While the goal of progressive relaxation training is to help the client achieve a deeply relaxed state, the initial use of tensing prior to relaxing is to help the client clearly discriminate feelings associated with those states. The client is often given an assignment to practice this and subsequent exercises at home.

As the client is able to achieve deep relaxation with the tension and release of the sixteen muscle groups, a series of procedures are used to decrease the time and effort needed to achieve relaxation. First, the sixteen muscle groups are combined into seven, and the client practices tensing and relaxing these combined groups as before (see Table 12-5). When proficient at achieving relaxation with this procedure, the seven muscle groups are further combined into four, and again tensing and relaxing are practiced until the client can consistently and deeply relax using the abbreviated procedure. At this point, the tensing portion of the practice cycle is dropped, and the client is trained to produce relaxation by focusing his attention on recalling the feelings associated with relaxation. Relaxation can be further elaborated by providing the person with a cue (the word *relax*, for example) when in the relaxed state. Via the association of relaxation with the cue, the client can then learn to elicit relaxation quickly by using the cue. The generalization or transfer to the nonclinical, natural environment is promoted by differential relaxation. The goal of differential relaxation is to help the client maintain the minimal amount of tension required to go about daily tasks and to relax muscles not required for those tasks. For example, as you read this book, some muscle tension is needed to hold your head up, to hold the book, and to turn the pages. But your legs and torso do not need to be tense. You would practice differential relaxation by relaxing the muscles in your legs and torso and by using only that amount of tension in your neck, hands, and arms needed to carry out the task. Teaching differential relaxation consists of a series of practice steps, beginning with relatively quiet activities (like reading a book) and progressing to more active tasks (like driving a car) as the client can maintain differential relaxation. Progressive relaxation, then, is a procedure for shaping

TABLE 12-5 Summary of Progressive Relaxation Training

INITIAL SESSIONS: TENSING AND RELAXING THE	COMBINED-7: TENSING AND RELAXING THE	COMBINED-4: TENSING AND RELAXING THE	COMBINED-4: RELAXING ONLY THE	CUED RELAXATION	DIFFERENTIAL RELAXATION
Dominant hand and forearm Dominant biceps	Dominant arm	Arms	Arms	Cue "relax" associated with relaxed state and used by the person to elicit that state quickly	Learning to relax muscles not necessary for a task and to maintain only needed tension in those muscles involved in that task
Nondominant hand and forearm Nondominant biceps	Nondominant arm				
Forehead Upper cheeks and nose Lower cheeks and jaws Neck and throat	Face, neck, and throat	Face and neck	Face and neck		
Chest, shoulders, and upper back Abdominal region	Torso	Torso	Torso		
Dominant thigh Dominant calf Dominant foot	Dominant leg	Legs	Legs		
Nondominant thigh Nondominant calf Nondominant foot	Nondominant leg				
(7 sessions)	(2 sessions)	(2 sessions)	(1 session)		

a relaxation response via instructions, practice, and feedback. The goal is to relax quickly and effectively in the natural environment.

Meditation

A client may also be taught to relax by providing instructions for meditation exercises adapted from yoga and transcendental meditation (Benson, 1976). Benson suggests that there are four necessary components in relaxation: (1) a quiet environment; (2) a mental device, usually a sound or a word repeated aloud or silently to shift attention from distracting external or internal stimuli; (3) a passive attitude that disregards distractions and avoids worry about performance; and (4) a comfortable position to reduce muscle tension.

The actual procedure used clinically is quite simple and stripped of its religious and cultic embellishments. Benson (1976, pp. 114–115) suggests the following instructions:

(1) Sit quietly in a comfortable position.
(2) Close your eyes.
(3) Deeply relax all your muscles, beginning with your feet and progressing up to your face. Keep them relaxed.
(4) Breathe through your nose. Become aware of your breathing. As you breathe out, say the word "one" silently to yourself. For example, breathe IN . . . OUT, "ONE," IN . . . OUT, "ONE," etc. Breathe easily and naturally.
(5) Continue for 10 to 20 minutes. You may open your eyes to check the time but do not use an alarm. When you finish, sit quietly for several minutes, at first with your eyes closed and later with your eyes opened. Do not stand up for a few minutes.
(6) Do not worry about whether you are successful in achieving a deep level of relaxation. Maintain a passive attitude and permit relaxation to occur at its own pace. When distracting thoughts occur, try to ignore them by not dwelling on them and return to repeating "ONE." With practice the response should come with little effort. Practice the technique once or twice daily, but not within two hours after any meal since the digestive processes seem to interfere with the elicitation of the Relaxation Response.

Effects

The effects of relaxation training have been studied using three broad classes of responses: motor and cognitive performance, physiological functions, and subjective levels of tension-anxiety. The physiological changes produced by progressive relaxation training, meditation, and other relaxation procedures are highly similar (Benson, 1976; Bernstein & Borkovec, 1973; Davidson & Schwartz, 1976). All these procedures result in reduced physiological activation, sympathetic nervous system activity, and skeletal-muscular tension (Shapiro, 1984).

Performance measures have been infrequently researched. When anxiety is so high that it interferes with performance, relaxation tends to enhance performance. However, the exact effect of relaxation on performance depends on the characteristics of the task and the tension level of the client. In terms of subjective reports of effect, all of the relaxation procedures result in a reduction in perceived anxiety or tension and in positive feelings of well-being. Again, data comparing the procedures are not available.

Clinical Applications

In terms of clinical procedure, the application of relaxation training is quite similar to that described for biofeedback. An adequate assessment is required, followed by teaching the relaxation skill via shaping, practice, and feedback and then transferring it to the client's natural environment. Relaxation training may be used to provide a client with an active strategy to gain control over a physiological function in biofeedback training. However, these procedures have also been used as a primary treatment modality for many disorders to which biofeedback is also applied, including headaches, high blood pressure, dysmenorrhea, asthma, and neuromuscular disorders (see Table 12-6).

The criteria for establishing the clinical effectiveness of relaxation training are similar to those of biofeedback. The current status of research on the effectiveness of relaxation training is comparable to that

TABLE 12-6 Summary of the Clinical Applications of Relaxation Training

DISORDER	PROGRESSIVE RELAXATION	MEDITATION	AUTOGENICS
Anxiety-related disorders	X	X	X
Insomnia	X		X
Essential hypertension	X	X	X
Muscle tension headache	X		
Migraine headache	X	X	X
Asthma	X		X
Stress reduction	X	X	X
Prepared childbirth	X		X
Gastrointestinal disorders			X
Neuromuscular reeducation	X		
Dysmenorrhea	X		

of biofeedback. The one exception is the application of progressive relaxation training to anxiety-related disorders, often in conjunction with modeling or systematic desensitization. Many data are available in this case, and the efficacy of the procedure is fairly well established, although not absolutely (Kazdin & Wilcoxon, 1976).

Although progressive relaxation training and meditation have been applied to similar types of disorders, it may be a mistake to think of them as interchangeable. The procedures may differ in the means by which they bring about relaxation and in the degrees to which they influence cognitive-affective, physiological, and behavioral expressions of tension, anxiety, and stress (Davidson & Schwartz, 1976; Schwartz, 1978).

Tension, anxiety, and stress are responses that occur at several levels in the person-environment system, and treatment needs to address the modalities in which the tension, anxiety, or stress is expressed. Effective treatment needs to be person as well as symptom oriented. Relaxation training requires the participation of the client to learn the skill, and thus the procedure used needs to be selected and modified to fit that person's characteristics and resources.

Relaxation Training: A Summary

Relaxation procedures represent another mode of altering physiological processes via behavioral methods. They may be used in conjunction with biofeedback or independently in the treatment of various clinical disorders and in prevention. While they are generally less costly than biofeedback, their effects may be less specific. Relaxation and biofeedback both promote active participation by the client to acquire the skill to self-control physiological, cognitive-affective, and behavioral responses.

SUMMARY

In this chapter, the methods, theory, and clinical use and evaluation of biofeedback and relaxation training have been described. The goals of such training are: (1) to enhance clients' sensitivity to physiological processes and to how those processes are influenced by thinking, behavior, and environment; and (2) to teach clients the psychophysiological skill of altering or controlling those processes to ameliorate symptoms or to prevent their occurrence.

Biofeedback and relaxation training are applicable to a wide variety of disorders either as an adjunct to more traditional medical interventions or other cognitive and behavioral methods or as a primary treatment modality. With a few exceptions, biofeedback and relaxation methods appear to have modest beneficial effects. The exact mechanisms that mediate these effects are unknown.

The advantage and potential of these methods entail teaching clients skills that utilize natural, built-in homeostatic mechanisms and processes. The methods are not magical; they are not a "quick fix." Just as with other highly skilled behaviors, if these skills are not well learned and consistently practiced, they will have only short-lived effects. Many clients do not persist in using these skills, and consequently, the beneficial effects do not persist.

The initial optimism about biofeedback and relaxation training and research is over. There is something useful in these procedures. What that something is needs to be more clearly identified, and the means to maximize and generalize these beneficial effects need to be developed. We are at the beginning and not the end.

REFERENCES

American Psychiatric Association. (1979). *Biofeedback: Report of the task force on biofeedback of the American Psychiatric Association*. Washington, DC: Author.

Anand, B. W. (1961). Studies on Shri Ramanandi Yogi during his stay in an air tight box. *Indian Journal of Medical Research, 49*, 82–89.

Basmajian, J. V. (Ed.). (1979). *Biofeedback: Principles and practice for clinicians*. Baltimore: Williams & Wilkins.

Benson, H. (1976). *The relaxation response*. New York: Avon Books.

Bernstein, D. A., & Borkovec, T. D. (1973). *Progressive relaxation training: A manual for the helping professions*. Champaign, Illinois: Research Press.

Birk, L. (1973). Biofeedback for therapeutics. In L. Birk (Ed.), *Biofeedback: Behavioral medicine*, 1–50. New York: Grune & Stratton.

Blanchard, E. B. (1979). Biofeedback and the modification of cardiovascular dysfunctions. In R. J. Gatchel & K. P. Price (Eds.), *Clinical applications of biofeedback: Appraisal and status*, 127–139. New York: Pergamon Press.

Blanchard, E. B., & Epstein, L. H. (1978). *A biofeedback primer*. Reading, MA: Addison-Wesley.

Davidson, R. J., & Schwartz, G. E. (1976). The psychobiology of relaxation and related states: A multiprocess theory. In D. I. Mostofsky (Ed.), *Behavior control and modification of physiological activity*, 467–493. Englewood Cliffs: Prentice-Hall.

Freeman, L. (1973). *Your mind can stop the common cold*. New York: Wyden.

Gatchel, R. J., & Price, K. P. (1979). *Clinical applications of biofeedback: Appraisal and status*. New York: Pergamon Press.

Hassett, J. (1978). *A primer of psychophysiology*. San Francisco: W. H. Freeman.

Kamiya, J. (1969). Operant control of the EEG alpha rhythm and some of its reported effects on consciousness. In C. Tart (Ed.), *Altered states of consciousness*, 507–518. New York: Wiley.

Kazdin, A. E., & Wilcoxon, L. A. (1976). Systematic desensitization and nonspecific effects: A methodological evaluation. *Psychological Bulletin, 83*, 729–758.

Lang, P. J. (1970). Autonomic control or learning to play the internal organs. *Psychology Today, 4*, 39–44.

Lindsley, D. B., & Sassomon, W. H. (1983). Autonomic activity and brain potentials associated with "voluntary control of the pilomotors." *Journal of Neurophysiology, 1*, 342–349.

Miller, N. E. (1969). Learning of visceral and glandular responses. *Science, 163*, 434–445.

Miller, N. E., & Dworkin, B. R. (1977). Critical issues in therapeutic applications of biofeedback. In G. E. Schwartz & J. Beatty (Eds.), *Biofeedback: Theory and research*, 129–162. New York: Academic Press.

Obrist, P. A. (1976). The cardiovascular-behavioral interaction as it appears today. *Psychophysiology, 13*, 95–107.

Olton, D. S., & Noonberg, A. R. (1980). *Biofeedback: Clinical applications in behavioral medicine*. Englewood Cliffs: Prentice-Hall.

Patel, C. H. (1975). Twelve-month follow-up of yoga and biofeedback training in the management of hypertension. *Lancet, 1*, 62–67.

Pepper, E., Ancoli, S., & Quinn, M. (Eds.), (1979). *Mind/body integration: Essential readings in biofeedback*. New York: Plenum.

Rugh, J. D. (1979). Instrumentation in biofeedback. In R. J. Gatchel & K. P. Price (Eds.), *Clinical applications of biofeedback: Appraisal and status*, 43–58. New York: Pergamon Press.

Schwartz, G. E. (1978). Psychobiological foundations of psychotherapy and behavior change. In S. E. Garfield & A. E. Bergin (Eds.), *Handbook of psychotherapy and behavior change: An empirical analysis*, 63–100. New York: John Wiley & Sons.

Schwartz, G. E., & Beatty, J. (1977). *Biofeedback: Theory and research*. New York: Academic Press.

Shapiro, D. H. (1984). Overview: Clinical and physiological comparison of meditation with other self-control strategies. In D. H. Shapiro & R. N. Walsh (Eds.), *Meditation: Classic and contemporary perspectives*, 5–13. New York: Aldine.

Shapiro, D., Crider, A. B., & Tursky, B. (1964). Differentiation of autonomic response through operant reinforcement. *Psychonomic Science, 1*, 147–148.

Shapiro, D., & Surwit, R. S. (1979). Biofeedback. In O. F. Pomerleau & J. P. Brady (Eds.), *Behavioral medicine: Theory and practice*, 45–74. Baltimore: Williams & Wilkins.

Shellenberger, R., & Green, J. (1986). *From the ghost in the box to successful biofeedback training*. Greely, CO: Health Psychology.

White, L., & Tursky, B. (1982). Conclusion: Where are we... where are we going? In L. White & B. Tursky (Eds.), *Clinical biofeedback: Efficacy and mechanisms*, 397–409. New York: Guilford Press.

Part IV
Applications of Behavior Change Principles to Specific Health Problems

13 Health- and Illness-Related Behaviors: Clinical and Preventative Interventions

This chapter begins the last part of the book, in which the principles considered in Part III are applied to the specific health-related behaviors and problems described in Parts I and II. In Chapter 13, strategies to alter health-impairing and health-promoting habits and illness-related decisions and actions are detailed. Chapter 14 focuses on stress management and coping skills training. In Chapters 15 and 16, more specific applications of behavior change strategies to heart disease, infectious diseases, cancer, and pain are described and evaluated. The development and utility of combined or multimodal cognitive-behavioral and medical-pharmacological interventions are emphasized.

INTRODUCTION

In Chapter 13, we will review the interventions used to alter health-impairing and health-promoting behaviors and illness-related decisions and actions. The characteristics and effectiveness of these interventions will be described and critically evaluated. Future developments that may enhance their effectiveness will be described. It is impossible to review comprehensively the application of behavior change programs to all health- and illness-related behaviors. Rather, three such behaviors will serve as the focus of this chapter: smoking, eating and exercise, and adherence to treatment recommendations. The first two are distal causes of several prevalent and serious diseases. The latter focus, adherence, is a major health care delivery problem. All three behaviors are critical targets in the prevention and treatment of disease. (For behavior change programs for other health-related behaviors, see Matarazzo, Weiss, Herd, Miller, & Weiss, 1984).

In our preview, we will see that current technologies for altering health-related behaviors are crude and modestly effective. It is more difficult to modify behavioral risk factors for chronic disease than factors that cause infectious disease. As suggested by Leventhal and Cleary (1980, p. 370): "There is no smoking swamp analogous to the breeding ground of the anopheles mosquito and no hypertension pump analogous to the Broad Street pump in London that helped identify contaminated water as the source of cholera." Behavioral risk factors for disease entail a mixture of social, psychological, behavioral, and physiological determinants.

SMOKING

As described in Chapter 2, smoking is a major risk factor for heart disease, cancer, emphysema, and other illnesses. Most smokers realize the danger and would like to quit. The clear risk of smoking and smokers' desire to quit indicate the need for programs that effectively help people stop smoking and that prevent the initiation of smoking. Let us look at interventions to help people stop smoking.

Two basic strategies have been used to help people stop smoking: behavioral and pharmacological. Smoking cessation programs have primarily been implemented in clinical settings with individuals or small groups. In a later section, the impact of community based antismoking campaigns, such as that initiated by the surgeon general's report on smoking, will be described and evaluated.

Smoking Cessation Programs: Clinical Settings

Aversion Programs. Aversion therapy has been the most common behavioral strategy to help clients stop smoking. Aversion entails pairing an aversive stimulus with the act of smoking. Via respondent conditioning or punishment, this pairing should result in an aversion to smoking and a consequent reduction in tobacco use. Several types of aversive stimuli have been used: electrical shock, imaginal nausea and vomiting, and cigarette smoke itself. The use of shock and imaginal aversive stimuli is not effective (Lichtenstein, 1982; Lichtenstein & Mermelstein, 1984).

Cigarette smoke is utilized as an aversive stimulus in two ways: satiation and rapid smoking. Satiation is a take-home procedure in which clients double or triple their usual rate of smoking. This dramatic increase results in highly aversive sensations and experiences and consequently effects a reduction in smoking. Outcome research suggests that satiation results in a reduction or cessation of smoking, but it is difficult to monitor and control clients' compliance with instructions to increase smoking dramatically. Rapid smoking is a clinical procedure in which clients smoke continuously and inhale every 6 to 8 seconds until they are unwilling to tolerate the procedure. Rapid smoking is quite effective in producing short- and long-term abstinence in a sizable number of clients. However, it may also impose risks. It leads to increases in heart rate and blood nicotine level and to changes in blood gases that may lead to cardiovascular problems. Currently, the extent of such risks is not clear (Lichtenstein, 1982).

Less dangerous variations of rapid smoking have been used: focused smoking and smoke holding. In focused smoking, clients are instructed to smoke at their normal rate but to concentrate on the negative sensations associated with smoking (e.g., the rasp of smoke in the throat, burning eyes, and the taste of cigarettes). In smoke holding, clients are instructed to hold smoke in their mouth for some specified period of time. The effectiveness of these less risky smoke aversion approaches is not yet clear. The few empirical reports available suggest that a sizable number of smokers become abstinent after involvement in these approaches.

Nicotine Fading and Controlled Smoking. Nicotine is a major factor in smoking. Persons may smoke to regulate the amount of nicotine in their body. Departures from optimal levels of nicotine stimulate smoking (Schacter, 1978). Nicotine fading is a procedure that involves the progressive reduction in nicotine intake and associated dependence. Clients work toward a quitting date by systematically switching to brands that are progressively lower in tar and nicotine. Such a strategy makes minimal demands of clients and results in an initial success experience. Clients appear to be quite willing to engage in the procedure. Research on the effectiveness of nicotine fading in producing long-term maintenance is mixed. Many individuals involved in nicotine fading programs continue to smoke, but use a lower tar and nicotine cigarette than their pretreatment brand and do not increase their smoking frequency. Although abstinence is the optimal goal, the less hazardous smoking that often results from nicotine fading may be a realistic alternative for persons who do not want to quit (Lichtenstein & Mermelstein, 1984).

Self-Control Programs. Self-control programs view smoking as a habit that is associated with specific environmental, physiological, cognitive, and affective cues and consequences. Self-control programs attempt to alter smoking by teaching clients to modify these cues and consequences. Initially, attempts are made to enhance participants' motivation and commitment to change. Clients are informed of the hazards of smoking and are asked to make a contingency deposit of money with the therapist. The money is then returned as the client implements self-control procedures. A target date is set for quitting but is often preceded by strategies to reduce the rate of smoking. The client is taught to self-monitor the number of cigarettes smoked and the temporal, interpersonal, environmental, and other salient stimuli associated with smoking. Self-monitoring often results in a short-term reduction in smoking.

Stimulus control procedures are then implemented. These procedures focus on altering or restructuring the antecedent stimuli associated with smoking. This may entail restricting or avoiding those situations in which smoking typically occurred. Clients are also taught to reduce the strength of smoking cues by associating smoking only with certain times and places (e.g., a smoking chair). Stimulus control is moderately effective but has a very gradual impact.

Contingency contracting and self-reinforcement are typically utilized to reinforce nonsmoking or to punish smoking. Contracts may, for example, entail response cost in which clients forfeit a certain amount of deposited money each time they smoke. Clients may provide themselves with preselected activity and material reinforcers contingent on nonsmoking. Reinforcement procedures are clearly effective in producing short-term change, but their effect in maintaining such change is uncertain.

Clients may also be taught alternate responses to smoking. The most commonly used alternate response is relaxation. The rationale is that tension and anxiety may be powerful occasions for smoking, and that relaxation provides both a means to reduce tension and a response incompatible with smoking. However, the evidence suggests that relaxation, as a sole intervention, does not effectively curtail smoking.

Pharmacological Interventions. Given smokers' dependence on nicotine and preference for effortless means to alter smoking behavior, it would seem logical that drug interventions would be a powerful tool in smoking cessation. The use of over-the-counter smoking deterrents and prescription tranquilizers and stimulants has not proved effective. Nicotine chewing gum, which prevents nicotine withdrawal and provides a substitute oral activity to smoking, may be useful. The limited evidence available suggests that it is a helpful aid in reducing and stopping smoking, but is probably most effective when used in conjunction with a behavioral program (Kozlowski, 1984).

Physician Warning and Instructions. Given the number of persons who seek medical services, it is important to assess whether physicians and other primary health providers can convince clients to quit smoking. The exact message utilized to effect client change has not been carefully specified in most studies. Typically, the intervention is very brief and relatively nonspecific. Despite this, physician intervention has a modest positive impact. This may be the result of intervention occurring at a critical time—when the client is sick. If these physician communications were coupled with specific information on how go about reducing or quitting smoking, a very powerful and economic intervention may be produced (Leventhal & Cleary, 1980).

Smoking Cessation Programs: A Summary. Up to this point, the various interventions for smoking have been evaluated in a relatively gross manner as effective, mixed, or not effective. Let us now get more specific. Those interventions indicated as effective resulted in greater reductions in smoking than placebo interventions. Those interventions that are effective result in a significant and relatively uniform reduction or cessation of smoking in 60 to 90% of the clients who complete treatment. However, there is also a relatively high dropout rate, often as high as 50%. If these dropouts are included in the results, the impressive outcomes are diminished. While intervention does appear to be effective for those who complete the programs, there is much recidivism in the year after completion of the programs. At six months, only 30 to 60% of those who completed the programs remain abstinent. At twelve months or longer, only 10 to 45% are still abstinent. Thus, current interventions for smoking result in relatively modest, positive short-term outcomes, but the benefits often do not persist over time (Glasgow & Lichtenstein, 1987; Leventhal & Cleary, 1980). These equivocal results have led to the development of new strategies whose goal is to effect greater and more lasting change. These new strategies entail combining several of the interventions described above and focusing more on the maintenance of change.

Multicomponent Smoking Cessation Programs. More recent smoking cessation programs have utilized a combination of the methods we have described in the hope that a combination will be more powerful than any one alone. This is a reasonable assumption given the complex determinants of smoking outlined in Chapter 2. Different variables control smoking in different people. Multiple-element programs may be more effective because of individual differences between smokers. On the other hand, more is not necessarily better (Franks & Wilson, 1978). Complex programs may confuse clients, demand too many changes, and contain incompatible elements.

A multicomponent smoking cessation program typically consists of three phases: preparation, quitting, and maintenance. An outline of such programs is shown in Table 13-1. Are these programs more effective? Most multicomponent programs have resulted in higher success rates and better maintenance (Hughes, Hymowitz, Ockene, Simon, & Vogt, 1981; Lando, 1981; Pomerleau & Pomerleau, 1978; Powell & McCann, 1981). Others have been no more effective and a few have even been less effective than single component programs.

Maintenance Strategies. Another recent trend in smoking cessation has been the development of strategies to enhance maintenance. Smoking programs enable clients to quit, but explicit, powerful strategies are needed to maintain this change. As listed in Table 13-1, booster sessions, social support, and coping skills training have been used to enhance maintenance. In booster sessions, clients meet with the health provider at specified intervals after treatment. In these sessions, behavior change strategies are reviewed to "inoculate" the client against a return to smoking. Such sessions have not resulted in improved maintenance, perhaps because they fail to occur when the client is experiencing an acute need to smoke and because clients fail to attend.

TABLE 13-1 Options in Multicomponent Programs for Smoking Cessation

Preparation

- Enhancement of client commitment and motivation
  - Contingency deposits
  - Review of risks of smoking and benefits of quitting
- Assessment
  - Self-monitoring to increase client awareness and identify situational cues and consequences for smoking
  - Set a target quitting date
- Self-management to reduce smoking frequency
  - Stimulus control
  - Stress management, relaxation
  - Use of substitutes for smoking

Quitting

- Aversive strategies
  - Imaginal sensitization
  - Rapid smoking or satiation
  - Focused smoking or smoke holding
- Nonaversive strategies
  - Nicotine fading
  - Nicotine chewing gum
  - Contracting

Maintenance

- Booster sessions and extended contracts
- Coping skills training
  - Cognitive-behavioral coping skills for high-risk situations
  - Avoiding abstinence violation effects
  - Careful transfer of self-management skills to the client
- Social support

Maintenance of nonsmoking is difficult and stressful for most clients. Social support may provide resources for coping with these stressors. Natural social supports are immediately available to clients when they are tempted to smoke. Persons who receive explicit and active support from family, friends, and coworkers are more likely to remain abstinent (Mermelstein, Lichtenstein & McIntyre, 1982; Ockene, Benfari, Hurwitz & Nuttall, 1982). Efforts to manipulate social support to enhance maintenance have been unsuccessful (Glasgow & Lichtenstein, 1987).

Cognitive and behavioral coping skills training has received the most attention as a method of enhancing maintenance. As detailed in Chapter 11, this approach entails identifying high risk situations for relapse and developing and rehearsing modes of self-instruction ("I knew this was going to be hard, but I don't want to smoke around my kids"), social behaviors (e.g., refusing temptation— "No thank you, I'm trying to quit"), and alternatives to smoking (e.g., chewing gum) to use in those situations. Similarly, if the person succumbs to the temptation to smoke, strategies to combat continued smoking (abstinence violation effects) are rehearsed and practiced. Although only limited data are available, such maintenance-promotion strategies appear to be effective.

Clinical interventions for smoking cessation have been only moderately successful and are relatively costly. Such interventions can address only a small segment of the present and future population of tobacco users. We also need to develop and test preventative and community interventions.

Prevention of Smoking

Prevention of smoking must begin very early in life and must address the variables that predispose persons to initiate smoking and to continue experimentation. Recall that these variables primarily entail positive attitudes toward smoking, peer influence, and rebelliousness and toughness.

A good example of such a prevention program was developed and implemented by Evans (1984) in the school system in Houston, Texas. The intervention had three primary components. First, the immediate negative financial, aesthetic, biological, and social effects of smoking were communicated. The emphasis on such immediate consequences is more powerful than on distal consequences like heart disease and cancer. Second, a positive image of nonsmokers was developed focusing on the need to be independent ("You decide for yourself") and associating nonsmoking with being self-reliant and attractive. The values of independence and attractiveness were emphasized because of their congruence with the developmental characteristics of the children and adolescents targeted in this study. This information was communicated via films, posters, and face-to-face communications. Third, high-status, slightly older peers were used to model and rehearse how to resist peer pressure to smoke and how to maintain the decision not to smoke. Thus, the program attempted to provide the audience with specific and relevant skills to reduce risk.

Evans's and others' similar programs have been found to instill antismoking attitudes and to reduce initiation of smoking. Several years will be required, however, before the long-term impact of these programs can be evaluated. At present, it is not clear whether the children never smoked or simply delayed initiation of smoking (Leventhal & Cleary, 1980).

Mass Communication and Smoking

Following the surgeon general's report on the risks of smoking, mass communication informational campaigns were implemented to convince people to stop or never start smoking. These nationwide efforts of the American Heart Association, the American Cancer Association, and the United States Department of Health, Education, and Welfare, using radio, TV, print media, and warnings on tobacco products, resulted in only a moderate decrease in consumption. Annual per capita consumption of cigarettes has dropped from a high of 4,200 in the early 1970s to 3,400 in 1984 (Ray & Ksir, 1987). However, these campaigns may have also led to increased motivation to quit and to the use of filtered and low tar and nicotine tobacco products (Warner, 1977). In addition, these informational programs have increased the social and ecological pressures against smoking (e.g., no smoking sections of restaurants) and the assertiveness of nonsmokers, and instilled general societal values of smoking as unattractive and dangerous.

Smaller-scale community interventions that have targeted at-risk populations and that have included more specific cognitive-behavioral suggestions on how to quit have proved to be modestly effective (Hughes et al., 1981; Maccoby & Farquhar, 1975). We will review these studies in depth in Chapter 15.

OBESITY, EATING, AND EXERCISE

The amount and type of food eaten play an important role in health. Obesity is associated with high blood pressure, cardiovascular disease, diabetes, pulmonary and renal problems, cancer, and increased risk during pregnancy and surgery. Being more than 30% overweight is clearly a distal risk factor for many types of disease. Obesity also has strong social consequences. Overweight individuals are less liked, face discrimination, and are blamed for their problem. Obesity is a psychological and social hazard in a society that values thinness (Brownell, 1982; Wilson, 1984).

Most overweight individuals want to lose weight. Over 400,000 people are involved annually in lay-administered weight reduction programs in the United States (Stunkard, 1979). New books on weight control are regularly on the best seller list. Most people who want to lose weight do so because of appearance rather than health concerns (Stuart & Jacobson, 1979).

Weight control strategies can be divided into four general categories: dieting and fasting, drugs and surgery, modification of eating behavior, and exercise. We will describe and evaluate each of these.

Dieting and Fasting

In dieting and fasting, individuals are instructed, in an educational format, to restrict their caloric, carbohydrate, and fat intake. Fasting is more severe than dieting and usually occurs in a hospital setting. Most dieting is either self-initiated and self-directed or run by lay individuals or organizations like Weight Watchers. Attrition in such programs is quite high, ranging from 20 to 80% (Stunkard, 1975). Weight losses produced are highly variable and inconsistently maintained (Straw, 1983).

Drugs and Surgery

Both over-the-counter and prescription drugs have been used to reduce appetite and restrict food consumption. Data suggest that drugs may be useful in effecting initial weight loss, but tolerance and side effects preclude their continued use and long-term effectiveness (Stuart, Mitchell, & Jensen, 1981). The most common surgical intervention, gastric surgery, involves stapling the stomach to reduce its food capacity. The procedure is expensive and risky, and not practical given the prevalence of obesity. Drugs and surgery are "quick and dirty fixes" that require little responsibility of the client and that address the symptoms rather than the cause of the problem.

Modification of Eating Behavior: Cognitive-Behavioral Programs. The goal of cognitive-behavioral strategies is to alter individuals' eating (and exercise; see below) to effect a negative energy balance and consequent weight reduction. Most behavioral strategies, originally derived from Stuart and Davis (1972), consist of four main strategies: self-monitoring and goal setting, stimulus control to restrict cues that evoke eating, change of the topography of eating, and reinforcement of these altered behaviors. Because the application of these procedures to eating were thoroughly described in the section on self-control in Chapter 11, they will not be described again here. With the exception of altering the topography of eating, each of the components appears to contribute to changes in eating behavior (Wilson, 1984).

More recently, cognitive-behavioral coping skills training has been added to these basic behavioral strategies. This training focuses on coping with urges to eat and with interpersonal situations and states that occasion eating. Thus, self-instructional training may aim at the development of self-statements to cope with eating urges and to self-reinforce changes in eating behavior. Social skills training could be aimed at helping clients refuse offers of food or involvement in food-related activities. If eating is evoked by anxiety, anger, or depression, programs that target these affective states (e.g., relaxation for anxiety) may also be included in the treatment package.

How effective are cognitive-behavioral programs for weight control? Only about 10 to 15% of those individuals who begin treatment drop out. Few of the negative side effects (e.g., irritability and depression) characteristic of dieting have been found in cognitive-behavioral programs. The average weight loss effected by these programs is 1 to 2 pounds per week, or 10 to 30 pounds over a standard eight- to sixteen-week program. This is a relatively modest effect for those who are grossly overweight, but may be enhanced by lengthening the duration of the program. These losses are frequently accompanied by positive changes in blood pressure, serum lipids, and psychological functioning. The amount of weight lost is highly variable, and this variability is poorly understood. The weight loss attained at the end of treatment is typically maintained for at least a year. Cognitive-behavioral programs to alter eating can be effectively implemented by trained paraprofessionals, and consequently can be easily integrated into popular and commercial weight loss programs (Brownell, 1982; Brownell & Jeffery, 1987).

More recently, cognitive-behavioral methods have been expanded to insure maintenance and to effect greater weight loss in persons who are severely overweight. As with smoking, booster sessions have been used to promote maintenance of weight loss without much effect. Because eating is often a social activity, the involvement of family, friends, and coworkers has the potential to enhance weight loss and maintenance. Several studies have found that the inclusion of parents or spouses has enhanced the efficacy of typical cognitive-behavioral weight control programs. Brownell (1982), for example, reports that maternal involvement in a cognitive-behavior program for obese adolescents resulted in greater weight loss. Relapse prevention strategies like those described for smoking have also led to enhanced maintenance of weight loss (Wilson, 1984). More recently, dietary restrictions and cognitive-behavioral programs have been combined to effect greater weight loss. The long-term success of this combination awaits further study (Brownell, 1982). Some persons may have physiological limits to healthy weight loss that are determined by fat cell number or size and by metabolic and other factors. Weight loss depends on a negative energy balance: Persons must use more calories than they ingest. Thus, exercise is an important part of any weight control program, as well as a desirable health habit in its own right.

Exercise

Exercise programs are designed to fit the individual using the principles of overload and progression. For exercise to be maximally health promoting, the individual needs to exercise in a manner that loads the body at a level greater than the current exercise level. For sedentary individuals, this may entail a relatively small amount of "work." As fitness improves, greater amounts of "work" are added to achieve overload and to stimulate change. Thus, overload is applied in a gradual, progressive fashion in accordance with current fitness to minimize the dangers and discomforts associated with exercise (Ribsal, 1984). In this approach, persons' exercise is slowly shaped in a manner that encourages exercise and that minimizes its perceived aversiveness. Exercise, especially when initiated by someone who is in poor condition or obese, should be preceded by a medical exam. The exercise plan should be congruent with an individual's age and current physical status (Haskell, 1984).

Motivating individuals to start an exercise program, to stay in such a program, and to maintain regular exercise over long periods of time is as difficult as achieving comparable goals for eating and smoking. Although most individuals think exercise is healthy, they are not very motivated to exercise. Beliefs are not turned into actions. Of those who start an exercise program, as many as 50 percent drop out within six months.

Several cognitive-behavioral methods have been used to recruit, involve, and maintain individuals' participation in exercise programs. The effectiveness of these methods has not been systematically evaluated. Convenient and affordable exercise settings motivate people to initiate and persist in an exercise regimen. The enlistment of natural social supports for exercise (e.g., exercising with someone) and the opportunity for social interaction as a part of exercise enhance recruitment, involvement, and maintenance. Goal setting, self-monitoring, contracting, and providing feedback about changes in weight and fitness also appear to be effective (Dishman, 1982; Oldridge, 1984). Much additional research is needed in this area.

Altering Food Preferences and Selection

Both what we eat and how much we eat strongly influence our weight and general health. The constituents of the food we ingest influence the probability of heart disease, stroke, certain types of cancer, Type II diabetes, and many other diseases. While dietary preferences are remarkably resistant to change, it is as important to alter *what* is eaten as *how much* is eaten.

Attempts to alter individual or family diets have borrowed heavily from cognitive-behavioral technologies. Self-monitoring, using forms like that shown in Table 13-2, have been used to help individuals keep a record of their daily food intake. Individuals are then taught to identify healthy foods (see Table 13-3). After a few weeks, they are asked to make small changes in their diets by substituting one or two healthy foods for a few unhealthy ones in a kind of shaping process. Stimulus control procedures could be utilized by providing these individuals with shopping lists of preferred and healthy foods. Social encouragement and reinforcement are useful in evoking and maintaining such changes, and may be supplemented with material and activity reinforcers (e.g, reductions in food bills) and with periodic physiological feedback about the benefits achieved (Wadden & Brownell, 1984). Modification of dietary preferences has not been the focus of much research, and deserves much more attention.

TABLE 13-2 Self-Monitoring Form for Lowering Cholesterol Intake[a]

DATE ____________

Food Group	*High Level*	*Moderate Level*	*Low Level*
Milk	Whole milk	Low fat milk	Skim or nonfat milk
Cheese	All firm or cheddar	Partly skim mozzarella	Cottage cheese
Cream	Whole cream, half-and-half	Powder cream substitute	Liquid cream substitute
Eggs	1 egg	1/2 egg	None
Meats	Liver, kidneys, cold cuts, fat meats	Choice steak, other fat meats	Very lean meat, veal, lean fillet or round
Fish	Shrimp, deep-fried fish	Shellfish other than shrimp	All nondeep-fried fish
Poultry	Duck, goose, deep-fried chicken	Chicken, turkey, game hens	Skinned chicken, turkey, game hens
Spreads	Butter, lard, margarine from palm oil	Margarine with hydrogenated oil	Polyunsaturated margarine
Oils	Lard, palm oil	Hydrogenated oil shortening	Corn, soybean, sesame, and sunflower oil
Total	___ X 3 = ___	___ X 2 = ___	___ X 1 = ___

[a]The client is asked to keep track of foods ingested and to tally total cholesterol use. The object is to lower the total score.

TABLE 13-3 Caloric Density and Salt, Sugar, and Saturated Fat Content of Common Foods[a]

HIGH CALORIE	MEDIUM CALORIE	LOW CALORIE
Typical American foods		
Commercial baked goods and cake mixes (SF, C, Sa, Su)	Buttermilk (SF, C, Sa)	Bouillon (Sa)
Hot dogs (SF, C, Sa)	Eggs (SF, C)	Consommé (Sa)
Bacon (SF, C, Sa)	Whole milk (SF, C)	Vegetable juice (Sa)
Ham, sausage, cold cuts (SF, C, Sa)	Shellfish (C)	Canned vegetables (Sa)
Regular cheeses (SF, C, Sa)	Canned soup (Sa)	Pickles (Sa)
Ice cream (SF, C, Su)	Canned corn, beans (Sa)	Sauerkraut (Sa)
Peanut butter (SF, Su)	Canned tuna (Sa)	Salted popcorn (Sa)
Red meat (SF, C)	Biscuits, muffins (Sa)	
Butter (SF, C)	Instant cereals (Sa)	
Candy (Su)	Bran flakes (Sa)	
Fruit in syrup (Su)	Soft drinks (Su)	
Potato and other chips (Sa)	Crackers, bread (Sa)	
Hard margarine (SF)	White rice	
	Spaghetti	
Alternate foods		
Vegetable oil	Whole grain breads	Sprouts
Avocado	Brown rice	Beets, broccoli
Honey	Chicken without skin	Carrots, celery
Natural peanut butter	Fresh fruit	Tomatoes, green beans
Sesame butter	Peas, beans, lentils	Squash
Soft margarine	Cottage cheese	
Unsalted nuts	Nonfat milk	
	Shredded wheat	
	Turkey	

[a]SF = saturated fats; C = cholesterol; Sa = salt; Su = sugar

Community-Based Preventative Applications: Eating, Exercise, and Diet. Several community-based preventative programs to reduce weight, increase exercise, and alter diet have been developed, implemented, and evaluated. These programs, as in smoking, use communication-informational and cognitive-behavioral principles. For example, cognitive-behavioral methods have been integrated with self-help programs for weight control, like TOPS (Take Off Pounds Sensibly), which address a very large audience (Stunkard, Levine, & Fox, 1970). In this study, four matched TOPS chapters were exposed to four different treatments: the standard TOPS program, TOPS plus behavioral methods led by a helping professional, TOPS plus behavioral methods led by a trained paraprofessional, and TOPS plus nutritional counseling. Adding the behavioral component to TOPS resulted in reduced attrition from the program and in significantly greater weight loss after twelve weeks of treatment and at a one-year follow-up. Thus, the use of cognitive-behavioral programs, even when implemented by lay individuals, holds great promise in the area of weight control.

In another example of a community approach, a national media program was used in Germany to foster weight reduction in the audience. A seven-month program, consisting of a forty-five-minute prime time program and 3-minute miniprograms, was presented to a nationwide audience, 35% of whom were thought to be overweight. The program described and modeled cognitive-behavioral methods like self-monitoring, goal setting, stimulus control, and incentive modification. In addition, considerable information was presented concerning the hazards of obesity, nutrition, and counting calories. The effects of the TV intervention alone and of the TV intervention plus written material compared to no intervention were assessed. The no intervention group lost an average of 2.2 pounds, the TV-only group lost 5.5 pounds, and the TV plus written material group lost 18.7 pounds. However, between 40 and 50% of the persons who began this weight control program dropped out (Stunkard, 1979). Multiple-impact mass communication that provides specific methods of changing behavior as well as general information about the benefits and reasons for change has the potential to be an economical means of weight reduction. However, additional program development and outcome assessment will be required before that potential will be fully realized.

Recognizing that dietary preferences are established at a young age, a Heart Healthy Eating Program was offered to primary school children by Coates, Jeffery, and Stinkard (1981). Before intervention, the children's lunch boxes were examined to determine their diet. A nutrition education program, which emphasized the consumption of more fruits and vegetables and less fats, salt, and sugar, was implemented. After the educational program, there was a nearly 40% increase in the amount of heart healthy food, and this change was sustained for four months.

Modification of food choice and consumption has also been implemented in the work place. Zifferblatt, Wilbur, and Pinky (1980) monitored food choices in a cafeteria at the National Institute of Health. They then introduced a Food for Thought program in which employees received one of fifty-two "playing cards" with each meal purchase. These cards contained information on the calories and constituents of the food served in the cafeteria. The cards could be made into poker hands and traded for prizes. As a result of this intervention, caloric intake decreased by 6 percent, primarily resulting from the decreased consumption of bread and desserts. Skim milk consumption increased, but there were no other significant shifts in purchases. Along these same lines, it would be possible for food services, restaurants, and institutions systematically to offer healthier food to their patrons (Brownell, 1982; Pomerleau, 1978).

Obesity, Eating, and Exercise: A Summary

Reducing the risk of disease often requires the simultaneous modification of several health-impairing and health-promoting habits. We have seen that health promotion or disease prevention focusing on weight control entails a focus on what is eaten (nutrition and food preferences), how much is eaten (eating behavior), and exercise. A summary of a comprehensive program for weight control is presented in Table 13-4. Several programs that have attempted to alter multiple health-promoting and health-impairing behaviors have been implemented in the work place (Naditch, 1984; Nathan, 1984) and in the community (Farquhar et al., 1984). We will review some of these studies in detail in Chapter 15.

TABLE 13-4 Options in a Multicomponent Program for Weight Control

Preparation
Enhance client commitment and motivation
  Contingency deposits
  Review risks of obesity and benefits of change

Alteration of Eating Behavior
Assessment
  Self-monitor eating to increase client awareness and to identify situation cues and consequences for eating
  Set short- and long-term goals for change in eating behavior

Self-management of eating behavior
  Stimulus control
  Incentive modification
  Coping skills training

(continued)

TABLE 13-4 Continued

Maintenance
- Relapse prevention training
- Enlisting natural social support systems

Alteration of Exercise
Assessment
- Self-monitoring of current exercise to increase client awareness and to identify situations and times in routine available for exercise
- Medical examination to determine current fitness and potential risks of an exercise program

Increasing exercise
- Identify convenient and affordable programs
- Stimulus control
- Enlisting natural social supports
- Progressive shaping of exercise using the principle of overload
- Structuring and modeling exercise session: type, length, and phases
- Feedback about the benefits of exercise and other incentive modifications

Alteration of Diet
Assessment
- Self-monitoring current food ingestion, amount, and type, using food chart

Dietary alteration
- Education to alter client's knowledge about "healthy" and "unhealthy" foods
- Dietary instruction and substitution to shape the amount and types of food eaten
- Stimulus control to develop "healthy" food shopping lists
- Incentive modification

ENHANCING ADHERENCE TO TREATMENT RECOMMENDATIONS

As discussed in Chapter 3, poor adherence to treatment recommendations is a frequent and serious health delivery problem. When clients fail to accurately and consistently follow recommended actions that promote health, reduce risk, or are an integral part of the treatment of an existing disorder, the efficacy of health care interventions is dramatically reduced. In this section, a number of strategies to enhance adherence will be described and evaluated. These strategies fall into three general categories: organizational, educational, and cognitive-behavioral (see Figure 13-1).

Organizational Strategies

Although most research focuses on the processes occurring in the client-health provider interaction, the nature of that interaction and the receptiveness of the client to influence depend on the organizational

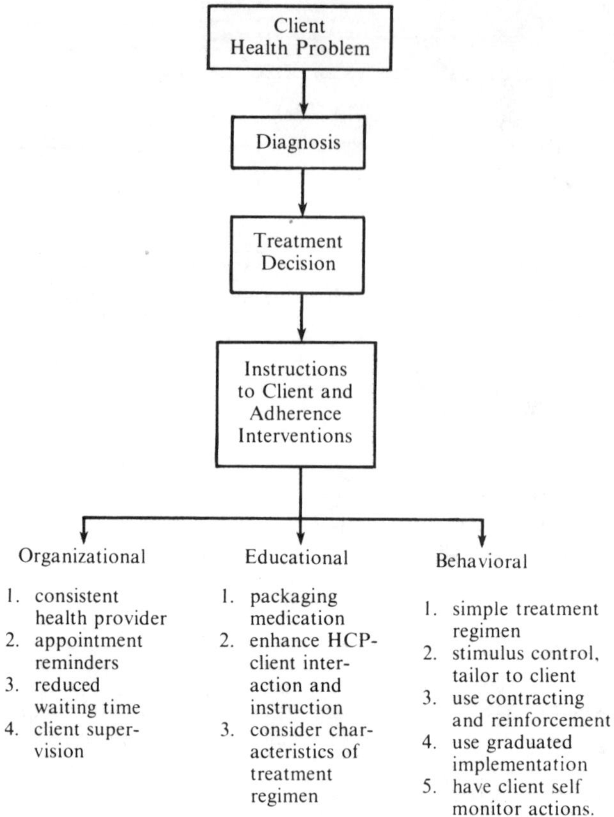

FIGURE 13-1 Strategies for Enhancing Adherence to Treatment Recommendations

qualities of the health care system. Adherence is better when clients are provided with a consistent source of care. Seeing the same provider facilitates client trust and satisfaction, and enables the health provider to know the client better and consequently to provide the interactional conditions congruent with the client's characteristics. Many of the educational interventions specified below are predicated on an ongoing relationship between the health provider and the client.

To prevent disease and to diagnose and treat disease once it occurs require the timely use of health care by clients. They must make and keep appointments, return for further work, and follow up on referrals. In general, the waiting time before appointments should be kept to a minimum. This may require specific as opposed to block appointment scheduling. Appointment keeping can be enhanced by sending postcard reminders or calling the client a few days before the appointment. This results in a 10 to 25% increase in appointment keeping and thus is likely to be cost effective (Haynes, 1979b.)

The strategies for improving adherence described below are time intensive. Given the press and cost of physician time, it may be necessary to utilize nurses, physicians' assistants, or other health professionals to provide the intensive educational and cognitive-behavioral strategies required to improve adherence. To do this in an economical fashion, judgments must be made concerning which clients need such additional attention. Research suggests that adherence is highly situational and cannot be predicted by the personality or demographic characteristics of the client. Means of assessing the situational probability of adherence are addressed in the next section. Research also suggests that persons with chronic disorders are less likely to adhere to treatment recommendations and thus should be targeted. The long-term cost effectiveness of intensive programs is unknown.

Educational Strategies

The nature of the recommended actions and the general context and specific manner in which they are communicated play a strong role in adherence. At a general level, adherence is improved when treatment recommendations occur within a client-health provider relationship in which the client is receptive to influence. It is useful to engage clients as active participants in information exchange and decision making (Eisenthal, Emery, Lazare, & Udin, 1979). Interaction characterized by a high proportion of positively to negatively toned statements increases adherence. Emotionally positive interactions in which the health provider communicates caring and concern, is sensitive to affective cues, and appears to be friendly and approachable enhance appointment keeping and client intentions to carry out treatment recommendations (Leventhal, Zimmerman, & Gutmann, 1984).

To carry out treatment recommendations, clients must understand and recall those recommendations, accept the recommendations as valid and useful, and have a plan for implementing the recommendations. These prerequisites for adherence can be facilitated by paying careful attention to the specific content of what is communicated to the client. Understanding and recall can be improved by the following principles (Ley, 1977; Ley & Spellman, 1967): (1) present the information about recommended actions near the beginning and end of the interaction; (2) stress the importance and benefits of the recommended actions; (3) use short words and sentences; (4) if several topics are discussed, explicitly categorize the topics; (5) repeat the instructions; (6) make specific, concrete, and detailed recommendations; and (7) ask the client to repeat and rehearse the instructions.

In addition to comprehending and remembering the information, the client must also feel that the recommendations are logical. Recall from Chapter 3 that clients develop a schema or self-diagnosis about their own symptoms. They also develop some notion about what ought to be done to address those symptoms. If there is a lack of congruence between the client's schema and the treatment recommendations that has not been adequately resolved in the clinical interchange, adherence is unlikely. Consequently, it is important to assess how the recommendations "fit" with client's schema of the illness. This may entail the close observation of a client's verbal and nonverbal reactions to the recommendations or an explicit question about how "sensible" such recommendations seem to the client or about the client's willingness to carry out the recommendations (Leventhal, 1984).

The nature and complexity of recommendations significantly influence adherence. Research suggests an inverse correlation between adherence and the number and difficulty of the behavior change requested (Haynes, 1976). In prescribing drugs, for example, the fewer number of drugs and the fewer times per day at which the client is asked to ingest the drugs, the better the adherence (Blackwell, 1979). Thus, there is some trade-off between maximizing efficacy by requesting multiple changes and the likelihood of adherence. The rule of thumb is to keep the recommendations as simple as possible while retaining the benefits resulting from the recommended actions. If complex, demanding regimens are necessitated by the nature of the problem, it is useful to implement components of the total regimen sequentially. As the client masters initial components, then additional components are added. The steps may be graded in order of difficulty or importance (Dunbar, Marshall, & Hovell, 1979).

It is also important to consider the aversive side effects of recommended actions. Obviously the selection of an effective treatment that has minimal aversive side effects is preferred. If aversive side effects are unavoidable, the nature and frequency of such side effects should be communicated to the client. This will enable the client to anticipate such effects and to develop, along with the health care provider, strategies to minimize their impact.

Cognitive-Behavioral Strategies

Individuals' day-to-day activities are usually highly predictable and routinized. These activities are strongly tied to recurring environmental, social, and behavioral cues. When making treatment recommendations, we are asking clients to change their routine, to do something different. These new behaviors may not be performed because they have no association with daily routine-generated cues. Thus, it is useful to tailor the recommended actions to fit a client's routine. A plan of action should be developed in which the recommended actions are tied to salient routine-generated cues or are scheduled to occur at times compatible with routine activities, or in which new salient cues that evoke the desired behavior are introduced into the natural environment.

Existing routines can be used to occasion the recommended action. For example, if medication is to be taken twice daily, in the morning and evening, the activity may be tied to routine tooth brushing. The medication container could even be taped to the toothpaste tube, or a written reminder could be placed on the bathroom mirror. If a client is asked to increase physical exercise, it would be useful to identify times and environmental opportunities congruent with the client's routine. This may entail taking the stairs rather than the elevator, or taking a walk on Monday, Wednesday, and Friday evenings, when the client's spouse is available and there are no strong competing activities like favorite TV programs. Medication packaging can also be used as a cue to action. This may entail a dated blister strip (like that used for oral contraceptives), medication calendars, or a dispenser containing an inexpensive signaling device that beeps when the client is to take the medication (Masur, 1981).

In Chapter 11, we learned that self-monitoring is reactive. It tends to promote desired behavior change. Self-observation of adherence behavior tends to enhance adherence because it focuses the client's attention on the regimen. It can also be used to provide the health provider with feedback concerning client's level of adherence (Dunbar et al., 1979). Self-observational data as a measure of actual compliance are, of course, subject to client distortion. However, self-observation is relaively inexpensive, and other measures of "actual" adherence are also problematic (Masur, 1981).

As with any behavior, the likelihood of adherence is affected by the consequences it engenders. In those cases in which the adherence behavior is not likely to result in immediate, perceivable positive consequences and/or is likely to result in aversive consequences, it is useful to build in a means of reinforcing adherence. Both contracting and self-reinforcement have been found to promote adherence (Dunbar et al., 1979; Masur, 1981).

Outcome research suggests that the strategies just described are moderately effective in increasing adherence. Generally, combinations of several of these strategies are more powerful than each alone. The most effective package may vary according to client, situation, and problem. Careful evaluation of these combined interventions has not yet occurred (Dunbar et al., 1979). Educational and cognitive-behavioral methods are generally sufficient to promote good short-term adherence for acute clinical problems. Insuring the long-term adherence necessitated by chronic health problems is much more difficult. After good adherence is initially attained, there is a persistent decline with time. Let us turn to strategies to promote long-term adherence.

Long-term adherence has been addressed using strategies similar to those elaborated in the earlier discussion of health habits: social support, continued monitoring (e.g., booster sessions), and cognitive-behavioral methods. Involving clients' natural social support systems appears to be particularly useful. Both familial and work- or school-related involvement of significant others has been found to enhance maintenance. In contrast to its application to health habits, continued monitoring of clients by a care provider has also proved to be useful (Haynes, 1979a).

The development of a conceptualization or schema that is shared by the client and the care provider is particularly critical to adherence in chronic disorders. Clients have a tendency to represent what may objectively be chronic disorders as acute. This is reasonable given most of their experience is with acute illness. An acute illness schema is also less threatening. Acute illness is more easily viewed as not part of oneself. A shared conceptualization of a health problem as chronic can be fostered by synthesizing cognitive-behavioral and educational methods. Self-monitoring of blood pressure, for example, could be used to help clients learn that their blood pressure is consistently rather than episodically elevated. The utility of reduced salt intake, increased exercise, and prescribed medication could be more directly accessed by the client via continued self-monitoring. Using the client as a collaborator in problem definition and problem solving may enhance the long-term adherence necessitated by chronic health problems.

SUMMARY

In this chapter, we have discussed methods to promote the performance of healthy behavior and to reduce the performance of unhealthy behavior. At a general level, the health care provider or organization is attempting to influence the thoughts, motives, and actions of clients. As described in Chapter 5, these targets of change are subject to client self-regulation. The thoughts, motives, and behaviors are influenced by a complex interaction of variables operating at many levels within the system. The relative success of health-promoting interventions to effect a large and lasting change depends on whether the change is compatible with and integrated into the self-regulating system that is the person. If it is not, the degree of change effected will be minimal and its duration short-lived. The change will only be engendered and sustained for as long as there is a strong and organized press from the external environment.

Health-promoting interventions must focus on incorporating the impetus for change on multiple levels of the regulating system so that when the intervention is withdrawn, the change will be sustained. The most effective means by which health-related behaviors can be altered vary according to the target of intervention, the personal and developmental characteristics of the individual, and the health problem. Current controlling factors regulating the target behavior must be understood, and, based on that information, multilevel interventions must be made to alter the antecedents and consequences of that behavior.

The numerous strategies and methods we have reviewed in this chapter begin to address this complex process. The most recent trend has been to target multiple behaviors and to use combinations of several methods to address the multiple determinants of these behaviors (e.g., effecting weight loss through exercise, alteration of eating behavior, and restrictive diets using cognitive-behavioral, nutritional, exercise physiology, and social-psychological principles). Although such combined interventions appear to produce greater and more sustained change, they are still relatively "gross." Further progress may require a combination of methods and targets selected to fit the often idiosyncratic factors that determine the target behavior.

REFERENCES

Blackwell, B. (1979). The drug regimen and treatment compliance. In D. L. Sackett & R. B. Haynes (Eds.), *Compliance with therapeutic regimens*, 144–156. Baltimore: The Johns Hopkins University Press.

Brownell, K. D. (1982). Obesity: Understanding and treating a serious, prevalent, and refractory disorder. *Journal of Consulting and Clinical Psychology, 50*, 820–840.

Brownell, K. D., & Jeffery, R. (1987). Improving long-term weight loss: Pushing the limits of treatment. *Behavior Therapy, 18*, 353–374.

Coates, T. J., Jeffery, R. W., & Stinkard, L. A. (1981). Heart healthy eating and exercise: Introducing and maintaining changes in health behavior. *American Journal of Public Health, 47*, 15–23.

Dishman, R. K. (1982). Compliance/adherence in health-related exercise. *Health Psychology, 1*, 237–267.

Dunbar, J. M., Marshall, G.D., & Hovell, M. F. (1979). Behavioral strategies for improving compliance. In R. B. Haynes, D. W. Taylor & D. L. Sackett (Eds.), *Compliance in health care*, 174–192. Baltimore: The Johns Hopkins University Press.

Eisenthal, S., Emery, R., Lazare, A., & Udin, H. (1979). "Adherence" and the negotiated approach to patienthood. *Archives of General Psychiatry, 36*, 393–398.

Evans, R. I. (1984). A social inoculation strategy to deter smoking in adolescents. In J. D. Matarazzo, S. M. Weiss, J. A. Herd, N. E. Miller, & S. M. Weiss (Eds.), *Behavioral health: A handbook of health enhancement and disease prevention*, 765–774. New York: John Wiley & Sons.

Farquhar, J. W., Fortman, S. P., Maccoby, N., Wood, P. D., Haskell, W. L., Barr Taylor, C., Flora, J., Solomon, D. S., Rogers, T., Adler, E., Breitrose, P., & Weiner, L. (1984). The Stanford five city project. In J. D. Matarazzo, S. M. Weiss, J. A. Herd, N. E. Miller & S. M. Weiss (Eds.), *Behavioral health: A handbook of health enhancement and disease prevention*, 1154–1165. New York: John Wiley & Sons.

Franks, C. M., & Wilson, G. T. (1978). *Annual review of behavior therapy: Theory and practice* (Vol. 6). New York: Brunner/Mazel.

Glasgow, R. E., & Lichtenstein, E. (1987). The long-term effects of behavior smoking cessation programs. *Behavior Therapy, 18*, 297–324.

Haskell, W. L. (1984). Overview: Health benefits of exercise. In J. D. Matarazzo, S. M. Weiss,

J. A. Herd, N. E. Miller & S. M. Weiss (Eds.), *Behavioral health: A handbook of health enhancement and disease prevention*, 409–423. New York: John Wiley & Sons.

Haynes, R. B. (1976). A critical review of the "determinants" of patient compliance with therapeutic regimens. In D. L. Sackett & R. B. Haynes (Eds.), *Compliance with therapeutic regimens*, 26–39. Baltimore: The Johns Hopkins University Press.

Haynes, R. B. (1979a). Determinants of compliance. In R. B. Haynes, D. W. Taylor & D. L. Sackett (Eds.), *Compliance in health care*, 49–62. Baltimore: The Johns Hopkins University Press.

Haynes, R. B. (1979b). Strategies to improve compliance with referrals, appointments and prescribed medical regimens. In R. B. Haynes, D. W. Taylor & D. L. Sackett (Eds.), *Compliance in health care*, 121–143. Baltimore: The Johns Hopkins University Press.

Hughes, G. H., Hymowitz, N., Ockene, J. K., Simon, N., & Vogt, T. H. (1981). The multiple risk factor intervention trial (MRFIT): Intervention on smoking. *Preventative Medicine, 10*, 476–500.

Kozlowski, L. T. (1984). Pharmacological approaches to smoking modification. In J. D. Matarazzo, S. M. Weiss, J. A. Herd, N. E. Miller & S. M. Weiss (Eds.), *Behavioral health: A handbook of health enhancement and disease prevention*, 713–728. New York: John Wiley & Sons.

Lando, H. A. (1981). Effects of preparation, experimenter contract, and a maintained reduction alternative on a broad spectrum program for eliminating smoking. *Addictive Behavior, 6*, 123–133.

Leventhal, H., & Cleary, P. D. (1980). The smoking problem: A review of the research and theory in behavior risk modification. *Psychological Bulletin, 88*, 370–405.

Leventhal, H., Zimmerman, R., & Gutmann, M. (1984). Compliance: A self-regulation perspective. In W. D. Gentry (Ed.), *Handbook of behavioral medicine*, 329–436. New York: Guilford Press.

Ley, P. (1977). Psychological studies of doctor-patient communication. In S. Rachman (Ed.), *Contributions to medical psychology* (Vol. 1), 9–42. Oxford: Pergamon Press.

Ley, P., & Spellman, M. S. (1967). *Communicating with the patient*. London: Staples Press.

Lichtenstein, E. (1982). The smoking problem: A behavioral perspective. *Journal of Consulting and Clinical Psychology, 50*, 804–819.

Lichtenstein, E., & Mermelstein, R. J. (1984). Review of approaches to smoking treatment: Behavior modification. In J. D. Matarazzo, S. M. Weiss, J. A. Herd, N. E. Miller & S. M. Weiss (Eds.), *Behavioral health: A handbook of health enhancement and disease prevention*, 695–712. New York: John Wiley & Sons.

Maccoby, N., & Farquhar, J. W. (1975). Communication for health: Unselling heart disease. *Journal of Communication, 25*, 114–126.

Masur, F. T. (1981). Adherence to health care regimens. In C. K. Prokop & L. A. Bradley (Eds.), *Medical psychology: Contributions to behavioral medicine*, 442–470. New York: Academic Press.

Matarazzo, J. D., Weiss, S. M., Herd, J. A., Miller, N. E., & Weiss, S. M. (Eds), (1984). *Behavioral health: A handbook of health enhancement and disease prevention*. New York: John Wiley & Sons.

Mermelstein, R. J., Lichtenstein, E., & McIntyre, K. Θ. (1982). Partner support and relapse in smoking cessation programs. *Journal of Consulting and Clinical Psychology, 51*, 465–466.

Naditch, M. P. (1984). The staywell program. In J. D. Matarazzo, S. M. Weiss, J. A. Herd, N. E. Miller & S. M. Weiss (Eds.), *Behavioral health: A handbook of health enhancement and disease prevention*, 1071–1078. New York: John Wiley & Sons.

Nathan, P. E. (1984). Johnson & Johnson's Live for Life: A comprehensive positive lifestyle change program. In J. D. Matarazzo, S. M. Weiss, J. A. Herd, N. E. Miller & S. M. Weiss (Eds.), *Behavioral health: A handbook of health enhancement and disease prevention*, 1064–1070. New York: John Wiley & Sons.

Ockene, J. K., Benfari, R. C., Hurwitz, I., & Nuttall, R. L. (1982). Relationship of psychosocial factors to behavior change in an intervention program. *Preventative Medicine, 11*, 13–28.

Oldridge, N. B. (1984). Adherence to adult exercise fitness programs. In J. D. Matarazzo, S. M. Weiss, J. A. Herd, N. E. Miller & S. M. Weiss (Eds.), *Behavioral health: A handbook of health enhancement and disease prevention,* 467–487. New York: John Wiley & Sons.
Pomerleau, O. F., & Pomerleau, C. S. (1978). *Break the smoking habit: A behavioral program for giving up cigarettes*. Champaign, IL: Research Press.
Powell, D. R., & McCann, B. S. (1981). The effect of multiple treatment and multiple maintenance procedures on smoking cessation. *Preventative Medicine, 10,* 94–104.
Ray, O. A., & Ksir, C. (1981). *Drugs, society and human behavior*. St. Louis: Times Mirror/Mosby.
Ribsal, P. M. (1984). Developing an exercise prescription of health. In J. D. Matarazzo, S. M. Weiss, J. A. Herd, N. E. Miller, & S. M. Weiss (Eds.), *Behavioral health: A handbook of health enhancement and disease prevention,* 448–466. New York: John Wiley & Sons.
Schacter, S. (1978). Pharmacological and psychological determinants of smoking. *Annals of Internal Medicine, 88,* 104–114.
Straw, M. K. (1983). Coping with obesity. In T. G. Burish & L. A. Bradley (Eds.), *Coping with chronic disease,* 337–351. New York: Academic Press.
Stuart, R. B., & Davis, B. (1972). *Slim chance in a fat world.* Champaign, IL: Research Press.
Stuart, R. B., & Jacobson, B. (1979). Sex differences in obesity. In E. S. Gomberg, & V. Franks (Eds.), *Gender and disordered behavior: Sex differences and psychopathology,* 318–336. New York: Brunner/Mazel.
Stuart, R. B., Mitchell, C., & Jensen, J. A. (1981). Therapeutic options in the management of obesity. In C. K. Prokop & L. A. Bradley (Eds.), *Medical psychology: Contribution to behavioral medicine,* 321–354. New York: Academic Press.
Stunkard, A. J. (1975). From explanation to action in psychosomatic medicine: The case of obesity. *Psychosomatic Medicine, 37,* 195–236.
Stunkard, A. J. (1979). Behavioral medicine and beyond: The example of obesity. In O. F. Pomerleau & J. P. Brady (Eds.), *Behavioral medicine: Theory and practice,* 279–298. Baltimore: Williams & Wilkins.
Stunkard, A. J., Levine, H., & Fox, S. (1970). The management of obesity: Patient self-help and medical treatment. *Archives of Internal Medicine, 125,* 1067–1072.
Wadden, T. A., & Brownell, K. D. (1984). The development and modification of dietary practices in individuals, groups, and large populations. In J. D. Matarazzo, S. M. Weiss, J. A. Herd, N. E. Miller & S. M. Weiss (Eds.), *Behavioral health: A handbook of health enhancement and disease prevention,* 608–631. New York: John Wiley & Sons.
Warner, K. E. (1977). The effects of the anti-smoking campaign on cigarette consumption. *American Journal of Public Health, 67,* 645–650.
Wilson, G. T. (1984). Weight control treatments. In J. D. Matarazzo, S. M. Weiss, J. A. Herd, N. E. Miller & S. M.Weiss (Eds.), *Behavioral health: A handbook of health enhancement and disease prevention,* 657–670. New York: John Wiley & Sons.
Zifferblatt, S. M., Wilbur, C. S., & Pinky, J. (1980). Changing cafeteria eating habits. *Journal of the American Dietetic Association, 76,* 15–23.

14

Stress Management: Clinical and Preventative Applications

INTRODUCTION

In Chapter 4, we learned that stress has a strong influence on individuals' psychosocial and biological adaptation. Via indirect psychophysiological effects, stress can serve as a distal cause of disease. Disease and associated diagnostic, treatment, and rehabilitative procedures may also serve as sources of stress and consequently influence the progression, recurrence, and prognosis of disease. The affective arousal and cognitive and behavioral disorganization that may accompany stress can also evoke health-impairing palliative coping responses (e.g., drinking, smoking, and drug use) and interfere with appropriate illness-related decisions and actions (e.g., recognition of symptoms, timely use of health care, and adherence to treatment recommendations). Interventions to reduce stress and to enhance coping are, then, important facets of health care and education.

In this chapter, methods used to reduce stress and enhance coping will be described and evaluated. The first two sections will provide general guidelines for coping skills training and potential targets of such training. The subsequent three sections will focus on specific applications: (1) reducing of stress in "at risk" populations;

(2) minimizing stress associated with threatening or aversive diagnostic, treatment, and rehabilitative procedures and settings; and (3) enhancing the skills of individuals experiencing chronic or acute disorders to promote recovery or reduce the probability of the recurrence of the problems.

COPING SKILLS INTERVENTIONS: GENERAL GUIDELINES

Programs to teach coping skills consist of a series of sequential steps or tasks: assessment and collaborative conceptualization, skills acquisition and rehearsal, and skills application and generalization (Meichenbaum & Cameron, 1983). An overview of these tasks is shown in Table 14-1. The specific skills to be taught are more variable and depend on the problem, the client, and the situation. Content domains will be elaborated after the procedural outline is described.

TABLE 14-1 Procedural Guidelines for Stress Management Training

Assessment and collaborative conceptualization

Identify the situational determinants, psychological and physiological manifestations, and the consequences of stress using

- Interviewing
- Imaginal recall and role playing
- Direct observation
- Questionnaires and tests

Help the client develop skills in problem identification and analysis

Develop with the client a shared conceptualization of the problem and plans for treatment

Skills acquisition and rehearsal

Use instruction and modeling of instrumental and coping skills

Client rehearsal of instrumental and coping skills

Provide constructive, positive feedback for client rehearsal

- In all three steps use
  - Multiple trials
  - A flexible approach to problems
  - Multiple skills—an instrumental and coping menu

Skills application and generalization

Promote the use of an experimental attitude

Arrange the application of skills to real-life stressors in a hierarchical manner

Engage in continuing practice with feedback

Encourage a sense of self-efficacy

Fade clinical contact with success

Evaluate and train new skills as needed

Assessment and Collaborative Conceptualization

The purpose of assessment is to (1) identify the source of stress, (2) identify the manner in which the client currently copes with stress, (3) determine whether the client lacks the necessary coping skills or fails to utilize existing skills, and (4) identify the types of skills needed to cope more effectively.

Several methods can be used to acquire these data. Problem-oriented interviews with the client and significant others often provide useful information concerning the manifestations of stress, the situations that are stress evoking, and the factors that alleviate or exacerbate the problem. This information should be elaborated by a detailed description of the thoughts, feelings, behavior, and physiology of the client in specified stressful situations (Kanfer & Saslow, 1969). The recall of such specific information can be enhanced by imagery-based recall and role playing. In imagery-based recall, the client is asked to relive the experience descriptively in a detailed manner. In role playing, the situation is reconstructed and reenacted as realistically as possible.

Self-monitoring also provides a valuable source of information. The immediate observation and recording of experiences by a client offer a fine-grained analysis of the problem and enhance a client's awareness of situations that are stress evoking and of the manner in which they respond to stress. In some cases, it may be possible for the clinician to directly observe client responses to stressful situations in the natural environment. Such observations provide information that is less subject to client distortion and thus a more objective view of the problem and of the client's current means of coping (Hartmann, 1982; Nelson, 1977).

There are also a number of questionnaires and objective tests that may provide relevant information. Instruments are available that assess the frequency and severity of stress (e.g., the hassles scale: DeLongis, Coyne, Dakoif, Folkman, & Lazarus, 1982), characteristic styles of appraising situations (e.g., the irrational beliefs test: Jones, 1968), affective responses (e.g., the multiple affect adjective checklist: Zuckerman & Lubin, 1965), social support (e.g., the social support questionnaire: Sarason, Levine, Basham, & Sarason, 1983), and coping strategies (Folkman & Lazarus, 1980).

A flexible approach to assessment is important. Not all of the methods and targets just specified are necessary. In some situations, limited time is available for an assessment. However, assessment is critical to tailoring a relevant and effective intervention. Clients should be actively involved in the assessment process. Such involvement provides clients with a sense of understanding and control where they may have previously experienced a sense of victimization. Active involvement also facilitates the development of a general set of problem-solving skills.

Growing out of this collaborative assessment is an explicit shared conceptualization of the presenting problem. The exact conceptualization depends on the client and the presenting problem, but may use notions like the transactional model of stress (Chapter 4) or the gate control theory of pain (Chapter 8). This collaborative framework enables the client to understand, monitor, and respond to stress-provoking experiences more effectively. It also reassures the client that the problem is "real" and sets the stage for intervention.

Skills Acquisition and Rehearsal

Based on the assessment data, the focus of intervention turns to the acquisition and practice of coping skills relevant to the presenting problem, the situational determinants of the problem, and client characteristics. The goal is to develop an extensive, flexible repertoire of coping skills in behavioral, cognitive, affective, and physiological domains. The skills to be taught can be instrumental or palliative. Instrumental coping skills refer to responses that are directed at altering the distressing event. Palliative coping refers to responses focusing on the regulation of the impact of the stressor on the person.

The methods used to teach and practice coping skills are directive and problem oriented. Skill acquisition typically entails a "tell-show-do" approach. The desired coping skill is described and modeled. The client then rehearses the skill, and positive and corrective feedback are provided to shape the response. This sequence is repeated until the client's performance is proficient (Goldfried, 1980; Thoreson, 1984).

A number of coping skills are taught and practiced so that effective coping responses appropriate to situational demands are available to the client. Target skills are selected to be relevant to the presenting problem and are practiced in situations and settings progressively similar to the real-life context in which they are needed. Multiple trials are used to promote flexibility and overlearning. The ultimate goal is to instill a problem-solving set in the client. This set will enable the client to identify and analyze future problems and to select and enact coping responses to deal with those problems. Rote, mechanical learning, and application of coping skills are insufficient.

Skills Application and Generalization

Once the client is proficient at coping, she is asked to use those skills in the natural environment. The transition from practice to use is not abrupt. During practice, the client has utilized the skills under conditions that increasingly approximate the natural environment. When transferring their use to the natural environment, it is useful to have the client initially apply the skills to stressors that are time limited and of moderate intensity. As these initial attempts are successful, the client can then use the skills in progressively more difficult situations.

Learning to ride a bicycle provides a good analogy for this transition. Initially, training wheels and close supervision are used to facilitate learning (acquisition and early practice). As the rider becomes more proficient, the training wheels are raised and then removed, but the rider still operates the bicycle on the sidewalk or a quiet street (practice under more demanding conditions). When the skills are well developed, automatic, and responsive to prevailing conditions, the rider is allowed to venture farther from home and on busier streets (early application). With continued proficiency and practice, the person is able to ride with increasing independence under even more demanding conditions.

During initial application, the clinician maintains regular contact and, along with the client, evaluates the utility and performance of the coping skills. Further training, practice, and feedback are provided as needed. During this time, the client's sense of self-efficacy is enhanced in terms of both being able to produce a positive response and effecting a positive outcome when that response is produced (Bandura, 1977). Failures are treated as opportunities to learn or as indications that additional skills need to be acquired or that already acquired skills need further refinement.

Adaptability of These Procedural Guidelines

These guidelines for coping skills training may appear to be very complicated, time consuming, and formidable. The degree to which each of these tasks is implemented in a detailed, extensive manner depends on the problem, the client, and the realistic constraints of the intervention setting. For pervasive, chronic, stress-related problems (e.g., migraine headaches, cancer, or diabetic self-care), effective intervention may require a detailed, careful, and intensive progression through each of the tasks. For acute, situational stress-related problems (e.g., aversive medical procedures like endoscopy, coronary catheterization, and tooth extraction), the process may be truncated and abbreviated.

TARGETS OF COPING SKILLS TRAINING

The exact content of coping skills training programs is variable and individualized according to the client and the problem. An extremely wide variety of cognitive, affect-management, physiological, motor, and interpersonal skills are relevant to coping with stress. In a sense, there is a "menu" of coping skills, and targets for training appropriate to the client and the problem are selected from this menu. A full description of each item on the menu is not possible. Rather, some of the more frequently used and more generalized targets used in coping skills training will be described.

Social Skills Training

The ability to develop and maintain mutually rewarding relationships with others is central to successful adaptation. Problematic interpersonal transactions are among the most frequent sources of stress: dealing with difficult supervisors or subordinates at work, parenting a difficult child or adolescent, coping with marital conflict and discord, and effectively communicating feelings, needs, and opinions in routine daily contacts with other persons. Individuals who lack adequate social skills are at risk for greater stress (Eisler, 1984). Interpersonal skills are also an integral aspect of developing a strong social support system. As we saw in Chapter 4, such a system provides emotional and material supports that act as buffers against stress (Heller, Swindle, & Dusenbury, 1986).

If a lack of social skills is identified as an important source of stress, cognitive-behavioral interpersonal skills training can be initiated. The cognitive component entails providing information about the types of behavior that are socially acceptable and effective in various problematic situations (e.g., how to express anger and how to say "no" to unreasonable requests) (Lange & Jakubowski-Specter, 1976). It also entails the ability to attend to and accurately perceive signals displayed in social encounters. Some persons may be insensitive to such signals (e.g., the host yawning and looking at his watch means it is time to leave), whereas others may be oversensitive to these signals (e.g., a neutral gesture or word is viewed as a threat or attack) (Argyle & Kendon, 1967).

The behavioral component of social skills training focuses on the acquisition and practice of behavioral responses. This includes both the content of the response (what to say) and its style of delivery (speed, volume, and pitch). The cognitive and behavioral skills to be trained must be flexible since no one set of responses is acceptable and effective in all situations. Both the cognitive and behavioral facets of social skills are taught via the use of instructions, modeling, response practice, shaping, and feedback reinforcement (Eisler & Frederiksen, 1980).

Time Management

The so-called Protestant ethic is a central tenet of American society: Individuals must work hard to succeed and to be respected. Productivity and effective use of time are keys to economic success and recognition. Thus, a large number of demands are placed on a person's time and energy. Attempts to meet these multiple demands may result in worry, pressure, vacillation between activities, and dissatisfaction. This pressure is also associated with negative health outcomes, including increased blood pressure, elevated serum cholesterol levels, increased risk of accidents, and a failure to engage in health-promoting habits like exercise and rest (Everly, 1984).

Time management training provides individuals with skills to self-regulate their activities more effectively in relation to time. Time management focuses on the acquisition and practice of three categories of behavior: (1) setting priorities, (2) increasing the amount of "functional" time, and (3) reducing the sense of time urgency. Initially, clients are asked to self-monitor how they use their time. These data are then summarized by calculating the total amount of time spent in each of several activity categories. The content and number of these categories are individualized according to clients' roles and goals. For a traditional college student, these categories could be study, class, labs, recreational, and interpersonal. The amount of time expended in each category is then compared to the client's personal goals and objectives (Davis, Eshelman, & McKay, 1982).

Often, individuals have not clearly delineated their goals. Another aspect of time management entails helping clients clarify, identify, and prioritize their goals. Goals can be interpersonal, educational, vocational, or recreational. Long-term goals can then be specified. These goals refer to desired long-term accomplishments (e.g., graduation, promotion, or finding a mate). These goals should be realistic and genuinely important to the individual. If there are many goals, it may be useful to rank order them in terms of importance.

The concrete actions required to achieve one or two of these goals are specified. This may entail establishing subgoals (e.g., getting a C in algebra to graduate) and paths to these subgoals (e.g., spending 6 hours per week studying algebra). Short-term objectives are specified in terms of actions to be taken on a daily or weekly basis. It is often helpful to make daily and weekly "to do" lists with items identified in terms of importance. These lists cue time allocation according to one's priorities. Of course, long- and short-term goals and the behavioral means of achieving these goals are redefined in a manner compatible with accomplishments and genuine shifts in long-term objectives.

The amount of time available for high priority actions depends on decreasing time spent on less important but seemingly demanding activities. Clients are taught to identify and reduce sources of "wasted" time and activity that contribute only minimally to their own important goals. These may then be assigned or "hired out" to other people. Clients also have to learn to say "no" to requests that are incompatible with their goals. High priority activities should be scheduled. Low priority items come last.

It may often seem that demands and deadlines are imposed on us. They seem real and cannot be avoided. Not all demands and deadlines are warranted, however. Many are arbitrary and self-imposed. It is useful to distinguish between those that are self- versus environmentally imposed and those that have valid reasons versus those that are needless (Everly, 1984). For those demands and deadlines that are self-imposed or needless, it is useful to ask whether they are functional. Demands and deadlines are verbal rules (e.g., "I have to get an A"; or "I have to get this done by Friday"). When such rules lead to unproductive worry and action, they are not functional. Clients can be taught to identify dysfunctional demands and deadlines and to respond in a manner that is congruent with their arbitrariness (Hayes, 1987).

Procrastination is a common problem. It is often the result of a reluctance to make mistakes or an inability to know how to start. Fear of mistakes is really another form of an unreasonable demand ("I have to be perfect") and can be addressed by focusing on the relativity and functional value of verbal rules as just described. Not knowing how to start can be addressed by breaking a large, complex task into smaller, more manageable parts (Everly, 1984).

Altering Cognitions

As discussed in Chapter 4, stress entails the appraisal of an event and one's own capabilities and resources. In addition, problem solving, planning, and self-generated directives are central to successful coping. Because both stress and coping involve a number of cognitive processes, it is possible to reduce stress and enhance coping by helping clients alter their own cognitive processing.

Persons who are at risk for or who have already developed stress-related diseases often engage in dysfunctional appraisals of themselves and their environments. These individuals may have developed a habitual style of appraisal that places excessive demands on themselves or emphasizes their lack of ability and control. Dysfunctional appraisals maintain and exacerbate stress. Individuals may also lack problem-solving and planning skills necessary to take effective action. Intervention entails identifying and altering these maladaptive appraisals or other cognitive processing deficits, and providing the client with instructions, modeling, corrective experiences, and practice to develop more effective cognitive skills.

Chronic disease and its treatment confront individuals with a wide variety of challenging tasks. Successfully coping with these challenges entails a realistic but hopeful appraisal of the situation, a scanning of one's response repertoire to select responses to manage emotional reactions, to manage the disease effectively, and to adjust to the demands of treatment. Once potentially effective palliative and direct coping responses are identified, clients need to direct those responses cognitively so that they are enacted in a skillful way. Chronic disease and its treatment often confront individuals with novel or extreme adaptive tasks (e.g., aversive treatment procedures, catastrophic diagnoses, enduring disabilities, or complex self-care regimens) that seem overwhelming and beyond their control. Successful adaptation, rehabilitation, and recovery can be enhanced by providing clients with adequate cognitive coping skills. Self-instructional training and cognitive therapy, as described in Chapter 11, provide clients with a more productive set of cognitive skills to cope with stress.

STRESS MANAGEMENT: ALTERING THE ENVIRONMENT

Up to this point, our discussion of stress management has focused on providing individuals with coping skills relevant to the situation and the problem. The person is the target of change. Stress represents a mismatch between the person and the environment. It is also possible to alleviate stress by changing the environment. This can be done in several ways. Health providers make up an important facet of the treatment environment. Their style of interaction and communication may be more or less stress evoking. Health providers also exert control over the physical characteristics and rules and regulations of the treatment setting (e.g., a hospital). Ease of adaptation may vary according to the ecology in which treatment occurs. Thus, stress may be partially alleviated by altering the treatment-specific environment.

Health professionals may also be able to influence important facets of clients' environment outside of the treatment setting, such as family involvement, work site adjustments, and enlistment of economic or social service resources. These ecological as compared to person-directed interventions foster an environment that minimizes the adaptive demands made of clients, provides coping resources, fosters the acquisition of coping skills by clients. We will consider three such ecological interventions: providing information to clients, enlisting and creating social support systems, and planning the treatment environment.

Providing Information

Successful coping is enhanced when individuals have information about the timing and nature of stressful events. This information enhances persons' sense of control and enables them to select and utilize coping responses that are effective in managing the stressful situation. Health professionals are often in a position to offer information about diagnostic and treatment procedures and settings, the implications of a diagnosis, the effectiveness of treatment, and the degree of expected rehabilitation and recovery. They can also involve clients in decision making.

An overview of control-enhancing interventions is shown in Table 14-2. Two types of information can be offered: procedural and sensory. Procedural information entails a relatively objective description of what will happen, when and where it will occur, and how long it will last. A

TABLE 14-2 Control-Enhancing Interventions

TYPE OF CONTROL	DEFINITION	EXAMPLES
Behavioral control	Taking action to alter the timing, duration, or intensity of an event or to control the occurrence of termination of an event	Breathing exercises during prepared childbirth; signaling the termination of a painful dental procedure
Cognitive control	Thinking differently about an event, distraction, problem solving, or self-instruction	Using a focal point in prepared childbirth; listing coping strategies while waiting for an aversive medical procedure to begin
Decisional control	Making decisions about the onset, timing, occurrence, or type of an event	Choosing between several alternative medical procedures; allowing an expectant mother to determine whether an anesthetic will be used during birthing
Informational control	Providing information about the nature and impact of an event	Learning about the different phases of labor and associated sensations; having the steps in a medical procedure described in detail

dentist, for example, might provide procedural information in the following way: "First, I'm going to give you a shot of procaine. It will take about five minutes for it to deaden any pain associated with the procedure. After it takes effect, I will use a high-speed drill and porcelain to repair the cavity. That will only take a few minutes. The procaine will wear off in three or four hours." Sensory information, on the other hand, focuses on the sensory and affective experiences of the client. The description focuses on experiences from the client's rather than an outside observer's point of view. A dentist might say:

> The topical anesthetic will taste rather bitter. But it will reduce the slight pang that you may feel when I use the needle to give you a shot of procaine. The procaine will make the side of your mouth numb in five or ten minutes.

> Often, this is an odd feeling, but it will recede in two or three hours. After the procaine takes effect, I'll start drilling. The drill is rather aversive sounding, and you'll feel some vibration and pressure as I work on your tooth. But you'll probably feel very little actual pain.

Sensory information appears to be more useful than procedural information, but in practice it is common to provide both. Such information has been found to have a modestly beneficial effect on distress and tolerance before, during, and after a stressful event (Taylor, 1986).

Decisional control refers to providing clients with the opportunity to make decisions about the nature, timing, duration, or occurrence of some stressful event. The capacity of clients to make good decisions assumes that they have been given adequate information. The health provider may describe several options and their likely consequences and indicate which option she feels is optimal. The client, however, is involved in the choice. The dentist may suggest that the procedure may be done any time in the next two weeks (timing), may offer the choice between two procedures (nature), or may allow the client to stop a procedure when it becomes uncomfortable or painful (duration).

Reviews suggest that providing clients with information and involving them in decisions have beneficial effects (Turk, Meichenbaum, & Genest, 1983), but that these benefits are not uniform across clients, target problems, and situations. Some individuals tend to respond to stress with avoidance (like the proverbial ostrich who sticks its head in the sand). These individuals, called repressers, tend to react negatively to control-enhancing efforts and may need intensive practice and exposure to benefit from information and involvement in decision making. On the other hand, there are persons whose typical response to stress is vigilance. These persons, called sensitizers, are more responsive and obtain greater benefit from information and involvement in decision making. In a similar vein, individuals who have had a very negative experience with some stressor (e.g., past dental work that has been very painful) may benefit less from these interventions. It is important to be accurate when providing information and involving persons in decisions. If the information is inaccurate, they are unable to select and use effective means of coping. The disconfirmation of expected control may actually enhance the distress and promote a negative reaction toward the health provider.

Enlisting and Creating Social Supports

The adjustive demands associated with disease, diagnosis, treatment, and rehabilitation have an impact on the quality of clients' relationships with family and friends. Because family and friends are important resources for clients, this impact may reciprocally influence clients' adjustment and recovery. There are three ways in which family and friends may influence coping. First, they are often involved in providing care and implementing treatment. Second, they are a source of information and support that influence clients' motivation and mode of coping. Third, both disease-specific and nonspecific interactions between clients and family or friends can exacerbate or reduce stress. Negative interactions characterized by conflict and rejection at one extreme or by indulgence and overprotection at the other extreme may exacerbate stress and interfere with adjustment. Avoidance, neglect, and a lack of communication between clients and their family members and friends are similarly problematic. Interactions characterized by acceptance, support, recognition of the realistic limitations imposed by the problem, and mutual problem solving and adjustive orientation reduce stress and facilitate recovery and adaptation (Masters, Cerreto, & Mendlowitz, 1983).

Health professionals should be sensitive to the contribution of natural social systems to client coping. The degree and nature of this involvement should be assessed (see, e.g., Stein & Reisman, 1980). Based on this assessment, intervention to enhance the quality of interaction between the client and significant others may be formulated and implemented. These interventions may focus on caring for the client, reducing conflict, increasing involvement, or promoting a supportive, problem-solving atmosphere.

In some cases, natural support systems can be supplemented by involving the client in new, problem-oriented support groups. In such groups, the client can meet other persons who are experiencing similar problems. Interaction with these peers may provide the client with support, and an opportunity to discuss the problem, to learn specific self-care and general coping skills, and to identify resources. Group members learn that other people are struggling with similar problems and serve as coping models from whom other members acquire relevant information and coping skills. These groups may be led by a professional, or they may consist of only nonprofessional peers. Although such groups appear to have potential, their effectiveness has not been adequately researched.

Planning the Treatment Environment

There are many approaches to assessing and altering environments. A social-ecological approach will be used in this discussion. This approach, which suggests that the environment shapes behavior, focuses on the impact of the environment from the perspective of the individual. Some forms of coping are constrained and others are facilitated by the characteristics of the environment (Moos, 1984).

On the basis of an environmental assessment, steps can be taken to alter the treatment environment systematically. For example, studies suggest that the environmental characteristics of nursing homes may shape passivity and hopelessness, which have deleterious effects on clients. Langer and Rodin (1976) attempted to increase client control and activity by altering a nursing home environment. Clients on one floor were given plants to care for and choice concerning when to participate in activities. Clients from another floor were given plants, but the staff cared for the plants. They participated in the same activities as the other clients, but were given no choice in terms of their timing. When compared with the clients who were given no control, clients who were given control were more active, displayed more positive affect, and reported a greater sense of well-being both one month and then one year after intervention. There were also fewer deaths among clients who were given enhanced control. The powerful effects engendered by such a simple and economical intervention suggest that alteration of the treatment environment holds great promise.

STRESS MANAGEMENT: APPLICATIONS

Coping with Aversive Medical Procedures

Many diagnostic and treatment procedures used in medicine and dentistry are aversive or painful. Cardiac catheterization, chemotherapy, radiation therapy, debridement of burns, postsurgical pain, dental work, injections, kidney dialysis, and many other procedures are effective and necessary biological interventions but also challenge clients' coping resources. The stress evoked by these procedures results in discomfort, worry, tension, decreased client cooperation, and physiological arousal. These reactions in turn may result in negative physical symptoms, exacerbation of the disease, and increased recovery time. To maximize physical and psychological comfort and recovery, interventions to prepare clients to cope with aversive procedures have been developed and tested.

A wide variety of strategies have been used to prepare clients: (1) psychological support, (2) information, (3) procedure-specific skills training, (4) relaxation training, (5) filmed modeling, and (6) cognitive-behavioral coping skills training (Kendall & Watson, 1981). A classic work in this area utilized filmed modeling to reduce children's distress prior to hospitalization and surgery. One group of children who were scheduled for surgery watched a film that provided information about the procedures and showed operating and recovery rooms. The narrator in the film discussed likely concerns and provided coping strategies for the viewers. A control group of children who were also scheduled for surgery watched an irrelevant film. The children who received the information and coping skills preparation displayed less physiological arousal and anxiety, and fewer self-reported fears than children who saw the irrelevant film (Melamed & Siegal, 1975). Similar information and coping skills modeling films used to prepare individuals for dental procedures have also led to positive results. Filmed modeling and information appear to be effective and economical means of preparing persons for aversive medical procedures.

Cognitive-behavioral coping skills training attempts to provide clients with a set of procedure-relevant skills so that they are better prepared for aversive medical interventions. This training has been applied to a number of different procedures, but our discussion will focus on its application to the treatment of burns. Clients who are severely burned experience continuous pain that is often exacerbated by the procedures used to treat the burns. Two particularly aversive treatments are "tanking" and debridement. In tanking, the client is lowered into a tub of fluid where dressings and encrusted medications are removed by gentle scrubbing. Debridement entails cutting away dead tissue in severely burned areas of the body. Wernick (1983) describes a cognitive-behavioral coping skills intervention for burn patients. After providing a rationale for intervention, burn patients are taught several physiological coping techniques including modified muscle relaxation, mental imagery, and deep breathing. They are also taught to reappraise treatment cognitively (e.g., "The pain is necessary for healing," rather than "This is awful, I can't stand it anymore"), and to distract themselves from the pain. These coping skills are rehearsed prior to the procedure and actively coached during the procedure. Compared to clients receiving no intervention, those receiving coping skills training were rated by treatment personnel as more cooperative, requested less pain medication, and reported less physical and affective distress.

In problem-specific skills training, clients are taught behaviors that are specifically relevant to the distress or discomfort caused by the procedure. For example, Lindeman and Van Aerham (1971) taught surgical clients to cope with postsurgical pain and discomfort by using diaphragmatic breathing, leg and foot exercises, and special techniques for coughing and turning over in bed. This problem-specific skills training entailed instruction, modeling, and practice with feedback. The specific-skills training group did not differ from a control group in the amount of postsurgical pain medication requested, but were able to leave the hospital earlier.

It appears that a number of interventions can be used to reduce distress, recovery time, and physiological arousal in response to aversive diagnostic and treatment procedures. Preparing clients by providing sensory and procedural information and by training in procedure-specific behavioral coping skills, relaxation, and cognitive reappraisal and distraction appears to be effective. It also appears that these interventions can be implemented in a time-efficient manner. Much of the research in this area suffers from methodological flaws. Placebo control groups are not used, individual differences in clients are ignored, and outcome assessment is often based on single measures by biased observers.

At the same time, there are sufficient research data to support the continued use of client preparation in clinical settings. Kendall and Watson (1981) offered an overview of preparatory interventions as shown in Figure 14-1. When the client and the health provider agree to engage in a procedure, an assessment of the client's concerns and reactions should be made. Is this client at risk? Would the client benefit from more extensive preparation than is usually given? When the procedure is scheduled, the client should be given procedural and sensory information and be offered more intensive preparation if needed. If the client accepts the offer for more intensive preparation, the types of skills appropriate to the procedure and the client should be identified.

Prior to the procedure, the selected procedure-specific behavioral, relaxation, and cognitive coping skills are introduced, modeled, and practiced. The duration of this phase varies depending on the client, the procedure, and the scheduling. The client's actual affective, physiological, and behavioral responses before, during and after the procedure should be assessed.

Coping with Chronic Illness

Chronic diseases, ranging from mild to severe to life threatening, are experienced by 50 percent of the population at any given time. Chronic illness often cannot be cured but only managed. Depending on its severity, chronic illness may have a pervasive effect on many areas of a person's life and confront the individual with a host of adjustive demands (Turk, 1985). The specific nature of the adaptational tasks varies according to illness. A general outline of these tasks was given in Chapter 4.

Coping skills training can be used to enhance clients' ability to meet these adaptive demands, to promote psychosocial well-being, and to limit the progression, severity, and recurrence of the disease. To get a concrete sense of the application of coping skills training to chronic disease, let us examine diabetes mellitus. Diabetes is a chronic metabolic disorder that results from one of two types of deficits: the insufficient manufacture and release of insulin from the pancreas or the inability of body tissue to utilize insulin. Diabetes is the tenth leading cause of death in the United States and is a major contributor to blindness, vascular disease resulting in the loss of limb, cardiac disease, and kidney degeneration and failure. It also increases the risk of perinatal death and abnormalities. It is the fourth leading cause of physician visits (Lipsitt, 1980). Because of its nature and sequelae, persons with diabetes are confronted with a number of adjustive tasks. These tasks are shown in Table 14-3.

Self-care is an integral aspect of the management of diabetes. To engage in effective self-care, diabetic clients must acquire and consistently perform a complex set of decisional and behavioral skills. Diabetic

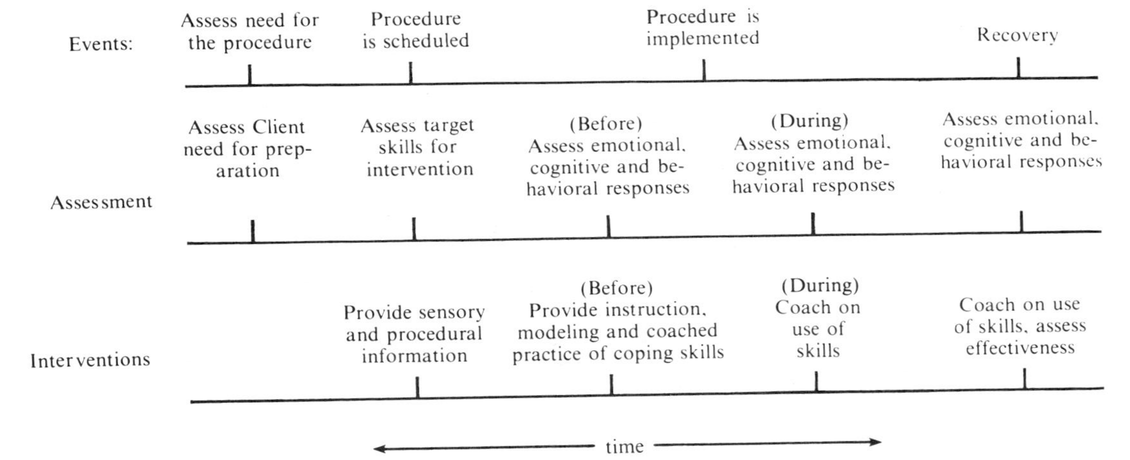

FIGURE 14-1 Guidelines for Preparation for Medical Procedures

TABLE 14-3 Adaptive Tasks Specific to Diabetes Mellitus

Self-care
- Monitoring
  - Urine and blood glucose
  - Discriminated insulin use, exercise, and eating based on monitoring
- Control
  - Insulin administration
  - Dietary adjustments in the frequency, amount, and type of foods
  - Exercise adjustments

Disturbances and adaptations
- Stress
- Reduced physical capabilities
- Social adjustments

Potential long-term sequelae
- Heart disease
- Kidney disease
- Retinal disease
- Peripheral vascular disorders
- Pregnancy complications

persons must accurately self-monitor their own blood sugar levels. This entails drawing blood and assessing blood sugar using home testing equipment. For severe diabetics, this monitoring must be done at several times during the day prior to injecting insulin, eating, and exercising. Modeling, shaping, and practice with feedback about accuracy can be used to teach these skills. Diabetics may also be taught to estimate their blood sugar levels more accurately using physiological cues rather than external monitoring devices (Wing, Epstein, Nowalk, & Lamparski, 1986).

If an error is detected between desired and actual blood sugar levels, the diabetic client must make an appropriate response. If blood sugar is too high or too low, appropriate adjustments must be made in eating, exercise, or insulin injections. The ability to make the controlling response (e.g., injecting insulin) and the appropriateness and accuracy of the response have been taught using chaining and reinforcement, modeling and rehearsal, and practice with feedback. Monitoring and controlling responses in self-care require knowledge and decisional as well as behavioral skills (Wing et al., 1986). The acquisition and consistent performance of these responses are critical to maintaining the quality of life and to reducing the likelihood of negative sequelae of the disease. As with other self-care behaviors, adherence is frequently a problem and may require intervention using the strategies described in the last chapter (see Wing et al., 1986, for a review of interventions to enhance adherence to diabetic self-care actions).

Research suggests that stress may, via indirect psychophysiological mechanisms, disrupt glucose and lipid metabolism in persons who are diabetic. These stressors may be disease specific (e.g., interpersonal conflict regarding self-care; unrealistic and realistic disease-related interference with recreational, vocational, and academic activities; and physiological complications created by diabetes) or more general (e.g., daily hassles, interpersonal conflicts, and major negative life events) (Turk & Speers, 1983; Wing et al., 1986). For individuals whose diabetic control and self-management are disrupted by stress, coping skills or environmental interventions may be useful. Relaxation training and EMG biofeedback training have been used with varied success in training diabetic individuals to cope more effectively with stress-induced changes in glucose and lipid metabolism. This training has resulted in improved metabolic control and a reduction in the frequency of diabetic crises in some but not all clients (Fowler, Budzinski, & VanderBergh, 1976; Rose, Firestone, Heick, & Faught, 1983; Surwit & Feinglos, 1983). Social skills and cognitive-behavioral coping skills training have also been utilized with some success (Gross, Johnson, Wildman, & Mullet, 1984; Hinkle & Wolf, 1952).

Attempts have also been to mitigate stress by enhancing the social support systems of diabetic clients (Tarnow, 1978) and by reducing family conflict (Minuchin, Rosman, & Baker, 1978; Snyder, 1987). Treatment focusing on stress management training for diabetics is in its infancy and has not been rigorously evaluated. The exact nature of the stressors and the requisite coping skills vary according to the client, situation, and severity of the diabetes. Many diabetic individuals adjust adequately. A careful assessment is required to identify diabetic individuals who could benefit from such training. The targets of the training need to be tailored according to the client.

This abbreviated excursion into coping skills training for individuals with diabetes only scratches the surface of the potential applications of coping skills training for persons experiencing chronic disease. The application of coping skills training to other disorders, including stroke, kidney disease, spinal cord injury, birth defects, and epilepsy, is beyond the scope of this book. Readers interested in applications to other chronic diseases should refer to Moos (1984) and Burish and Bradley (1983) for additional information. Descriptions of coping skills training for individuals experiencing coronary artery disease, cancer, and pain will be detailed in the next two chapters.

SUMMARY

Stress often contributes to the etiology of disease and may interfere with treatment and recovery. Disease, especially chronic disease, presents the individual with a diverse set of threats to their biological, psychological, and social well-being. Diagnostic and treatment procedures may also evoke distress and discomfort. Consequently, stress management and coping skills training represent potentially effective means of promoting health and recovery from disease. They can be applied in a preventative fashion to individuals who are at risk for stress-related disease but not yet symptomatic. It can be used to enhance psychosocial and physiological recovery from acute and chronic disease. Finally, it can be used to minimize the negative effects of aversive and painful diagnostic and treatment procedures.

Coping skills training can take many forms. It can focus on providing clients with cognitive, behavioral, and physiological skills to cope in a direct or palliative fashion with stress. It may also entail changing the environment so that it is less stress-provoking or so that informational, emotional, and material sources of support are more available. The exact nature of person- or environment-focused intervention varies according to the client, problem, and environmental context. The efficacy and cost effectiveness of such interventions are far from completely established. Data currently available suggest that stress management and coping skills training are potentially powerful weapons for health promotion and disease prevention.

An implicit theme in this chapter is self-regulation. There has been an emphasis on helping persons acquire and perform responses by which they can more adequately adapt to their environment, their own health status, and their recommended treatment. In each application, the goal is to foster individuals' capabilities so that they prosper psychologically, affectively, socially, and organically.

REFERENCES

Argyle, M., & Kendon, A. (1967). The experimental analysis of social performance. In L. Berkowitz (Ed.), *Advances in experimental social psychology* (Vol. 3), 55–99. New York: Academic Press.

Bandura, A. (1977). Self-efficacy: Toward a unifying theory of behavior change. *Psychological Bulletin, 84*, 191–215.

Burish, T. G., & Bradley, L. A. (1983). *Coping with chronic disease: Research and applications*. New York: Academic Press.

Davis, M., Eshelman, E. R., & McKay, M. (1982). *The relaxation and stress reduction workbook* (2nd ed.). Oakland, CA: New Harbinger.

DeLongis, A., Coyne, J. C., Dakoif, G., Folkman, S., & Lazarus, R. S. (1982). Relation of daily hassles, uplifts and major life events to health status. *Health Psychology, 1*, 119–136.

Eisler, R. M. (1984). Promoting health through interpersonal skills development. In J. D. Matarazzo, S. M. Weiss, J. A. Herd, N. E. Miller, & S. M. Weiss (Eds.), *Behavioral health: A handbook of health enhancement and disease prevention*, 351–362. New York: John Wiley & Sons.

Eisler, R. M., & Frederiksen, L. W. (1980). *Perfecting social skills: A guide to interpersonal behavior development*. New York: Plenum Press.

Everly, G. S. (1984). Time management: A behavioral strategy for disease prevention and health enhancement. In J.D. Matarazzo, S. M. Weiss, J. A. Herd, N. E. Miller, & S. M. Weiss (Eds.), *Behavioral health: A handbook of health enhancement and disease prevention*, 363–370. New York: John Wiley & Sons.

Folkman, S., & Lazarus, R. S. (1980). An analysis of coping in a middle-aged community sample. *Journal of Health and Social Behavior, 21*, 219–239.

Fowler, J. E., Budzinski, T. H., & VanderBergh, R. L. (1976). Effects of EMG biofeedback relaxation on the control of diabetes. *Biofeedback and Self Regulation, 1*, 105–112.

Goldfried, M. R. (1980). Toward a delineation of therapeutic change principles. *American Psychologist, 54*, 125–133.

Gross, A. M., Johnson, W. G., Wildman, H., & Mullet, N. (1984). Coping skills training with insulin dependent pre-adolescent diabetics. *Child Behavior Therapy, 6*, 183–196.

Hartmann, D. P. (1982). *Using observers to study behavior*. San Francisco: Jossey-Bass.

Hayes, S. C. (1987). A contextual approach to therapeutic change. In N. Jacobson (Ed.), *Cognitive and behavior therapies in clinical practice*, 123–149. New York: Guilford Press.

Heller, K., Swindle, R. W., & Dusenbury, L. (1986). Component social support processes: Comments and integration. *Journal of Consulting and Clinical Psychology, 54*, 466–470.

Hinkle, L. E., & Wolf, S. (1952). Importance of life stress in the course and management of diabetes mellitus. *Journal of the American Medical Association, 148*, 513–520.

Jones, R. (1968). *A factored measure of Ellis' irrational beliefs system with personality and maladjustment correlated*. Unpublished doctoral dissertation, Texas Technical College. Lubbock, TX.

Kanfer, F., & Saslow, G. (1969). Behavioral diagnosis. In C. Franks (Ed.), *Behavior therapy: Appraisal and status*, 417–444. New York: McGraw-Hill.

Kendall, P. C., & Watson, D. (1981). Psychological preparation for stressful medical procedures. In C. K. Prokop & L. A. Bradley (Eds.), *Medical psychology: Contributions to behavioral medicine*, 198–223. New York: Academic Press.

Lange, A. J., & Jakubowski, P. (1976). *Responsible assertive behavior: Cognitive / behavioral procedures for trainers*. Champaign, IL: Research Press.

Langer, E. J., & Rodin, J. (1976). The effects of choice and enhanced personal responsibility for the aged: A field experiment. *Journal of Personality and Social Psychology, 34*, 191–198.

Lindeman, C. A., & Van Aerham, B. (1971). Nursing intervention with the presurgical patient: The effects of structured and unstructured preoperative teaching. *Nursing Research, 20*, 319–331.

Lipsitt, L. F. (1980). Overview of diabetes mellitus. *Behavioral Medicine Update, 2*, 15–17.

Masters, J. C., Cerreto, M. C., & Mendlowitz, D. R. (1983). The role of the family in coping with childhood chronic illness. In T. G. Burish & L. A. Bradley (Eds.), *Coping with chronic disease: Research and applications*, 357–378. New York: Academic Press.

Meichenbaum, D., & Cameron, R. (1983). Stress inoculation training: Toward a general paradigm for training coping skills. In D. Meichenbaum & M. E. Jaremko (Eds.), *Stress reduction and prevention*, 13–47. New York: Plenum Press.

Melamed, B. G., & Siegal, L. J. (1975). Reduction of anxiety in children facing hospitalization and surgery by use of filmed modeling. *Journal of Consulting and Clinical Psychology, 43*, 511–521.

Minuchin, S., Rosman, B. L., & Baker, L. (1978). *Psychosomatic families*. Cambridge, MA: Harvard University Press.

Moos, R. H. (1984). *Coping with physical illness* (Vol. 2). New York: Plenum Press.

Nelson, R. O. (1977). Methodological issues in assessment via self-monitoring. In J. D. Cone & R. P. Hawkins (Eds.), *Behavioral assessment: New directions in clinical psychology*, 217–240. New York: Brunner/Mazel.

Novaco, R. W. (1978). Anger and coping with stress: Cognitive-behavioral intervention. In J. P. Foreyt & D. P. Rathjen (Eds.), *Cognitive behavior therapy: Research and application*, 135–174. New York: Academic Press.

Rose, M. I., Firestone, P., Heick, H. M., & Faught, H. K. (1983). The effects of anxiety management training on the control of juvenile diabetes mellitus. *Journal of Behavioral Medicine, 6*, 381–395.

Sarason, I. G., Levine, H. M., Basham, R. B., & Sarason, B. R. (1983). Assessing social support: The social support questionnaire. *Journal of Personality and Social Psychology, 47*, 127–139.

Snyder, J. (1987). Behavioral analysis and treatment of poor diabetic self-care and antisocial behavior: A single subject experimental study. *Behavior Therapy, 18*, 251–263.

Stein, R. E., & Reisman, C. K. (1980). The development of an impact-on-the-family scale: Some preliminary findings. *Medical Care, 18*, 465–472.

Surwit R. S., & Feinglos, M. D. (1983). The effects of relaxation on glucose tolerance in non-insulin dependent diabetics. *Diabetes Care, 6*, 176–179.

Tarnow, J. D. (1978). The psychological implications of the diagnosis of juvenile diabetes on the child and the family. *Psychosomatics, 19*, 487–491.

Taylor, S. E. (1986). *Health psychology*. New York: Random House.

Thoreson, C. (1984). Overview. In J. D. Matarazzo, S. M. Weiss, J. A. Herd, N. E. Miller, & S. M. Weiss (Eds.), *Behavioral health: A handbook of health enhancement and disease prevention*, 297–307. New York: John Wiley & Sons.

Turk, D. C. (1985). Factors influencing the adaptive process of coping with chronic illness: Implications for intervention. In I. Sarason & C. Spielberger (Eds.), *Stress and Anxiety*. (Vol. 6), 291–312. Washington, DC: Hemisphere.

Turk, D. C., Meichenbaum, D., & Genest, M. (1983). *Pain and behavioral medicine: A cognitive-behavioral perspective*. New York: Guilford.

Turk, D. C., & Speers, M. A. (1983). Diabetes Mellitus: A cognitive-functional analysis of stress. In T. G. Burish & L. A. Bradley (Eds.), *Coping with chronic disease: Research and applications*, 147–169. New York: Academic Press.

Wernick, R. L. (1983). Stress inoculation in the management of clinical pain: Applications to burn patients. In D. Meichenbaum & M. E. Jaremko (Eds.), *Stress reduction and prevention*, 337–359. New York: Plenum Press.

Wing, R. R., Epstein, L. H., Nowalk, M. D., & Lamparski, D. M. (1986). Behavioral self regulation in the treatment of patients with diabetes mellitus. *Psychological Bulletin, 45*, 78–89.

Zuckerman, M., & Lubin, B. (1965). *Manual for the Multiple Affect Adjective Checklist*. San Diego: Educational and Industrial Testing Service.

15

Coronary Artery Disease and Cancer: Preventative and Clinical Interventions

INTRODUCTION

In Chapters 6 and 8, the involvement of psychosocial and behavioral variables in the etiology, treatment, and recovery from coronary artery disease and cancer was described. Given their influence, interventions that systematically alter these variables may powerfully contribute to preventative and clinical health care. Figure 15-1 provides an overview of preventative and clinical interventions in the natural history of a disease. In that figure, intervals along the time line represent the progression of the disease process and its manifestations. As this progression occurs, there are consonant changes in the methods and goals of intervention.

At the prepathogenic stage, the goal is to reduce individuals' exposure to risk factors so that the disease process (biological onset) is not initiated. Interventions to achieve this goal are called primary prevention. Once the disease process begins, the goal is to detect early signs of the disease and to implement interventions to slow its progression and to delay or preclude its clinical onset. This is called secondary prevention. After the symptoms of the disease have become manifest, clinical and rehabilitative interventions are used to arrest the disease and to restore individuals' functional capacity.

Critical Points		Biological Onset		Clinical Onset		
Disease Process	prepathnogenesis		pathnogenesis		progression	
Manifestations	risk factors		signs		signs & symptoms	residual functional capacity
Type of Intervention	Primary Prevention		Secondary Prevention		Clinical Intervention	Rehabilitation
Goals	reduce risk of biological onset		reduce risk of clinical onset		arrest progression of the disease	

time →

FIGURE 15-1 An Overview of Preventative and Clinical Interventions in the Natural History of a Disease

Behavioral and psychosocial principles and methods are central to the preventative and clinical interventions used at the various stages of the disease process. In this chapter, behavioral and psychosocial strategies applicable to the preventative and clinical treatment of coronary artery disease and cancer will be described and evaluated. The discussion will cover a variety of assessment and intervention strategies targeting health habits, stress, health care utilization, preparation for medical procedures, and coping with the consequences of disease. These applications are quite recent and circumscribed. As you will learn, we are at the beginning of a promising and exciting endeavor (Agras, 1984).

CORONARY ARTERY DISEASE

Health Habit Modification: Risk Reduction and Prevention

A number of behaviors are associated with an increased risk for coronary artery disease (see Table 15-1). If the risk of coronary artery disease is related to specific behaviors, then the disease is potentially preventable given the modification of these behaviors. In particular, behaviors targeted for change in the prevention of coronary artery disease are: (1) smoking, (2) caloric intake, (3) consumption of cholesterol, saturated fat, salt, and sugar, and (4) aerobic exercise (Coates, Perry, Killen, & Slinkard, 1981).

Several large-scale efforts have been made to assess whether the risk of cardiovascular disease can be reduced by altering individuals' health habits. Most of these interventions have focused on adults who already show subclinical symptoms of coronary artery disease (i.e., secondary prevention). Only a few attempts have been made to alter behaviors associated with risk for cardiovascular disease in children and

TABLE 15-1 Behavioral Risk Factors for Coronary Artery Disease

PHYSIOLOGICAL RISK FACTOR	BEHAVIORAL CAUSE
Overweight	Excessive eating and drinking Lack of adequate exercise
Elevated blood cholesterol	High dietary consumption of fats High dietary consumption of saturated fats
Elevated blood pressure	High dietary consumption of salt Lack of adequate exercise Excessive eating and drinking
Acceleration of atherosclerosis	Smoking Type A behavior

adolescents (i.e., primary prevention). Let us begin by examining three large-scale secondary prevention studies: the Stanford Heart Disease Prevention Program (SHDPP), the North Karelia Project, and the Multiple Risk Factor Intervention Trial (MRFIT).

The objective of the SHDPP was to alter individuals' knowledge, attitudes, health behaviors, and physiological risk associated with cardiovascular disease (Farquhar et al., 1977). Measures of knowledge, health habits (smoking, diet, and exercise), and physiology (weight, blood pressure, and levels of serum cholesterol and saturated fats) were assessed in samples taken from three California communities prior to intervention and annually for three subsequent years. During those three years, one community received an intensive media campaign and individual counseling (called the media and counseling group), one received the media campaign only (called the media group), and the remaining community received no intervention (called the control group). The media campaign consisted of the wide and frequent dissemination of information concerning the causes of cardiovascular disease and the specific behaviors that influence its occurrence. It also provided specific information and recommendations about how to change those behaviors to reduce risk. Individual counseling entailed face-to-face intervention to foster behavior change using principles of self-control (self-monitoring, stimulus control, and self-reinforcement), modeling, and rehearsal. Both interventions were intensive during the first two years and then faded during the last year (Maccoby, Farquhar, Wood, & Alexander, 1977).

The media and counseling group experienced a 50% increase and the media only group a 25% increase in knowledge after the first year, compared to almost no change in the control community. These differences were maintained over time. Both the media only and the media and counseling interventions resulted in decreased dietary intake of fats compared to the control group. The media and counseling group showed a substantial reduction or cessation in smoking relative to the media only and control groups. No consistent and lasting changes were found in blood pressure or exercise. Using a multiple risk factor score based on age, gender, plasma cholesterol, systolic blood pressure, and weight, the media and counseling group reduced their risk score by 28% in the first year, and this reduction was maintained during the two subsequent years. The media only group showed a slower reduction in risk to about 25% after two years, but this change was not fully maintained during the third year. The control group's risk score did not change by more than 5% over the three-year period (Meyer, Nash, McAlister, Maccoby, & Farquhar, 1980). The primary sources of change in risk were reduced smoking and cholesterol.

At first glance, the results of the SHDPP are quite encouraging. This initial impression must be tempered by the consideration of several methodological and analytical weaknesses in the study. First, a number of individuals dropped out of the study, especially in the media and counseling group. When the data from these individuals are included in the outcome analysis, the beneficial effects of the program are much less powerful (Leventhal, Safer, Cleary, & Gutmann, 1980). Second, the multiple risk factor score may not be a good predictor of coronary heart disease in individuals (Kasl, 1980). Third, it is not clear whether changes in clients' knowledge and behavior effected change in physiological risk factors for heart disease. Finally, maintenance of the beneficial effects has not been established.

A similar community-based risk factor reduction program was implemented in North Karelia, Finland (McAlister, Puska, Salonen, Tuomilehto, & Koskela, 1982; Salonen, Puska, & Mustaniemi, 1979). Although this program, similar to the SHDPP, attempted to alter knowledge, habit, and risk factor targets, this intervention focused on producing changes in community organizations to effect ongoing and lasting individual change. The North Karelia project entailed a mass media campaign, health education, health services, the development of a communication and information network, training of local health providers, and alteration of the environment. Ten thousand persons from North Karelia were initially assessed on smoking, blood pressure, and serum cholesterol and compared to individuals from a control community. The North Karelia group was followed for nine years.

At the end of five years, North Karelia males showed a 17% and females showed an 11% reduction in multiple risk factor scores compared to controls. The greatest change was in smoking. After five years, there were 17% and 10% reductions in heart attacks for men and women, respectively. Strokes were reduced by 13% in men and 35% in women. This project demonstrated that efforts to alter the community in order to foster long-term changes in knowledge and health habits are a potent means of reducing the incidence of cardiovascular disease.

Taken together, these and other studies indicate that behavioral interventions can reduce behaviors associated with increased risk for cardiovascular disease. In the case of the North Karelia study, such a reduction also was associated with a decreased incidence of such disease. The relative effectiveness of media, community-focused, and personal interventions is not clear. Based on this first round of studies, more sophisticated interventions focusing on the secondary prevention of heart disease are currently under way (e.g., the Stanford Five City Project—Farquhar et al., 1984; the Minnesota Heart Health Program—Blackburn et al., 1984) that will provide more definitive information about the economy and effectiveness of such programs.

The projects just described are labeled secondary prevention efforts because in most adults the atherosclerotic process is evident in nonsymptomatic, subclinical forms. True primary prevention would have to target younger individuals. The atherosclerotic process begins early. Children and adolescents share with adults similar health habits and lifestyles that increase the risk for cardiovascular disease. They learn such behaviors from their adult counterparts. For example, normative surveys suggest that many American youths engage in relatively little sustained aerobic exercise, eat foods high in fats and calories, are overweight, and show evidence of elevated blood pressure and serum cholesterol (Coates, Perry, Killen, & Slinkard, 1981). Recall also from Chapter 2 that smoking begins in earnest in early adolescence. Approximately 5% of 12-year-olds and 25% of 17-year-olds are regular smokers (National Cancer Institute, 1977).

At first glance, it might be assumed that changing such risky behaviors of children and adolescents would be easier than changing those of adults. This may not be the case. Youth face no immediate health hazard. They reside in a social and cultural environment that promotes risky behaviors (e.g., fast foods and reduced activity requirements). In any case, efforts at prevention probably must use different tactics than those targeting adults. Intervention must be congruent with the developmental status of the target individuals. Let us review two programs relevant to the primary prevention of cardiovascular disease. Coates, Jeffery, and Slinkard (1981) implemented and assessed a school program to enhance exercise and alter the diet of 160 grade-school children. Paper and pencil measurements of knowledge, activity preferences, and home diet; phone interviews with parents about home diet; and observations of activity level at school and actual lunch constituents were obtained prior to and after intervention and after a three-month summer vacation. A nutrition education program that emphasized the identification of heart-healthy foods was initiated as a part of the science curriculum. Using behavioral commitment strategies, goal sheets, self-monitoring, feedback, extrinsic token reinforcement, and child negotiation with parents, students were taught to modify their lunches to contain more heart-healthy foods (more fruits and vegetables, less salt and fat). Parents were contacted by the PTA to provide further support. The intervention resulted in an increase in knowledge, a 40% increase in heart-healthy foods in school lunches, and beneficial parent-reported changes in home dietary practices. These changes were maintained at the follow-up.

This study is a relatively modest short-term demonstration project. It suggests that preventative interventions are potentially effective and emphasizes the importance of the active involvement of the social system of the target children (peers, family, and school) in attaining and maintaining change. Better controlled, more intensive interventions using physiological as well as behavioral measures are needed.

In summary, current research suggests that both the primary and secondary prevention of cardiovascular disease are attainable goals. Mass communication, health education, and the use of behavioral principles result in changes in risky behavior and may consequently alter the incidence of cardiovascular diseases. Continued research is needed to identify program components that are effective and economical and to establish more clearly their long-term impact on the occurrence of cardiovascular and other diseases. Because changes must be sustained over many years to have such an effect, interventions that engender individual change by altering the peer, family, school, and community systems in which persons reside may be particularly powerful.

Modification of Type A Behavior

Recall from Chapter 6 that Type A behavior is a risk factor for coronary artery disease and contributes to the prediction of that disease independent of other behavioral, demographic, and physiological risk factors. This hostile, competitive, hard-driving transactional style is thought to be associated with a psychophysiological response that facilitates coronary atherosclerosis. If this is the case, modification of Type A behavior may reduce the risk for coronary artery disease or the recurrence of a heart attack. Most of the existing interventions to alter Type A behavior attempt to reduce physiological arousal by altering clients' appraisal of themselves and the environment, by changing overt behavioral correlates of that arousal, or by reducing the arousal itself. Let us detail some of the efforts at modifying Type A behavior.

In an early study, Roskies, Spivack, Surkis, Cohen, and Gilman (1979) assigned twenty-nine healthy adult males to psychoanalytical or behavioral interventions for Type A behavior. In the psychoanalytical group, clients were taught to alter their need to master and control the environment by resolving childhood conflicts. The behavioral intervention entailed teaching clients to relax and to use this skill to avoid situational physiological arousal. After fourteen weeks of training, both groups showed significant reductions in systolic blood pressure, serum cholesterol, and self-reported time pressure but no change in serum triglycerides or diastolic blood pressure. These effects were maintained at a six-month follow-up. More recently, Roskies has broadened the focus of her behavioral treatment to include the alteration of cognitive and behavioral aspects of Type A behavior (Roskies & Avard, 1982).

In a recent study by Roskies et al. (1986), the effects of three short-term interventions (stress management, aerobic exercise, and weight training) on the modification of Type A behavior and cardiovascular reactivity were compared. The subjects were corporate executives who evidenced high levels of Type A behavior, high cardiovascular reactivity to stress, and no history of heart disease, diabetes, or high blood pressure. The stress management intervention entailed self-monitoring of stress and teaching, rehearsing and applying a number of coping strategies: relaxation, problem solving, cognitive relabeling, and communication training. Clients in the stress management group showed a substantial reduction in Type A behavior relative to the other two groups. There was no change in cardiovascular reactivity in any of the groups.

In perhaps the most sophisticated and ambitious study to date, Freidman et al. (1984) recruited 862 clients who had suffered at least one heart attack in the previous six months, who had not smoked for at least six months, and who did not have diabetes. These clients were randomly assigned to either a cardiac counseling group or cardiac and Type A behavioral counseling. These treatments are outlined in Table 15-2. Serum cholesterol, cardiovascular functioning, and general physical condition were assessed prior to and one and a half and three years after entry into the program. Type A behavior, assessed using a structured interview and spouse and coworker ratings, was measured prior to treatment and annually thereafter.

Clients receiving cardiac and Type A counseling showed greater reductions in Type A behavior than those in the cardiac counseling group. Nearly 50% of the clients in the former group evidenced significant reductions and 30% evidenced marked reductions in Type A behavior. Serum cholesterol levels dropped significantly in both groups during the first year and were maintained over the next two years. Most impressively, the cumulative three-year incidence of heart attacks was

TABLE 15-2 Intervention Program for Modifying Type A Behavior in Postmyocardial Infarction Patients

Cardiac Counseling
Information about the causes of heart attacks
Modification of standard risk factors for heart disease
  Blood pressure
  Weight
  Smoking
  Exercise
Information about surgical and medical management of heart disease
Information about avoiding activities that may precipitate heart attacks

Behavioral Counseling
Identification of behaviors descriptive of Type A behavior
Increasing awareness of personal responses to stress
Relaxation training
Cognitive relabeling
Behavioral rehearsal with feedback

7.2% in the group receiving cardiac and Type A counseling compared to 13% in the group receiving cardiac counseling (see Figure 15-2).

Taken together, these and similar studies suggest that Type A behavior is modifiable and that such modification may lead to a reduction in the physiological arousal associated with atherosclerosis and in the incidence of the recurrence of heart attacks. With the exception of the Freidman et al. (1984) study, most of the research is exploratory. Studies are characterized by small sample size, inadequate controls, and inadequate measurement of outcome. A large number of issues must be addressed before any strong statements can be made about the potential efficacy of interventions for Type A behavior.

One important issue involves assessment. Ideally, Type A behavior, physiological indicators of cardiovascular activation, and the prospective incidence of heart disease should all be measured. Measure-

FIGURE 15-2 Effects of Type A Counseling on Mortality. (From "Alteration of Type A Behavior and Reduction in Cardiac Recurrences in Postmyocardial Infarction Patients" by M. Freidman, C. E. Thoreson, J. J. Gill, L. H. Powell, D. Ulmer, L. Thompson, V. A. Price, D. D. Rabin, W. S. Breall, T. Dixon, R. Levy, and E. Bourg, 1984, *American Heart Journal, 108*, p. 244. Copyright 1984 by the C. V. Mosby Co. Reprinted by permission.)

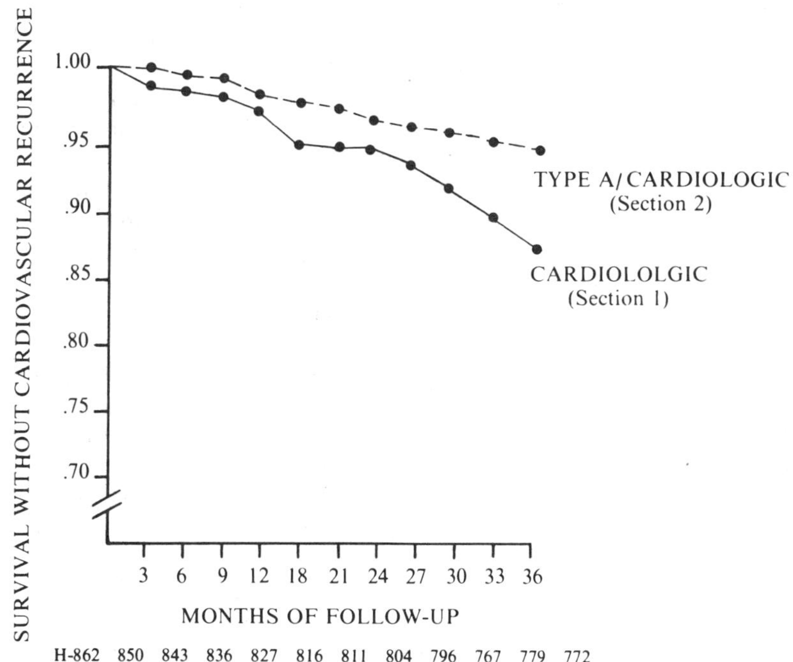

ment of the first two variables remains problematic. A second issue is what should be changed. Type A behavior, as described in Chapter 6, involves a broad range of behaviors that are moderately correlated, such as hostility, competitiveness, and time urgency. Recent research suggests that not all of these behaviors are associated with coronary artery disease. Only a subset (e.g., hostility) may show such an association. Interventions that focus on altering only those aspects of Type A associated with heart disease (i.e., coronary prone) may be more efficient and effective. These interventions would not alter other aspects of Type A behavior that may be adaptive (e.g., achievement striving). The third issue is how to alter coronary prone behavior most efficiently. A wide range of cognitive, behavioral, and physiological approaches have been used, but we have little knowledge about which is the most effective and efficient combination. Further, once change is effected, how can it be maintained? In clinical or preventative applications, sustained change is critical. The use of the maintenance strategies described in Chapter 11 or the involvement of clients' natural social systems (e.g., family and coworkers) may be necessary (Chesney, Eagleston, & Rosenman, 1981) (Carver, Diamond, & Humphries, 1985).

Psychosocial Interventions and the Clinical Treatment of Heart Disease

Heart disease and its treatment confronts individuals with a wide range of adaptive tasks: coming to terms with the implications of the disease for future psychosocial functioning and self-image; coping with diagnostic and treatment procedures, settings, and personnel; and becoming involved in rehabilitative actions and decisions. The procedures and technology used in the treatment of heart disease are truly remarkable. The drugs, surgical techniques, and diagnostic tests and equipment used to identify and repair damage and to sustain life have greatly enhanced survival and recovery. The effectiveness of these procedures can be further enhanced by appropriate behavioral and psychosocial interventions. In this section, we will describe several of these interventions.

Heart disease and its treatment threaten individuals' sense of control and efficacy. Attempts to enhance clients' sense of control and efficacy may reduce emotional distress and consequently enhance psychophysiological recovery. Medical procedures used to diagnose and treat heart disease may be quite distressing. One example is cardiac catheterization, a diagnostic procedure used to visualize the chambers of the heart and the great arteries to determine blood flow, obstruction, and arteriole structure. In this procedure, the client is laid supine and strapped to a table during the 2- to 3-hour procedure. Only a mild tranquilizer is used because the procedure requires client involvement. A catheter, or long, narrow tube, is inserted into the femoral artery near the groin and is moved to the heart. A camera is situated above the chest to take pictures of the heart and surrounding vessels as dye is injected via the catheter. The client is asked to breathe deeply to reduce obstruction of the view by the lungs. The client is also periodically asked to cough to remove the dye from cardiac circulation. The client may experience heart palpitations and warmth as the dye is injected. The procedure may produce discomfort, pain, and nausea. Finally, findings from the procedure have important implications for future treatment and recovery. In short, the procedure is stressful.

Kendall et al. (1979) assessed the effectiveness of stress management training and preparatory information on clients' response to catheterization. Clients were assigned to one of three interventions: stress management, preparatory information, or nonspecific attention. Each intervention was implemented in one 45-minute session prior to the procedure. In stress management, clients discussed the aspects of the procedure they considered stress provoking, observed a model coping with stress, rehearsed preferred existing coping strategies, and received feedback about that practice. Clients in the preparatory information group were taught about heart disease and catheterization using verbal descriptions and a model catheter and heart. They were also given a four-page informational pamphlet. Both procedural and sensory information were provided. Clients in the third group discussed their feelings with a nondirective counselor. No group differences in anticipatory anxiety prior to treatment were found. Clients receiving stress management and preparatory information reported less stress during the procedure. Health providers implementing the diagnostic procedure (who were blind to the type of intervention) rated the stress management and prepared clients as less anxious and more cooperative during the procedure than clients receiving nondirective attention. However, stress management was superior to preparatory information in reducing anxiety and enhancing cooperation. This study suggests that a very brief intervention can substantially reduce client distress and increase cooperation with aversive medical procedures.

Stress management and information are similarly beneficial for clients during acute hospital treatment for heart attacks. Cromwell, Butterfield, Brayfield, and Curry (1977) assigned clients hospitalized for heart attack to varied combinations of the following interventions: information, participation, and attention diversion. Information entailed educating clients about the causes, physiology, and treatment of heart attacks. Participation entailed offering clients some control and choice in treatment actions. Attention diversion entailed providing clients enhanced access to TV, reading materials, and visitors. Physiological variables were not differentially influenced by these interventions. Hospital stay was affected. High information combined with low participation or diversion was associated with increased length of hospitalization. High information with high participation or diversion led to reduced length of hospitalization. A complex interaction among the interventions and client characteristics was found. It would appear that too much information, responsibility, and control may be as bad as too little.

Gruen (1975) assessed the effects of a brief psychosocial intervention on heart attack victims' sense of control and coping abilities. The intervention entailed listening, identifying and rehearsing of coping strategies, problem solving, and prompting to seek information from health providers. Compared to those receiving normal cardiac care, those receiving the psychosocial intervention spent less time in the coronary care unit and hospital, were less depressed and anxious according to both staff- and self-report, demonstrated greater physical strength, and were less likely to experience congestive heart failure. They also displayed better rehabilitative progress four months after hospitalization. The intervention appeared to increase clients' sense of control and self-efficacy, reduce distress, enhance physiological recovery, and counteract the chronic sick role that occasionally occurs after a heart attack.

In summary, these and other studies suggest that involving the client in diagnostic and treatment activities, providing information, and mobilizing coping strategies and resources may have beneficial behavioral, psychosocial, and physiological effects. Further, the interventions can be brief and economical and may reduce hospitalization and health provider time. To be effective, the interventions must be sensitive to client differences and must selectively provide information and foster coping congruent with those differences. Not all clients may need such intervention. There currently exists no standardized screening procedure to identify clients who would benefit. Bar-On (in press) suggests that clients who attribute the cause of their heart attack to modifiable factors (e.g., being overweight, lack of exercise, and smoking) are more likely to initiate action plans for recovery and to resume work and other normal activities than those who attribute the heart attack to forces beyond their control.

Adherence in Preventative and Clinical Interventions for Coronary Heart Disease

The effectiveness of primary and secondary prevention programs depends on whether the audience engages in the recommended changes in lifestyle and health habits and then maintains those changes for a long period. The clinical treatment of clients with coronary heart disease similarly requires a number of behavior changes. These may include stopping tobacco use, beginning a graduated program of physical exercise, reducing dietary intake of calories and fats, and regularly ingesting one or more of several medications (e.g., diuretics, antihypertensive agents, or drugs to reduce serum cholesterol). The successful treatment of heart disease depends on adherence (Herd, 1981).

Such adherence is not always forthcoming. Although adherence to drug treatment is often relatively high (approximately 80%) in post-myocardial infarction clients, it is lower for exercise and dietary restrictions (Carmody, Fey, Pierce, Conner, & Matarazzo, 1982; Carmody, Sinner, Malinow, & Matarazzo, 1980). This suggests that cognitive-behavior change principles found to enhance the adherence to other types of actions in other client populations (see Chapter 4) may be useful in treating clients with heart disease.

The importance of adherence is evident in an ambitious study assessing the effectiveness of drugs that lower serum lipids in the secondary prevention of heart disease (Coronary Drug Project Research Group, 1980). In this study, clients were given either drugs that lowered serum lipids or a placebo. Both adherence and mortality rate were measured. The mortality rates of good adherers in the drug group was 15.7% compared to 22.5% for nonadherers. This finding is of course expected. Interestingly, adherers to the placebo also showed a lower mortality rate (16.4%) than nonadherers (25.8%). Adherence itself seemed to have a critical effect, because the placebo group did not receive any active pharmacological agent. However, the placebo may have enhanced clients' sense of control and well-being or evoked changes in other health habits (Epstein & Chess, 1982).

Behavioral programs appear to enhance adherence to treatment regimens for essential hypertension. Nessman, Carnahan, and Nugent (1980), for example, had hypertensive clients monitor their own blood pressure and utilize a self-control program to facilitate drug ingestion. These clients demonstrated an average decrease in diastolic blood pressure of 16 mmHg over six months, and the blood pressure of twenty-four of the twenty-five clients was under clinical control (diastolic blood pressure less than 90 mmHg). In summary, data on the adherence to preventative and clinical recommendations in the area of cardiovascular disease are sparse. The existing research suggests that cognitive-behavioral programs to enhance adherence are successful and that adherence is associated with positive health outcomes.

Psychosocial and Behavioral Methods in the Prevention and Treatment of Coronary Heart Disease: A Summary

Psychosocial and behavioral interventions are applicable to a wide range of targets in the prevention, treatment, and rehabilitation of coronary heart disease. These interventions hold particular promise in the prevention of coronary heart disease by targeting changes in health habits, coronary prone behavior, and coping. For individuals who suffer from heart disease, these interventions also have the potential to reduce the distress evoked by the disease and by the procedures used in its diagnosis and treatment and to enhance recovery by facilitating adherence to treatment regimens.

At the present time, the potential of such interventions has not been fully realized. A limited number of methodologically adequate, controlled studies have assessed the application of cognitive-behavioral procedures in the prevention and treatment of heart disease, especially in treatment and rehabilitation. However, the most effective and economic means of intervention, the mechanisms by which change is effected, and the technology to promote the maintenance of change remain to be explored. Cognitive-behavioral methods could contribute in other ways to the treatment of heart disease. Self-monitoring and self-observation, for example, are ideally suited to assess the psychosocial and behavioral outcomes of the treatment of heart disease, thus complementing more traditional medical and physiological indicators of recovery. Additional research on the psychophysiology of heart disease may provide the basis for more effective preventative and clinical interventions focusing on the alteration of health habits and coronary prone behavior.

CANCER

In Chapter 8, the nature, causes, course, treatment, and adjustive demands of cancer were described. In the remaining portion of this chapter, we will study the application of psychosocial, cognitive, and behavioral principles in the prevention and treatment of cancer. As discussed in Chapter 8, the incidence of cancer is associated with exposure to certain environmental agents such as tobacco, radiation, industrial chemicals, and dietary constituents, that are the product of our personal behavior or collective socioeconomic actions and policies. Given these epidemiological data, primary intervention entails altering personal behavior or collective actions and policies. Some risk factors are modifiable.

Secondary prevention entails identifying those individuals whose cancer is at an early stage in order to deter its progression and to increase survival by early intervention. Such preventative actions include screening of high risk groups to detect cancer at a nonsymptomatic stage and teaching individuals to recognize early signs and symptoms of cancer (Lilienfeld, 1980). Finally, cancer and its treatment confronts victims with an array of adjustive demands. Psychosocial and cognitive-behavioral interventions may be used to enhance clients' sense of control, knowledge, participation, and personal and social coping resources. The goals are to reduce client distress, to improve cooperation and adherence, and perhaps thereby to enhance prognosis and recovery. Let us begin our discussion with primary prevention.

Psychosocial and Behavioral Interventions in the Primary Prevention of Cancer

Risk factors vary according to the type of cancer. Because of limited space, we will focus on lung cancer as an exemplar in our discussion of primary prevention. The risk factors for cancer of the lung are smoking, exposure to asbestos, arsenic, and other chemicals, and vocational or medical exposure to radiation. It is obvious that these risk factors are modifiable to varying degrees. A continuum of potential modifiability is shown in Figure 15-3. Naturally occurring carcinogenic agents (e.g., ultraviolet radiation) would be extremely difficult to modify (but consider the effect of fluorocarbons on the Van Allen belt). Some host characteristics are currently unmodifiable (e.g., multifactorial genetic predisposition). Some more modifiable risk factors are personal behaviors (e.g., smoking) or environmental carcinogens that occur as a result of social and economic choices (e.g., nuclear weapons, asbestos, and PCBs).

Primary prevention can focus on reducing the occurrence or availability of carcinogenic agents or on altering personal behavior to reduce contact with those agents. Let us consider lung cancer. Smoking is clearly a causal factor in lung cancer (Higgins, Lilienfeld, & Last, 1980). There is a clear dose-response relationship between the number of cigarettes smoked and the mortality rates from lung cancer. However, persons who stop smoking can substantially reduce their risk. Continuing smokers have eight to fifteen times the risk as persons who have never smoked. Exsmokers who have abstained for five years halve that risk, and those who have abstained for fifteen years are only twice as likely to develop lung cancer as individuals who have never smoked.

Reduction in smoking can be achieved in two ways: by altering individuals' behavior or by reducing the availability of tobacco. Methods to prevent smoking or to alter smoking behavior, once it has occurred, have been described and evaluated in Chapters 11 and 13. In those chapters we learned that programs focusing on individual behavior are moderately effective but relatively costly given the scope of the problem. A more efficient approach may be to reduce the availability of tobacco. Let us examine this option.

FIGURE 15-3 Continuum of Modifiability of Risk Factors for Cancer

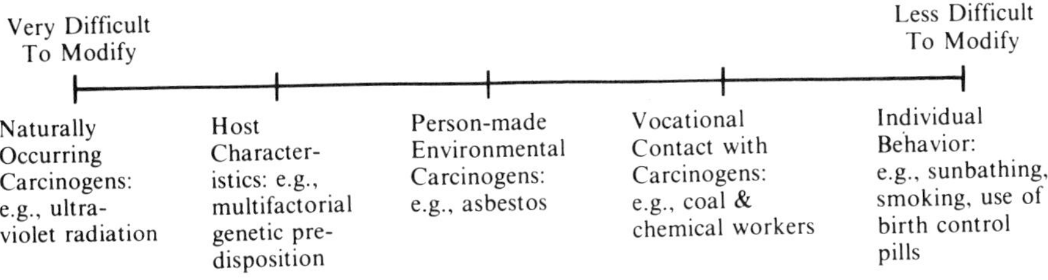

Personal freedom is highly valued in the United States. The decision to smoke is considered a personal right, but evidence on the negative effects of passive smoking (i.e., inhaling others' tobacco smoke) suggests that personal decisions to smoke may infringe on the rights of others. This has resulted in the development of a public policy that emphasizes the education of the public concerning the dangers of smoking (e.g., media education, the surgeon general's reports, and warning labels on tobacco products) and some restrictions on the access to tobacco products (e.g., age restrictions on tobacco purchase and limitations on media advertising). Various governmental agencies also provide funding for basic preventative and clinical research on tobacco use. These actions appear to have a beneficial effect in terms of both effecting some reduction in tobacco use and changing societal attitudes concerning the acceptability of that use (see Chapter 13 for research in this area). Legislation has also been passed that limits smoking in some public areas. The other major deterrent action by the government is to tax tobacco products heavily. The impact of such "sin taxes" on tobacco consumption is currently unclear. At the present time, legislation to ban tobacco sales and use is unlikely. As argued in Chapter 1, such an enlightenment approach has not been successful in the past (e.g., Prohibition).

Government policy, however, is not totally constructive. The tobacco industry has a powerful lobby and considerable economic clout. It employs over 2 million people and makes an annual contribution to the gross national product of over 50 billion dollars. The federal government, as a consequence, provides price supports for tobacco crops and makes loans to facilitate the sale of tobacco leaves. At the same time, tobacco use is very costly. The annual health costs of smoking in the United States are estimated to be over 40 billion dollars. This does not include the indirect costs of smoking, such as accidents, fires, increased insurance rates, and reduced work efficiency (Bell & Levy, 1984).

The private sector has also become involved. Some insurance companies offer lower policy rates to nonsmokers. Some businesses are paying bonuses to employees who stop smoking or are making nonsmoking a prerequisite to hiring or maintaining employment. Such social, political, and economic actions have a cumulative impact. As such, they are important targets of change, for changing the larger system rather than individual behavior may be more efficient and effective in the long run.

Primary prevention of cancer is in its infancy. While epidemiological research has identified carcinogenic agents and associated health habits, many of these risk factors are extremely difficult to modify. Of those that are modifiable, very few interventions (other than statutory bans on some carcinogenic substances or strict regulations on their use) have reduced the contact with carcinogens or the incidence of cancer.

The one exception is smoking and lung cancer. Primary prevention of cancer is extremely difficult because of the complexity of its etiology (multiple "hits" from divergent sources) and its development (the neoplastic process occurs over years) and the relative lack of knowledge about the basic physiological mechanisms and processes related to cancer. This is not to say that efforts at primary prevention should not be continued, but progress in primary prevention will go hand in hand with progress in basic research.

Psychosocial and Behavioral Interventions in the Secondary Prevention of Cancer

The secondary prevention of cancer primarily involves encouraging persons to utilize screening tests provided by health providers or teaching persons to engage in self-administered examinations to detect cancer or its precursors at an early stage. Early detection at nonsymptomatic stages facilitates medical intervention to limit the progression of cancer and to increase survivorship (Lilienfeld, 1980). Examples of such tests are chest x-rays, Pap smears, mammography (x-rays of the breast); and breast self-examination. Evidence suggests that early detection is beneficial, at least for some types of cancer (e.g., breast, cervix, and skin).

The success of secondary prevention depends on two factors. First, a reliable, sensitive, and economic means of early detection must be available. Second, individuals must utilize such detection methods. As detailed in Chapters 2 and 3, it is often difficult to motivate individuals to seek preventative services or, in the case of self-administered detection, to engage in nonroutine behaviors. This difficulty is probably amplified as a result of persons' fear of cancer. Such fear promotes avoidance: "What you don't know can't hurt you." Not only must effective screening tests be made available, but educational efforts using mass communication and individual health provider-client communication (using the principles of the health beliefs or conflict theory models described in Chapter 3, and the education model described in Chapter 13) must be made to stress the availability, importance, and benefits of screening.

Let us use the secondary prevention of breast cancer as an example as to how this might be accomplished. Breast self-examination is a cost-effective and widely acceptable method for the early detection of breast cancer. It entails the systematically self-administered palpation of one's breast. Ninety percent of all breast cancers are discovered by the victim, but only 35% of all women do breast self-examinations regularly, and many of those do not do it correctly (National Cancer Institute, 1980). Many women indicate that they do not know how to do it and that they fear finding something (Trotta, 1980).

How can women be motivated to engage in regular breast self-examination, and how can they be trained to do so correctly? Motivation may be engendered by indicating the risk of breast cancer (it strikes 1 out of 11 women) and by indicating that early detection leads to successful treatment in 85 to 95% of the cases (American Cancer Society, 1982). Verbal instructions on how to do breast self-examination appear to be inadequate. Training using modeling and rehearsal with feedback is more effective. Hall et al. (1980), for example, provided a group of women with practice on a realistic breast model embedded with simulated tumors of varying size, shape, and location. The ability of these women and a group of women who had not received training to detect benign breast lesions in other women was assessed before and after training. Relative to untrained women, trained participants were more able to correctly detect lesions, were more systematic, spent more time on the breast examination, and indicated greater confidence in their ability. Trained women also showed an increase in false-positive identifications (finding a lesion when none existed). This was not unexpected because of the normal nodularity of breast tissue, but indicates that training for even finer discriminations may be necessary. The training was relatively brief (30 minutes) and quite effective. Such training may also enhance participants' motivation to engage in regular breast self-examination as a result of increased feelings of confidence and competence.

But training in breast self-examination and communicating the benefits of this practice is not sufficient to promote routine adherence (Strauss, Solomon, Costanza, Worden, & Foster, 1987). This is evident in a study by Craun and Deffenbacher (1987). They compared combinations of three types of intervention to promote breast self-examination: education about breast cancer, demonstration and practice of self-examination, and monthly prompts to engage in self-examination. The education and demonstration formats resulted in increased knowledge, but had no effect on actual monthly use. The demonstration condition increased proficiency and self-confidence in doing self-examination, but also had no effect on actual monthly use. Only when monthly reminders were sent did subjects engage in regular breast self-examination. It appears that the regular performance of an infrequent, nonroutine behavior like breast self-examination requires not only knowledge and skills but also continued prompts from health providers.

While the secondary prevention of cancer awaits the discovery of reliable and economic means of detecting many kinds of cancer in their early stages, some screening tools and preventative actions are currently available. Relatively little research has focused on motivating individuals to use such services. Investigations in this area are fertile ground.

Psychosocial and Behavioral Methods in the Clinical Treatment and Rehabilitation of Cancer

As detailed in Chapter 8, cancer confronts its victims with a variety of threats and challenges to their survival, physical integrity, self-esteem, social relationships, and normative roles. The degree to which persons with cancer can cope in direct or palliative fashions with these threats may play an important role in their subsequent psychosocial adjustment and physical prognosis. Health providers are in a position to provide psychosocial and behavioral interventions to enhance clients' "safe passage" through the maze of events beginning with the discovery of cancer through treatment, recovery, rehabilitation or through recurrence and death (Weisman, 1979). This helping process may entail very general supportive actions by health providers, may focus on enhancing clients' ability to cope with specific issues, or both. Let us examine how this can be done.

Assessment. A client's psychosocial adaptation and physical prognosis following the discovery of cancer are the net result of a number of factors, as shown in Figure 15-4. They depend on the client's premorbid adjustment, current coping strategies and resources, interaction with health providers, nature of the treatment, and characteristics of the cancer and the biology of the client (Barofsky, 1981).

Assessment of the client should be directed at psychosocial and behavioral as well as physiological functioning. Such an assessment must be flexible because of variations in the disease, the treatment, and the client. Meyerowitz, Heinrich, & Schag (1983) propose that assessment focus on the client's coping competence. In this approach, stressors or adaptive tasks facing the client are identified, the client's current and potential modes of coping are assayed, and targets of intervention to enhance coping are listed.

At least two assessment devices have been developed to aid in this task. One is a structured interview (Gordon et al., 1980), which assesses 122 psychosocial problems in 13 areas of functioning. Perhaps more practical is a client self-reporting measure, the Cancer Inventory of Problem Situations, which lists 131 problems commonly experienced by persons with cancer (Schag, Heinrich, & Ganz, 1983). The items cover a very wide range of situations, such as sleeping, eating, finances, self-care, anxiety, communications with health providers, family relationships, appearance, employment, and sexuality. Clients are asked to indicate the degree to which these situations are problems for them. This assessment approach is advantageous because it is flexible and specifies particular problems that can be targeted for intervention. As we will see

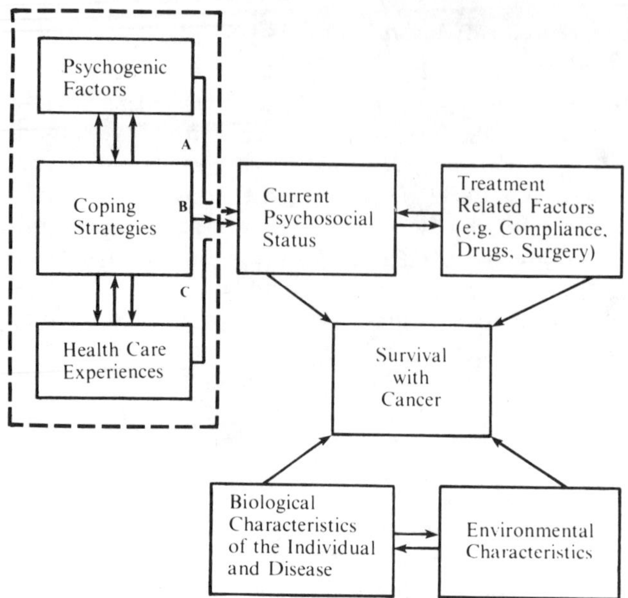

FIGURE 15-4 Multiple Determinants of Psychosocial and Physiological Outcomes of Persons with Cancer. (From "Issues and Approaches to the Psychosocial Assessment of the Cancer Patient" (p. 62) by I. Barofsky, 1981, in C. K. Prokop and L. A. Bradley (Eds.), *Medical Psychology: Contributions to Behavioral Medicine*, New York: Academic Press. Copyright 1981 by Academic Press. Reprinted by permission.)

shortly, problem-specific interventions appear to be more effective than global interventions. These assessment devices may also serve as sensitive outcome measures for estimating the effectiveness of various kinds of interventions.

Guidelines for Health Professionals. Health professionals who treat persons with cancer are in a unique position to promote safe passage. They can provide clients with information about the meaning of findings, anticipated procedures and treatments, and the sensations, thoughts, and feelings that are likely to accompany such events. They may also involve clients in decisions based on such information. Such actions reduce distress and enhance client cooperation and control. Health providers are often able to assess how clients are coping and consequently make referrals for more intensive psychosocial and behavioral interventions. In addition to providing information and social and emotional support, care providers may also encourage adaptive interactions between clients and persons forming their natural social system (Wortman & Dunkel-Schetter, 1979).

General Coping Interventions. The targets of psychosocial and cognitive-behavioral interventions for persons with cancer vary from very global to very specific. In global interventions, clients are provided with a variety of strategies and experiences thought to be relevant to coping with the wide range of adaptive tasks associated with cancer. Problem-oriented or specific interventions focus on enhancing coping and adjustment to specific, situational challenges. We will first explore the global approach.

We learned in Chapter 4 that social support mitigates the negative effects of stress. It also enhances the recovery of persons who are already ill, including those who have cancer (Taylor, Falke, Shoptaw, & Lichtman, 1986). Natural social support systems (family, friends, and co-workers) are very important sources. However, these natural sources of support may be strained or unavailable. An alternate or additional source of support may come from peer social support groups.

Peer social support groups typically involve small group meetings in which individuals sharing a common problem interact to solve a problem, cope with an illness, and provide information and emotional support. Attendance is voluntary, and the degree of participation varies according to participants' needs. Although these groups may include a professional helping agent, peer assistance or self-help is the primary vehicle for delivering aid. Peer self-help groups offer a number of potentially effective opportunities and resources. First, clients interact with other persons experiencing similar problems. This provides an opportunity for open communication, which engenders emotional support, clarification of problems, and feedback about the meaning and utility of various feelings and actions. Second, practical information about how to cope with treatment, where to seek financial and other kinds of aid, what to tell people at work, and a host of other issues is available. Third, peers who share the same disease and who experience similar problems may serve as particularly potent coping models and consequently enhance learning effects (Wortman & Dunkel-Schetter, 1979).

A number of self-help social support programs have been developed for clients with cancer, including Make Today Count, I Can Cope, Reach for Recovery, and We Can Do. Who uses these groups? How effective are they? Current research suggests that only a limited number of all persons with cancer participate in peer support groups. These participants are typically middle and upper class white women. Self-help groups are infrequently used by males, minorities, and persons of lower socioeconomic standing (Gordon et al., 1980). Participants, then, are a relatively select group, and consequently any benefits found to result from support groups may not apply to participants with different characteristics.

Are these groups helpful? Spiegel, Bloom, and Yalom (1981) compared women with breast cancer who did and did not participate in a social support group. One year later, the participants reported less anxiety, confusion, and fatigue, fewer phobias and maladaptive coping responses, and more vigor relative to the nonparticipants. Jacobs, Ross, Walker, and Stockdale (1983) found that male clients with Hodgkin's disease who participated in an educational intervention evidenced more knowledge, less anxiety, and fewer treatment-related problems than their counterparts who did not participate. However, other studies have found that social support groups have little impact (Watson, 1983).

Self-help social support groups have the potential to serve as an economical means to foster individuals' adjustment to cancer and its treatment. The effectiveness of such groups has not been established. To provide definitive answers concerning their effectiveness, several questions must be answered. For whom are such groups effective? Up to now, the groups may have been utilized by those who are likely to have good coping resources already. Are there any negative effects associated with participation in such groups? If so, for which people? What kinds of interaction and information are most helpful?

In contrast to general support groups, a number of professionally led interventions have been developed that attempt to teach a general set of coping skills applicable to a broad range of issues related to cancer and its treatment. These groups are more time limited and structured than self-help support groups. An exhaustive review of such programs will not be attempted. Rather, a pioneering project (Gordon et al., 1980) and two recent, controlled interventions (Heinrich & Schag, 1985; Telch & Telch, 1985) that have used cognitive-behavioral principles will be used as examples of this research.

Gordon et al. (1980) assigned 157 persons with cancer to a cognitive-behavioral intervention and 151 to a control group. These clients were assessed upon hospital admission, at discharge, and three and six months after discharge. The assessment entailed a structured interview detailing the presence and severity of over one hundred psychosocial problems, client ratings of life quality, and client self-reported affect, stress, psychiatric problems, and daily activities. As shown in Table 15-3, the intervention had three components: (1) education about the disease, (2) counseling to facilitate affective expression, provide support, and to teach coping strategies such as relaxation, instructions, and role playing concerning interaction with health providers, and (3) develop and utilize social support. The number and severity of problems decreased in both groups; there was no differential treatment effect. Clients who received the intervention reported less negative effect and less physical discomfort and were more active and vocationally involved after treatment compared to their no treatment counterparts. The response to the intervention depended on the clients' type of cancer. Be-

TABLE 15-3 Principles of Psychosocial Intervention for Cancer

Educational
Clarify and give information about the medical system—procedures, insurance, services, and patient rights
Provide clarifying information about the client's condition—the type of cancer and its progression and prognosis
Teach about cancer treatment and its side effects—procedural and sensory information and interference with normative roles
Teach relief and coping methods for physical and emotional distress—relaxation, distraction, and cognitive relabeling
Promote adherence to the treatment regimen

Counseling
Promote and empathize with the client's expression of feelings
Provide the client with emotional and verbal support
Encourage the client to act on the environment—asking questions, seeking information, and expressing needs and feelings

Environmental
Work with family and friends of the client
Seek appropriate financial and other resources needed by the client
Work with health professionals providing services to the client

cause different issues are associated with different types of cancer, interventions may be more effective if they are individualized.

In more recent work, Heinrich and Schag (1985) randomly assigned fifty-one cancer patients to either usual medical care or usual medical care and a stress management program. Prior to, immediately after, and four months after treatment, clients were assessed on their knowledge of cancer, coping activities, daily activities, adjustment specific to cancer-related problems, quality of life, and general psychosocial problems. In the stress management program, cognitive-behavioral strategies were used to teach clients problem solving, relaxation, and behavioral skills specific to cancer-related problems. The clients were also provided with information and education concerning cancer and its treatment. Relative to clients receiving usual medical care only, clients receiving the additional stress management intervention demonstrated more knowledge about cancer and coping and more satisfaction with medical care. No differences were found in adjustment and daily activity.

Telch and Telch (1985) randomly assigned forty-one cancer clients to receive one of three interventions: coping skills training, support group therapy, or no psychosocial treatment. Measures of distress in a number of areas—mood, frequency and severity of problems associated with cancer, and perceived self-efficacy—were assessed before and after treatment. Coping skills training focused on the development of several problem-specific coping skills using instruction, modeling, and feedback.

These skills included relaxation, stress management, communication and assertiveness, problem solving, affect management, and activity planning. After treatment, the coping skills group showed more improvement on all measures than the support group therapy and no treatment groups. However, group therapy was more effective than no treatment. This project suggests that social support is helpful, but that the systematic provision of problem-oriented coping skills is even more effective.

In summary, these and other studies suggest that problem-oriented interventions that are structured to enhance knowledge and the acquisition and performance of coping behaviors reduce distress, negative mood, and physical discomfort. They may also enhance the continued performance of normal vocational, social, and recreational activities, communication with health providers, and a sense of self-efficacy. The impact of these interventions on physical prognosis has not been systematically evaluated. Given that these studies use relatively time-limited group interventions, benefits may be achieved in an economical fashion. Many questions are still to be answered. How long do the benefits last? Are the benefits similar for persons with different kinds of cancer or cancer at different stages? Given a sizable participation refusal and dropout rate, are these programs addressing those most in need of help? The focus of psychosocial interventions may also be expanded. For example, psychotropic medications are frequently prescribed for persons with cancer to reduce anxiety and depression (Derogatis, 1986). How do pharmacological and psychosocial interventions interact?

Specific or Problem-Oriented Interventions. As an alternative to using a "shotgun" approach to enhancing coping skills to deal with cancer, it may be more effective and economical to develop interventions focusing on very specific problems. In this section, two such problem-focused interventions will be described: coping with the aversive side effects of chemotherapy and coping with pain.

As described in Chapter 7, chemotherapy often results in a number of aversive side effects, including nausea and vomiting. After several chemotherapy treatments, 20 to 60% of cancer victims experience anticipatory nausea and vomiting (i.e., prior to the chemotherapy session), probably as a result of classical conditioning. These anticipatory side effects are different than direct, pharmacological effects. Anticipatory nausea and vomiting often increase in severity with continued sessions. Anticipatory and direct pharmacological nausea and vomiting are highly distressing, exacerbate existing nutritional problems, and in some cases may lead to refusal of further treatment.

Antiemetic drugs have been used in an attempt to control nausea and vomiting associated with chemotherapy. These drugs are not consistently effective, however, and often produce their own aversive side effects (Harris, 1978). Given the psychological involvement (learning) in at least anticipatory nausea and vomiting, a number of investigators have attempted to develop and assess the effectiveness of cognitive-behavioral treatment of nausea and vomiting. Several treatment protocols have been used: progressive muscle relaxation, guided imagery (hypnosis), systematic desensitization, biofeedback, and stress inoculation. These protocols make relatively similar and congruent assumptions about the problem and how to treat it. They assume that autonomic arousal associated with anxiety fosters gastrointestinal distress, nausea, and vomiting. Consequently, attempts are made to reduce arousal and anxiety using progressive muscle relaxation (alone or as part of systematic desensitization), imagery, or biofeedback. All of the procedures either implicitly (e.g., by providing the client with a competing task) or explicitly (e.g., by using a focal point) teach clients to distract themselves from environmental, cognitive, and affective stimuli that may contribute to nausea and vomiting. Some procedures, especially systematic desensitization, may also extinguish the conditioned emetic response by imaginally exposing the person to the conditioned stimuli in the absence of the unconditioned stimuli (the chemotherapy drug). All of the procedures also enhance clients' sense of control and self-efficacy and provide sensory and procedural information to some degree (Redd & Andrykowski, 1982).

Several experimental studies have demonstrated that these treatment protocols are effective. Redd, Andresen, and Minagawa (1982) taught clients who experienced anticipatory nausea and vomiting to relax and distract themselves by using imagery. This eliminated anticipatory nausea in all clients and also reduced nausea during chemotherapy. When the clients stopped using imagery, the nausea returned. Burish and his colleagues (Burish & Lyles, 1979, 1981; Lyles, Burish, Krozely, & Oldham, 1982) assigned clients experiencing anticipatory nausea and vomiting to either a relaxation and guided imagery treatment or no treatment. After intervention, clients receiving treatment relative to controls demonstrated decreases in physiological arousal and self-reported anxiety during chemotherapy and decreases in anticipatory nausea and vomiting. These benefits persisted at the follow-up, when clients used the strategies without the aid of the therapist but at a reduced level. Morrow and Morrell (1982) compared chemotherapy clients assigned to either systematic desensitization, counseling support, or no treatment. Clients receiving systematic desensitization displayed less anticipatory nausea and vomiting than clients in the other two groups. This suggests that the treatment was procedure specific and not just the result of nonspecific attention from the clinician.

The use of relaxation and guided imagery may also prevent the development of conditioned side effects during chemotherapy. Burish,

Carey, Krozely, and Greco (1987) provided relaxation and guided imagery to twelve clients prior to the initiation of chemotherapy. Relative to twelve control clients, those in the treatment group evidenced significantly less frequent and severe vomiting and nausea and less anxiety and physiological arousal during chemotherapy.

Relaxation, imagery, and desensitization procedures appear to have a substantial impact on anticipatory nausea and vomiting and to reduce distress associated with chemotherapy. In fact, the various procedures are remarkably similar in effectiveness. There are several issues, however, that await resolution. First, the mechanism by which these procedures produce a beneficial effect is not clear. Second, the degree to which these procedures may also reduce the direct, pharmacological aversive effects of chemotherapy drugs (in addition to anticipatory nausea and vomiting) is unclear. These side effects are certainly pharmacological in nature, but nevertheless may be modulated by cognitive-behavioral interventions (recall the research that documents the actual reversal of the pharmacological effects of drugs by placebo interventions in Chapter 8). Third, these interventions currently require two to six hours of professional time. This is relatively costly. It may prove feasible to train paraprofessionals or family members to implement the treatment, but attempts to do so have failed (Carey & Burish, 1987). Fourth, it is not clear that all clients need or benefit from this treatment to the same degree. Anticipatory nausea appears to be particularly associated with high levels of anxiety and affective distress; it may be useful to target only these clients for intervention. Fifth, efforts are needed to enhance the maintenance of the beneficial effects. The current data suggest that the benefits are reduced when clients are asked to use the coping skills on their own. More emphasis on client practice of the skill may enhance persistence. Despite these shortcomings, it appears that cognitive-behavioral interventions can have an appreciable impact on client distress during chemotherapy and the anticipatory nausea and vomiting associated with chemotherapy.

Pain is another specific problem associated with cancer that may be amenable to modification using psychosocial and behavioral methods (Jay, Elliott, & Varni, 1986). Cancer-related pain may result from the cancer itself, usually because of its infiltration or compression of other tissue. This pain ranges from mild to excruciating. Pain may also result from cancer treatments such as surgery, radiation, chemotherapy, or other invasive diagnostic and clinical procedures. Cancer-related pain can be acute or chronic or respondent or operant (see Chapter 8).

The management of pain (see Chapter 16 for more detail) is one of three types: (1) definitive—eliminating the source of the pain, as in the excision of a tumor; (2) symptomatic—using narcotic or nonnarcotic analgesics, nerve blocks, or psychotropic drugs to reduce anxiety and depression; and (3) psychosocial or cognitive-behavioral. Here we will focus on cognitive-behavioral interventions. Relatively little controlled investigation concerning the management of cancer-related pain has been done using any of these perspectives. In part, this is the result of the nature of cancer. It encompasses as many as one hundred variations, each occurring at various body sites and differing in progression. As well as the fluctuating nature of the disease, constant alterations in medical treatment confound efforts to assess systematically the effectiveness of interventions to reduce pain (Jay et al., 1986).

The application of cognitive-behavioral methods to manage cancer pain is similarly in its infancy. Some systematic interventions focusing on preparatory coping have been described (Turk & Rennert, 1981) but not evaluated. Jay, Elliot, Katz, and Siegel (1987) used such a cognitive-behavioral intervention to treat fifty-six children and adolescents with cancer who were undergoing bone marrow aspiration. Bone marrow aspiration is most often performed in cases of leukemia. It entails inserting a long needle into the hip bone and suctioning out bone marrow to ascertain the presence of cancer cells. The procedure is very painful and is not adequately addressed by pain-killing medication. The intervention consisted of a filmed model demonstrating positive coping behaviors, rehearsal of breathing exercises, imagery, distraction strategies, and a positive incentive for coping. A behavioral coach helped the youths use these strategies during the procedure. The clients receiving the intervention self-reported less pain and showed less behavioral distress and physiological arousal prior to and during the procedure relative to those receiving no treatment. Those who received Valium (an antianxiety agent) were less distressed than those receiving no treatment before the procedure, but the drug was not as effective as the cognitive-behavioral intervention in reducing distress during the procedure. The effects do not generalize to future bone marrow aspiration procedures in the absence of the behavioral coach.

Other psychosocial interventions such as hypnosis and the provision of sensory and procedural information have also been used to manage cancer-related pain in children and adults. Most studies of these procedures are uncontrolled case studies. At present, little progress has been made, but much potential exists.

Psychosocial and Behavioral Interventions and Cancer: A Summary

The current status of psychosocial and behavioral interventions in the prevention, early detection, diagnosis, and treatment of cancer has been described. As elaborated in Chapter 7, psychosocial and behavioral variables may play an important role at all of these stages. Interventions focusing on altering individual or collective behavior (e.g., smoking, manufacture of and exposure to environmental carcinogens, breast self-examination, and coping with adverse side effects of chemotherapy) appear to have promise. The focus of these interventions take many forms, from providing information and altering specific health habits to prevent cancer to providing general emotional and informational support (safe passage) and problem-specific coping strategies for individuals who develop cancer. These interventions complement basic research on the causes of cancer and medical procedures used in the diagnosis and treatment of cancer.

Currently, the research on the preventative and clinical applications of psychosocial and behavioral interventions is relatively gross and unsophisticated. Adequate controls are often lacking, good measures are not available, and intervention strategies have not been replicated and refined. Advancement will simply require continued and more careful work. To a degree, however, the efficacy of such interventions may be limited by basic knowledge about the multiple causes and mechanisms of cancer and the varying challenges associated with having cancer. The interface between physiology and psychosocial variables exists, but we need to explore and expand it (Derogatis, 1986).

REFERENCES

Agras, W. S. (1984). The behavioral treatment of somatic disorders. In W.D. Gentry (Ed.), *Handbook of behavioral medicine*, 479–530. New York: Guilford.

American Cancer Society. (1982). *Cancer facts and figures*. New York: Author.

Barofsky, I. (1981). Issues and approaches to the psychosocial assessment of the cancer patient. In C. K. Prokop & L. A. Bradley (Eds.), *Medical psychology: Contributions to behavioral medicine*, 57–67. New York: Academic Press.

Bar-On, D. (in press). Causal attributions and the rehabilitation of heart attack patients. *Psychosomatic Medicine*.

Bell, C. S., & Levy, S. M. (1984). Public policy and smoking prevention. In J. D. Matarazzo, S. M. Weiss, J. A. Herd, N. E. Miller, & S. M. Weiss (Eds.), *Behavioral health: A handbook of health enhancement and disease prevention*, 775–788. New York: John Wiley & Sons.

Blackburn, H., Luepker, R., Kline, F., Bracht, N., Carlaw, R., Jacobs, D., Mittlemark, M., Stauffer, L., & Taylor, H. (1984). The Minnesota Heart Health Program. In J. D. Matarazzo, S. M. Weiss, J. A. Herd, N. E. Miller, & S. M. Weiss (Eds.), *Behavioral health: A handbook of health enhancement and disease prevention*, 1171–1179. New York: John Wiley & Sons.

Burish, T. G., Carey, M. P., Krozely, M. G., & Greco, F. A. (1987). Conditioned side effects induced by cancer chemotherapy: Prevention through behavioral treatment. *Journal of Consulting and Clinical Psychology, 55*, 42–48.

Burish, T. G., & Lyles, J. N. (1979). Effectiveness of relaxation training in reducing the aversiveness of chemotherapy treatment of cancer. *Behavior Therapy and Experimental Psychiatry, 10*, 357–361.

Burish, T. G., & Lyles, J. N. (1981). Effectiveness of relaxation training in reducing adverse reactions to cancer chemotherapy. *Journal of Behavioral Medicine, 4*, 65–78.

Carey, M. P., & Burish, T. G. (1987). Providing relaxation training to cancer chemotherapy patients: A comparison of three delivery techniques. *Journal of Consulting and Clinical Psychology, 55*, 732–737.

Carmody, T. P., Fey, S. G., Pierce, D. K., Conner, W. E., & Matarazzo, J. D. (1982). Behavioral treatment of hyperlipidemia: Techniques, results and future directions. *Journal of Behavioral Medicine, 5*, 91–116.

Carmody, T. P., Sinner, J. W., Malinow, M. R., & Matarazzo, J. D. (1980). Physical exercise rehabilitation: Long term drop-out rates in cardiac patients. *Journal of Behavioral Medicine, 3,* 163–168.

Carver, C. S., Diamond, E. L., & Humphries, C. (1985). Coronary prone behavior. In N. Schneiderman & J. T. Tapp (Eds.), *Behavioral medicine: The biopsychosocial approach,* 66–82. Hillsdale, NJ: Lawrence Erlbaum.

Chesney, M. A., Eagleston, J. R., & Rosenman, R. H. (1981). Type A behavior: Assessment and intervention. In C. K. Prokop & L. A. Bradley (Eds.), *Medical psychology: Contributions to behavioral medicine,* 20–37. New York: Academic Press.

Coates, T., Perry, C., Killen, J., & Slinkard, L. (1981). Primary prevention of cardiovascular disease in children and adolescents. In C. K. Prokop & L. A. Bradley (Eds.), *Medical psychology: Contributions to behavioral medicine,* 157–197. New York: Academic Press.

Coates, T. J., Jeffery, R. W., & Slinkard, L. A. (1981). Heart healthy eating and exercise: Introducing and maintaining changes in health behavior. *American Journal of Public Health, 71,* 15–23.

Coronary Drug Project Research Group. (1980). Influence of adherence to treatment and response of cholesterol on mortality in the Coronary Drug Project. *New England Journal of Medicine, 303,* 1038–1041.

Craun, A. M., & Deffenbacher, J. L. (1987). The effects of information, behavioral rehearsal and prompting on breast self exams. *Journal of Behavioral Medicine, 10,* 351–365.

Cromwell, R. L., Butterfield, E. C., Brayfield, F. M., & Curry, J. J. (1977). *Acute myocardial infarction and recovery.* St. Louis: C. V. Mosby.

Derogatis, L. P. (1986). Psychology in cancer medicine: A perspective and overview. *Journal of Consulting and Clinical Psychology, 54,* 632–638.

Epstein, L. H., & Chess, P. A. (1982). A behavioral medicine perspective on adherence to long-term medical regimens. *Journal of Consulting and Clinical Psychology, 50,* 950–971.

Farquhar, J. W., Fortmann, S. P., Maccoby, N., Wood, P., Haskell, W., Taylor, C., Flora, J., Solomon, D., Rogers, T., Adler, E., Breitrose, P., & Weiner, L. (1984). The Stanford Five City Project. In J. D. Matarazzo, S. M. Weiss, J. A. Herd, N. E. Miller, & S. M. Weiss (Eds.), *Behavioral health: A handbook of health enhancement and disease prevention,* 1154–1165. New York: John Wiley & Sons.

Farquhar, J. W., Maccoby, N., Wood, P. D., Alexander, J. K., Breitrose, H., Brown, B. W., Haskell, W. L., McAlister, A. L., Meyer, A. J., Nash, J. D., & Stern, M. P. (1977). Community education for cardiovascular health. *Lancet, 1,* 1192–1195.

Freidman, M., Thoreson, C. E., Gill, J. J., Powell, L. H., Ulmer, D., Thompson, L., Price, V. A., Rabin, D. D., Breall, W. S., Dixon, T., Levy, R., & Bourg, E. (1984). Alteration of Type A behavior and reduction in cardiac recurrences in postmyocardial infarction patients. *American Heart Journal, 108,* 237–248.

Gordon, W. A., Freidenberg, I., Diller, L., Hibberd, M., Wolf, C., Levine, L., Lipkens, R., Ezrachi, O., & Lucido, D. (1980). Efficacy of psychosocial intervention with cancer patients. *Journal of Consulting and Clinical Psychology, 48,* 743–759.

Gruen, W. (1975). Effects of brief psychotherapy during the hospitalization period on the recovery process in heart attacks. *Journal of Consulting and Clinical Psychology, 43,* 223–232.

Hall, D. C., Adams, C. K., Stein, G. H., Stephenson, H. S., Goldstein, M. K., & Pennypacker, H. S. (1980). Improved detection of human breast lesions following experimental training. *Cancer, 46,* 408–414.

Harris, J. G. (1978). Nausea, vomiting and cancer treatment. *Ca—A Cancer Journal for Clinicians, 28,* 194–201.

Heinrich, R. L., & Schag, C. C. (1985). Stress and activity management: Group treatment for cancer patients and spouses. *Journal of Consulting and Clinical Psychology, 53,* 439–446.

Herd, J. A. (1981). Treatment of cardiovascular disorders. In C. K. Prokop & L. A. Bradley (Eds.), *Medical psychology: Contributions to behavioral medicine,* 142–156. New York: Academic Press.

Higgins, I., Lilienfeld, A., & Last, J. M. (1980). Ill effects of tobacco smoking. In J. M. Last (Ed.), *Public health and preventative medicine*, 1066–1076. New York: Appleton-Century-Crofts.

Jacobs, C., Ross, R. D., Walker, I. M., & Stockdale, F. E. (1983). Behavior of cancer patients: A randomized study of the effects of education and peer support groups. *American Journal of Clinical Oncology, 6*, 347–353.

Jay, S. M., Elliot, C. H., Katz, E. R., & Siegel, S. E. (1987). Cognitive- behavioral and pharmacological interventions for children's distress during painful medical procedures. *Journal of Consulting and Clinical Psychology, 55*, 860–865.

Jay, S. M., Elliott, C. & Varni, J. W. (1986). Acute and chronic pain in adults and children with cancer. *Journal of Consulting and Clinical Psychology, 54*, 601–607.

Kasl, S. V. (1980). Cardiovascular risk reduction in a community setting: Some comments. *Journal of Consulting and Clinical Psychology, 48*, 143–149.

Kendall, P. C., Williams, L., Pechacek, T. F., Graham, L. E., Shisslak, C., & Herzoff, N. (1979). Cognitive-behavioral and patient education interventions in cardiac catheterization procedures: The Palo Alto medical psychology project. *Journal of Consulting and Clinical Psychology, 47*, 49–58.

Leventhal, H., Safer, M. A., Cleary, P. D., & Gutmann, M. (1980). Cardiovascular risk modification by community-based programs for life-style change: Comments on the Stanford Study. *Journal of Consulting and Clinical Psychology, 48*, 150–158.

Lilienfeld, A. M. (1980). Cancer. In J. M. Last (Ed.), *Public health and preventative medicine*, 1147–1167. New York: Appleton-Century-Crofts.

Lyles, J. N., Burish, T. G., Krozely, M. G., & Oldham, R. K. (1982). Efficacy of relaxation training and guided imagery in reducing the aversiveness of cancer chemotherapy. *Journal of Consulting and Clinical Psychology, 50*, 509–524.

Maccoby, N., Farquhar, J. W., Wood, P. D., & Alexander, J.K. (1977). Reducing the risk of cardiovascular disease: Effects of a community-based campaign on knowledge and behavior. *Journal of Community Health, 3*, 100–114.

McAlister, A. L., Puska, P., Salonen, J., Tuomilehto, J., & Koskela, K. (1982). Theory and action for health promotion: Illustrations from the North Karelia Project. *American Journal of Public Health, 72*, 43–50.

Meyer, A. J., Nash, J. D., McAlister, A. L., Maccoby, N., & Farquhar, J. W. (1980). Skills training in a cardiovascular health education program. *Journal of Consulting and Clinical Psychology, 48*, 129–142.

Meyerowitz, B. E., Heinrich, R. L., & Schag, C. C. (1983). A competency-based approach to coping with cancer. In T.G. Burish & L.A. Bradley (Eds.), *Coping with chronic disease: Research and applications*, 274–298. New York: Academic Press.

Morrow, G. R., & Morrell, B. S. (1982). Behavioral treatment of anticipatory nausea and vomiting induced by cancer chemotherapy. *New England Journal of Medicine, 307*, 1018–1029.

National Cancer Institute. (1977). *Cigarette smoking among teenagers and young women.* (U.S. Department of Health, Education and Welfare, DHEW Publication No. NIH 77–2203). Washington, DC: U.S. Government Printing Office.

National Cancer Institute. (1980). *Breast cancer: A measure of progress in public understanding.* (DHHS/NIH Publication No. 81–2291). Washington, DC: U.S. Government Printing Office.

Nessman, D. G., Carnahan, J. E., & Nugent, C. A. (1980). Increased compliance: Patient operated hypertension groups. *Archives of Internal Medicine, 303*, 1038–1041.

Redd, W. H ., Andresen, G. V., & Minagawa, R. Y. (1982). Hypnotic control of anticipatory emesis in patients receiving cancer chemotherapy. *Journal of Consulting and Clinical Psychology, 50*, 14–19.

Redd, W. H., & Andrykowski, M. A. (1982). Behavioral intervention in cancer treatment: Controlling aversive reactions to chemotherapy. *Journal of Consulting and Clinical Psychology, 50*, 1018–1029.

Roskies, E., & Avard, J. (1982). Teaching healthy managers to control their coronary-prone

(Type A) behavior. In K. Blankstein & J. Polivy (Eds.), *Self-control and self-modification of emotional behaviors*, 218–236. New York: Plenum.

Roskies, E., Saraganian, P., Oseasohn, R., Hanley, A., Collu, R., Martin, C., & Smilga, R. (1986). The Montreal Type A intervention project: Major findings. *Health Psychology, 5*, 45–69.

Roskies, E., Spivack, M., Surkis, A., Cohen, C., & Gilman, S. (1979). Changing the coronary-prone (Type A) behavior pattern in a non-clinic population. *Journal of Behavioral Medicine, 2*, 195–207.

Salonen, J. T., Puska, P., & Mustaniemi, H. (1979). Changes in morbidity and mortality during comprehensive community programme to control cardiovascular diseases during 1972–77 in North Karelia. *British Medical Journal, 2*, 1178–1183.

Schag, C. C., Heinrich, R. L., & Ganz, P. A. (1983). Cancer inventory of problem situations: An instrument for assessing cancer patients' rehabilitation needs. *Journal of Psychosocial Oncology, 1*, 11–24.

Spiegel, D., Bloom, J., & Yalom, I. (1981). Group support with patients with metastatic cancer. *Archives of General Psychiatry, 38*, 327–333.

Strauss, L. M., Solomon, L. J., Costanza, M. C., Worden, J. K., & Foster, R. S. (1987). Breast self-examination practices and attitudes in women with and without a history of breast cancer. *Journal of Behavioral Medicine, 10*, 337–350.

Taylor, S. E., Falke, R. L., Shoptaw, R. L., & Lichtman, R. R. (1986). Social support, support groups and the cancer patient. *Journal of Consulting and Clinical Psychology, 54*, 608–615.

Telch, C. F., & Telch, M. J. (1985). Group coping skills instruction and supportive group therapy for cancer patients: A comparison of strategies. *Journal of Consulting and Clinical Psychology, 54*, 802–808.

Trotta, P. (1980). Breast self-examination: Factors influencing compliance. *Oncology Nursing Forum, 7*, 13–17.

Turk, D., & Rennert, K. (1981). Pain and the terminally ill cancer patient. In H. J. Sobel (Ed.), *Behavior therapy in terminal care: A humanistic approach*, 95–124. Cambridge, MA: Ballinger.

Watson, M. (1983). Psychosocial intervention with cancer patients: A review. *Psychological Medicine, 13*, 839–846.

Weisman, A. D. (1979). A model for psychosocial phasing in cancer. *General Hospital Psychiatry, 1*, 187–195.

Wortman, C. B., & Dunkel-Schetter, C. (1979). Interpersonal relationships and cancer: A theoretical analysis. *Journal of Social Issues, 35*, 120–155.

16

Pain and Infectious Diseases: Preventative and Clinical Interventions

INTRODUCTION

In this chapter, the treatment of two common health problems, pain and infectious diseases, will be considered. In our everyday experience, the treatment of these disorders entails the simple use of pharmacological and other types of biological interventions. We will learn that psychosocial and behavioral interventions are important adjunctive and sometimes central means of preventing and treating these disorders.

Pain refers to the subjective experience of distress associated with a simultaneous interaction of cognitive, behavioral, physiological, and environmental events and processes. A detailed description of the etiology, manifestations, and course of pain was offered in Chapter 9. In this chapter, psychosocial strategies used for the prevention and clinical treatment of pain will be described and evaluated. Particular attention will be given to the manner in which cognitive-behavioral interventions complement medical interventions. We will learn that cognitive-behavioral interventions often play a more central role in the clinical treatment of pain than in the treatment of heart disease and cancer. On the other hand, relatively little work has been done on the primary and secondary prevention of pain. We will examine this research primarily in terms of what needs to be done to develop such preventative programs.

PAIN

Pain is a distress signal from the body that indicates that something is wrong and that a regulatory response is needed to correct the problem. The expression and experience of pain involve the whole system: biochemical, physiological, cognitive-affective, behavioral, and socioenvionmental. Consequently, cognitive behavioral treatments may effectively complement pharmacological, surgical, and physical therapy approaches to clinical pain, whether it occurs in acute, chronic, or operant forms. The contribution of cognitive-behavioral approaches to the assessment and treatment of pain will be described and evaluated, with a special emphasis on operant pain. First, medical interventions will be described. This provides us with a context in which to understand the complementary nature of cognitive-behavioral strategies.

Pain is an adaptive response that is critical to survival. This seems to preclude any role for secondary prevention. If we think carefully about the meaning of secondary prevention, this is not the case. Recall that secondary prevention refers to slowing or stopping the progression of some pathological process before it is clinically manifested. However, if we think of acute pain as an adaptive and not a pathological process, pain that persists after it has signaled some damage (i.e., chronic and operant pain) is pathological. Secondary prevention, in this sense, entails taking steps to preclude the progression of acute to chronic and operant forms of pain.

Medical Treatment of Pain

Medical interventions in the treatment of pain, as summarized in Table 16-1, can be classified as either definitive or symptomatic. Definitive interventions focus on removing or correcting the "cause" of pain. Symptomatic treatments focus on reducing the amount of pain experienced by the client or on compensating for losses in functional capacity. These treatments are very powerful. They strongly influence system status, typically for the better. However, these treatments are not always or uniformly effective for all types of pain. Because they are so powerful, they may also cause negative side effects and, in some cases, inadvertently contribute to the development and maintenance of chronic and operant pain. These risks and side effects will be described, especially in terms of their relevance to the secondary prevention of chronic pain.

TABLE 16-1 Medical Interventions in the Treatment of Pain

Definitive
Surgical
  Removal of offending agent or correction of an injury
Mechanical
  Casts, braces, or other devices to immobilize the body to promote healing
Pharmacological
  Drugs that alter the source of the pain (e.g., antibiotics for inner ear infections)
Behavioral
  Selected exercise to strengthen some portion of the body
  Rest or reduced activity to promote healing

Symptomatic
Pharmacological
  Aspirinlike analgesics
  Narcotic analgesics
  Antidepressants
  Sedative-hypnotics
  Antianxiety agents
Surgical
  Section or destruction of nervous system pathways or nuclei to disrupt transmission of information about pain
Sensory modulation
  Transcutaneous electrical nerve stimulation
  Application of thermal or mechanical stimuli

Definitive Treatment of Pain

Definitive treatment of pain can be surgical, mechanical, pharmacological, or behavioral. Definitive treatment is not always available if the source of pain eludes identification or if the treatment to remove the source of pain is not available. Chronic (and operant) pain are, by definition, a failure in definitive treatment. But definitive treatment may directly or indirectly contribute to the development of chronic pain. Surgical, pharmacological, and mechanical interventions may accidentally lead to an injury or disruption in physiology that evokes pain. Along with behavioral prescriptions, they may indirectly lead to muscle weakness, body disuse, and reduced sensory input, which exacerbate existing pain. Further, these treatments legitimize illness behaviors and may discourage well behaviors. Given inappropriate environmental contingencies and/or a predisposition to hypochondriac illness schema, depression, and anxiety, the stage may be set for the development of operant components to the pain problem. This does not mean that definitive treatment should not be used. That is obviously absurd. However, these treatments are powerful and should be used carefully and judiciously.

Symptomatic Treatment of Pain

Pharmacological Control of Pain. Pharmacological agents are frequently used to alter biochemical or neurophysiological processes involved in encoding, transmitting, or decoding of information about pain (analgesics); pain-related physiological processes (muscle relaxants); or affective states that contribute to pain (antidepressants, antianxiety agents, or sedative-hypnotics). Two types of drugs account for 90% of the medications used for pain: aspirinlike drugs and opiates. Aspirinlike substances, more formally called acetylsalicylic acids, come in two forms: aspirin and acetaminophen (Tylenol). Both act peripherally to reduce pain, decrease inflammation, and ease fever. They have their effect by inhibiting the production of prostaglandins, which are chemicals released by the cells after injury. Prostaglandins sensitize neural receptors to damage and produce the swelling and redness associated with inflammation.

Aspirin and Tylenol are effective analgesics for slow, prolonged pain, whatever its location. A broken leg, an extracted tooth, and an arthritic joint all involve the release of prostaglandins and consequently are sensitive to aspirinlike substances. Aspirin is not analgesic when there is no tissue damage, however. It is useful in the treatment of acute and chronic but not operant pain (Aronoff, Wagner, & Spangler, 1986; Melzack & Wall, 1983). Aspirin does have a ceiling effect, or a dosage beyond which there is no increase in analgesia. This dose is about 1,000 mg every four hours (Aronoff & Evans, 1985).

Aspirin has a number of side effects, such as gastric irritation and bleeding and suppressed blood coagulation. Less common side effects include liver and kidney problems. The range between the effective analgesic dose and the onset of side effects is relatively small. Aspirin is, then, potentially iatrogenic. Tylenol does not have the adverse gastrointestinal and renal side effects associated with aspirin (Kantor, 1984).

The second major class of analgesic drugs is the narcotics (opiates). The opiates include naturally occurring (e.g., morphine and codeine), semisynthetic (e.g., Dilaudid and Percodan), and synthetic (e.g., Demerol and Darvon) compounds. All act on the central nervous system, probably effecting analgesia by imitating naturally occurring endorphins and enkephalins to activate endogenous, pain-modulating systems. Narcotic (or opiate) analgesics are the treatment of choice for rapid-onset, acute pain, and for chronic pain associated with terminal illness. Their use for other chronic pain and for operant pain is very limited (Aronoff & Evans, 1984). The analgesic effectiveness of the various narcotic drugs is similar if they are given in equivalent doses.

Narcotic drugs have a number of side effects: sedation, mental clouding, reduced contraction of smooth muscles, and nausea. They also produce physiological tolerance and addiction. Tolerance refers to the need for increasingly higher doses, after repeated administration, to achieve the same analgesic effect. Tolerance is unavoidable. Physical addiction refers to the habituation of the body to the presence of the drug such that withdrawal symptoms occur when ingestion of the drug is stopped. Psychological dependence may also develop.

Narcotic analgesics may actually exacerbate chronic pain and contribute to the development of operant pain. The mental clouding and confirmation of the sick role associated with narcotic use may interfere with learning nonmedication-related strategies to deal with the pain (McNairly, Maruta, Ivnik, Swanson, & Ilstrup, 1984). Because anxiety and depression are often associated with pain, the sedation and euphoric effects of narcotic use may result in drug-seeking behavior that is independent of pain and that may interfere with the performance of normative roles (Brena, 1983). Research suggests that clients with acute pain usually do not become addicted and that narcotics are more likely to be addictive and problematic when used by persons who already evidence serious adjustment problems, lack skills, and experience anxiety or depression. This is descriptive of many persons with chronic pain.

A number of drugs are used as adjuncts to analgesics in the treatment of pain; including antidepressants, antianxiety agents, and sedative-hypnotics. Antidepressants have a long history of use for chronic pain, but have little effect on acute pain. Based on a small number of controlled studies, antidepressants have a beneficial effect in 60 to 80% of the cases of chronic pain (Lindsay & Olsen, 1985). Antidepressants may exert a therapeutic effect in two ways. First, depression is a frequent concomitant of chronic pain and may serve to exacerbate or maintain pain. Insofar as antidepressants alleviate depression, they may also reduce pain. Antidepressants may also have a more direct effect on pain. Pain and depression are associated with similar neurochemical substrates: relative functional deficits in adrenergic neurotransmitters (norepinephrine, dopamine, and seratonin). Antidepressants increase the functional levels of adrenergic transmitters and consequently may relieve depression and inhibit pain (Ward et al., 1982). Although antidepressants have adverse side effects, they do not seem to present a particular risk of progression to operant pain.

Sedative-hypnotics and antianxiety agents are frequently used in the treatment of pain. They produce drowsiness, sedation, and sleep by depressing the central nervous system. Pharmacologically, these drugs are like alcohol. They have no demonstrated analgesic effect. In fact, some of these drugs may deplete adrenergic neurotransmitters and actually exacerbate depression and pain and increase anger and hostility (Kantor, 1984). These drugs also produce physical and psychological dependence. They are clearly not useful in the treatment of chronic and operant pain, and should be used very judiciously in the treatment of acute pain.

Several points should be clear from this brief review. A number of powerful drugs can be used in the treatment of pain. They can be both beneficial and dangerous. These drugs have a number of side effects as well as interacting and sometimes opposing pharmacological properties. These drugs are not equivalently effective for all types of pain. Aspirin-like substances are potentially beneficial for acute and chronic pain. Narcotics are potentially useful for acute but not chronic pain, and antidepressants for chronic but not acute pain. Antianxiety agents and sedative-hypnotics seem to have very limited utility in the treatment of any type of pain. Drugs should be used in a judicious manner, and their effects and side effects should be carefully monitored. The dose and combination of analgesic drugs should be clinically sensible. Their use is legitimate and often effective, but they present a risk of progression from acute to chronic pain. They are but one treatment modality and are often overemphasized as the primary means of intervention.

Surgical sectioning of sensory pathways results in disruption of the pattern of sensory input and neural firing, which may lead to the long-term exacerbation rather than relief of pain. In short, these procedures may often exacerbate chronic pain and contribute to the development of operant pain. They probably are only justified in cases of terminal illness (Melzack & Wall, 1983).

Sensory Control of Pain. As described in Chapter 9, the experience of pain is associated with alterations in the pattern of sensory input to the gate. Theoretically, interventions that alter this pain-evoking pattern may close the gate and consequently diminish the pain.

One method of sensory control of pain entails the electrical stimulation of peripheral or central nerves. Mild electrical stimulation is thought to stimulate large-diameter neurons selectively and thus close the gate. A popular method of electrical stimulation is called transcutaneous electrical nerve stimulation (TENS). In TENS, electrodes are placed on the skin and attached to a battery-powered, pocket-sized stimulator that generates a series of electrical pulses (Wall & Sweet, 1967). The frequency and duration of the pulses and the location of the electrodes are varied according to their empirical effects on the pain. TENS appears to be more effective than placebos in the treatment of chronic pain, but the long-term benefits have not been established (Fox & Melzack, 1976; Jeans, 1979; Taylor, Hallet, & Flaherty, 1981). However, it is a noninvasive procedure that has few documented side effects.

Sensory modulation is applicable to acute and chronic pain but has been applied primarily to chronic varieties of pain. The effectiveness of sensory modulation is highly variable, and its application often uses a "let's see if this works" approach. The mechanism that mediates sensory modulation is relatively unknown. Existing research suggests that, given judicious use, these procedures are devoid of negative side effects and do not increase the risk of progression to operant pain.

Secondary Prevention of Pain

Secondary prevention of pain refers to reducing the likelihood that acute pain will progress to chronic or operant forms. Obviously, effective definitive and symptomatic medical treatment of acute pain is central to such efforts. But some clients do progress to chronic and operant types of pain. How can this progression be minimized or prevented? There is a lack of epidemiological, longitudinal research in this area. No studies have followed a number of clients with acute pain in order to identify factors associated with such a progression. Only data from retrospective studies are available. Consequently, the subsequent discussion must be considered in a tentative fashion (Keefe, 1982).

Let us recall variables associated with the progression to chronic and operant pain (see Chapter 9 for a more complete discussion and Table 16-2 for a summary). During acute pain, persons engage in adaptive behaviors to deal with their pain. They decrease physical activity and other well behaviors, take medication, make adjustments in movement, use supportive devices, seek health care, and verbalize their pain to remediate damage and promote healing. However, some clients may continue such actions in the relative absence of tissue damage (i.e., after healing has substantively occurred) and enter a prechronic state in

TABLE 16-2 Conditions Promoting the Progression from Acute to Chronic and Operant Pain

Client characteristics
Unwillingness or inability to resume normal activities and roles
Abruptly resuming normal activities and roles incongruent with physiological recovery
Predisposition toward depression or a preexisting depressive disorder
Predisposition toward anxiety or a preexisting anxiety disorder
Guarded body movement and body-protective behaviors disproportionate to tissue damage
Reinforcement of pain behavior by either social and material rewards or avoidance or escape from unwanted roles and responsibilities
History of drug dependence or drug-seeking behavior
Nature of the tissue damage
Severe injury
Long-duration injury
Characteristics of the treatment regimen
Inappropriate use of analgesics and other psychoactive drugs
Neurosurgery for symptomatic treatment of pain
Failure to educate the client about pain and to monitor the client's responses at emotional, cognitive, and behavioral levels

which pain behavior maintains or exacerbates the experience of pain. Clients who gradually return to their normal roles and responsibilities congruent with healing are less likely to progress into this prechronic state. Clients who are unable or unwilling to return to normative activities and roles because of a lack of skills or opportunity are at risk for chronic pain. Individuals who attempt to return to normative activities and roles too early or abruptly may occasion further injury and pain and consequently return to pain and illness behavior. In the latter case, the repeated performance of illness behavior may result in reinforcement and maintenance of that behavior. Acute pain, particularly if severe and of long duration, may evoke depression, especially in those who are already predisposed. We have noted the neurophysiological similarities between depression and pain. The lack of recovery may also evoke anxiety and, via psychophysiological arousal, increase muscle tension and visceral disturbance, which exacerbate the pain problem. As clients guard their movements, muscle weakness and reduced normal sensory input may result, further reinforcing the pain process (Keefe, 1982).

In the previous discussion of medical treatment, we have noted treatment regimens for acute pain that increase the risk of the progression to chronic and operant pain, especially when working with at-risk clients: inappropriate use of analgesic and other drugs, neurosurgery for symptomatic pain relief, and a failure to educate clients and to closely monitor recovery on behavioral, cognitive, and affective as well as physiological levels. At a practical level, how can secondary prevention be implemented? First, clinicians should identify persons who are at risk for developing chronic pain in terms of both the parameters of the acute pain (severity and duration) and client characteristics. Second, a good client-clinician relationship should be established to monitor recovery and to modulate negative behavioral, affective, and cognitive responses to pain. Third, drug interventions should not be overemphasized as the sole way of dealing with pain. An educational approach can be used in which the responsibility and cognitive-behavioral participation of the client are considered important facets of treatment. This may include approaches to pain management like relaxation, biofeedback, stress management, sensory modulation, and appropriate exercise and activity (Gottlieb et al., 1977; Turk, Meichenbaum, & Genest, 1981). Fourth, the issue of the legitimacy of a pain complaint is very important. Suggestions by clinicians that pain has psychosocial components or may be treated with cognitive-behavioral modalities may trigger anger and resistance in the client (Katon, 1984). To a degree, this issue is mitigated by the use of an educational approach to acute pain, by the establishment of a good working relationship, and by reframing the problem and interventions in biological terms (see Chapter 11). Antidepressants, for example, have effects on the neurophysiology of pain as well as depression. Relaxation, graded exercise, and a modulated return to normal activities can be explained by focusing on their muscle-strengthening and spasm alleviating effects. In short, the treatment of acute pain is not a "one-shot," "fix-it" affair. Good treatment requires attention to behavior, affect, socioenvironmental contingencies, and thinking as well as physiology.

Cognitive-Behavioral Assessment of Pain

Pain is a multidimensional phenomenon that requires a multilevel assessment to include subjective experience (pain, affect, and cognitions), overt behavior, socioenvironmental contingencies, and medical status. Such an assessment may be useful in treating acute pain and is essential in treating chronic and operant pain. In this section, methods to assess the psychosocial and behavioral aspects of pain will be described. Medical assessment is central to this process but will not be examined in any depth. Let us begin with assessing the subjective experience of pain.

The Subjective Experience of Pain. At a gross level, clients can simply be asked to rate the severity of pain on a numerical scale (e.g., from 0, indicating no pain, to 10, indicating excruciating pain). There are two problems with this approach. First, only intensity is rated. Second, distances between numbers on the scale are probably not equal (Tursky, Jamner, & Friedman, 1982). Efforts have been made to develop pain perception measures that tap into multiple dimensions of pain in a quantifiable and valid manner. Probably the best known and most widely used instrument for this is the McGill Pain Questionnaire, or MPQ (Melzack, 1975). The MPQ consists of a series of adjectives describing pain along three dimensions: sensory, affective, and evaluative (see Figure 16-1). Within each category, the client is asked to select the adjective that is most descriptive of their own experience of pain. These adjectives are rank ordered in severity and thus allow some scaling of the pain. The MPQ is reliable and valid, but provides a qualitative rather than a quantitative measure of pain (Keefe, 1982).

Another promising device to measure subjective pain is the Pain Perception Profile (Tursky, 1976; Tursky et al., 1982). The profile has four parts. First, sensation, discomfort, and tolerance thresholds are measured in a psychophysical manner, providing information about individual differences in sensitivity. Second, clients are asked to judge the intensity of a series of stimuli to determine hypo- and hyperresponsiveness to pain. Third, clients complete a psychophysical rating scale of pain descriptors on dimensions of intensity, unpleasantness, and feeling. This results in a quantitative measure of pain as experienced by the client. Fourth, this pain descriptor scale can be used to self-monitor pain in relation to environmental and other events and to various types of

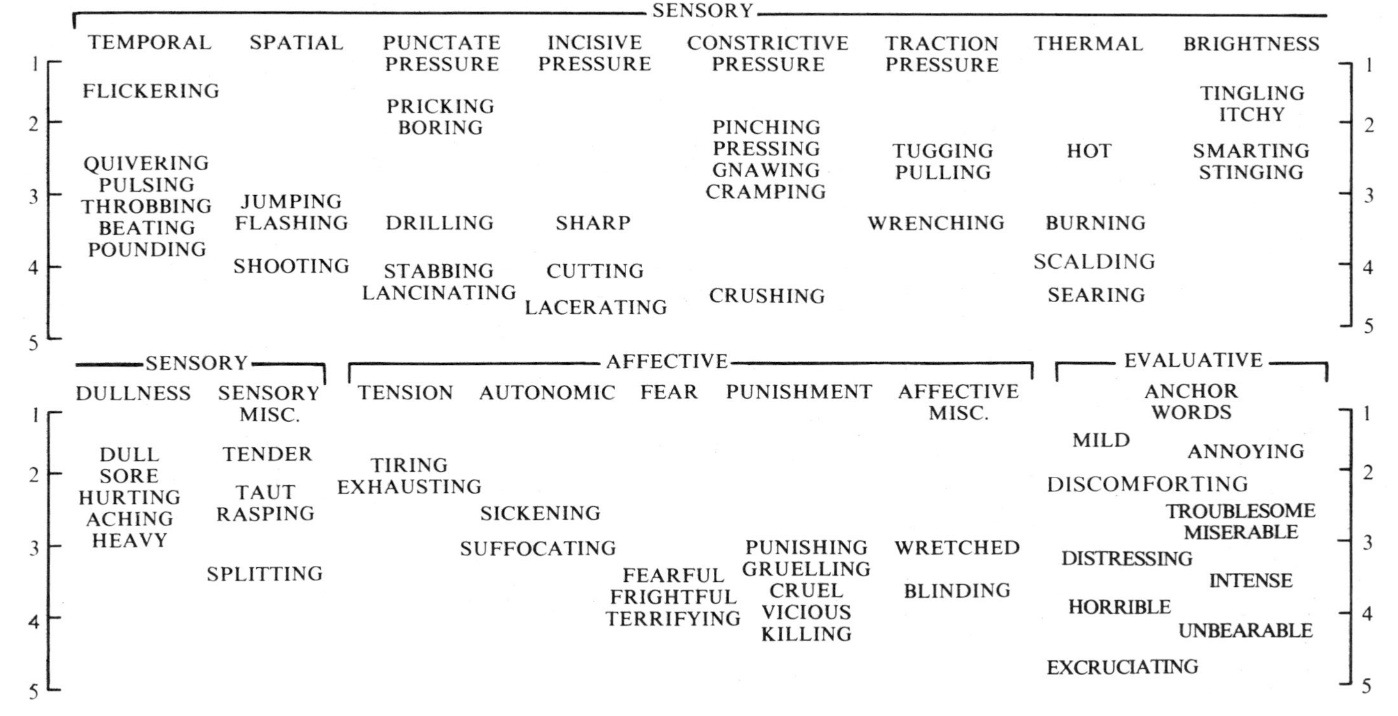

FIGURE 16-1 Pain Descriptors Used in the McGill Pain Questionnaire. (From "On the Language of Pain" by R. Melzack and W. S. Torgeson, 1971, *Anesthesiology*, *34*, pp. 56–57. Copyright 1971 by J. B. Lippincott Co. Reprinted by permission.)

treatment. Although quite complicated, the profile is valid, reliable, and clinically useful (Keefe, 1982).

Behavioral Responses to Pain. Both well behaviors (e.g., activity level and normative role actions) and pain behaviors (e.g., medication use, time in bed, verbal complaints and guarded movement) are important targets for assessment, especially in the operant treatment programs described later in this chapter. Behavioral interviews with the client and spouse can be used to identify critical target behaviors and the situational, temporal, and reinforcement parameters associated with those behaviors (Fordyce, 1976). Interviews are quite economical but may be suspect in terms of reliability and validity.

Because of these problems, several observational approaches to pain and well behavior have been developed: self-monitoring, participant observation, and structured observation. In self-monitoring, the client is given a daily log and asked to self-observe and self-record concretely specified behaviors such as medication use, time spent in bed, and time spent walking or standing. As shown in Figure 16-2, targets of self-monitoring may also include affect, subjective experience of pain, and socioenvironmental events associated with these behaviors and subjective experiences (Fordyce, 1976). In participant observation, family members of the client serve as observers. Of course, only overt behaviors can be assessed in this case. These approaches have the advantage of economy and provide data that are less based on recall and less subject to distortion. They are also useful in identifying variables that control pain and pain behavior in the natural setting. Both methods are subject to bias and distortion by the client or the participant observer (Kremmer, Block, & Gaylor, 1981).

Finally, it is often useful to observe pain and well behaviors using trained observers. This is usually done while clients are engaged in a structured task. The occurrence of some specified set of behaviors is coded at preset intervals while the client is exercising (Keefe & Block, 1982; Richards, Nepomuceno, Riles, & Suer, 1982) or during social interaction in a limited setting such as a hospital ward or the family dining room (Kremmer et al., 1981). These procedures provide highly reliable and valid results but are costly.

Affect. Another important target is subjective emotional experience. The most common approach has been to use the Minnesota Multiphasic Personality Inventory (MMPI) to assess the degree to which clients are characterologically predisposed to depression, anxiety, and somatization (Bradley, Prokop, Gentry, VanDer Heide, & Prieto, 1981). Clients with chronic pain typically show elevations on scales measuring these characteristics, but the causal status of these findings is questionable. The MMPI is often used in litigation to determine whether the pain is functional or organic. Such a question, however, is counter-

Time:	______	______	______
Pain Present	yes no	yes no	yes no
Severity	no pain / very severe	no pain / very severe	no pain / very severe
Interference	none / total	none / total	none / total
medication	type amount	type amount	type amount
	__ ____	__ ____	__ ____
	__ ____	__ ____	__ ____
	__ ____	__ ____	__ ____

location:
(shade in areas where you currently experience the pain)

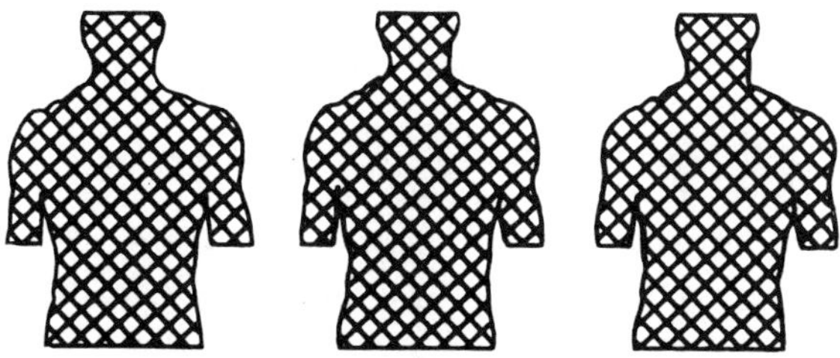

FIGURE 16-2 Self-Monitoring of Daily Plan

productive in terms of treatment. The MMPI may be used to assess whether a person is at risk for progression to chronic pain, but has not consistently predicted the effectiveness of treatment for such pain (Bradley et al., 1981; Sternbach, 1973).

Most research on the role of affect in pain has taken a trait approach. It may be more useful to assess the covariation of pain and affective states, which requires state measures of depression and anxiety such as the Multiple Affect Adjective Checklist (Zuckerman & Lubin, 1965) and the Beck Depression Inventory (Beck, Ward, Mendelson, Moch, & Erbaugh, 1961). This permits a determination of the situational role of pain and affect.

Cognition. Pain is stressful. Therefore, it may prove useful to assess appraisal and coping strategies used by clients to respond to pain. Cognitive errors in processing information may maintain and exacerbate chronic pain (Turk & Genest, 1979; Turk & Rudy, 1986). Questionnaires have been developed to assess the cognitions of clients experiencing chronic pain (LeFebvre, 1981). The questionnaires contain items specific to cognitive distortions associated with chronic pain as well as those relevant to more general appraisal.

There are also questionnaires that assess clients' response to pain. One such questionnaire is the Coping Strategy Questionnaire (Rosenstiel & Keefe, 1983), which assesses clients' response to pain along six cognitive (e.g., diverting attention and reinterpreting sensations) and two behavioral (activity level and pain behavior) dimensions. Scores on this questionnaire correlate with emotional and behavioral adjustment to chronic pain. The validity and reliability of these questionnaires on appraisal and coping in chronic pain are not clearly established (Turk & Rudy, 1986).

Assessment of Pain: A Summary. A broad battery of sophisticated assessment devices has been developed to measure the various aspects of pain. A multimodal assessment of pain is congruent with its multiaxial nature and complements medical findings. Psychosocial and behavioral assessment may be useful in treating acute pain and is central to the effective treatment of chronic and operant pain. An extensive battery of testing is expensive and time-consuming. A multiple gating approach to assessment can be used to address this problem. In multiple gating, assessment begins with broad, relatively inexpensive methods like an interview. If psychosocial variables appear to play a potential role in the pain based on information from the interview, the assessment of relevant variables is pursued using more specialized and expensive devices like self-report tests, behavioral observation, and similar intensive methods.

Cognitive-Behavioral Treatment of Pain

A number of related cognitive-behavioral interventions have been developed to treat pain: operant-contingency management programs, cognitive self-control programs, psychophysiological methods (biofeedback and relaxation), and behavioral skills training. Although these methods will be described separately, they are compatible and often combined. These methods are used for clients whose pain involves varying degrees of physical pathology and necessitates a genuine integration with medical forms of treatment. A total intervention program often entails various forms of definitive and symptomatic medical treatment as well as cognitive-behavioral modalities. It is important to recognize that clients in pain are not a homogeneous group. They evidence varying degrees of physical pathology, their pain arises from different causes, and they bring different coping resources to treatment. Medical and cognitive-behavioral interventions need to be individualized to fit these differences. General strategies concerning screening clients, preparing them for intervention, developing individualized programs, and promoting maintenance of change over time will be discussed. In addition to describing psychosocial interventions for pain, we will evaluate their utility. Do they really alleviate pain and restore normative functioning? How long do these effects last?

Contingency Management. Contingency management programs focus on changing pain behaviors rather than clients' subjective experiences of pain. Treatment has three goals: (1) decreasing pain behavior, (2) increasing well behavior, and (3) modifying natural environmental contingencies to maintain these changes (Fordyce, 1976). After assessment, clients and their spouses are provided a clear description of the program and its goals and rationale. A learned behavior conceptualization of pain is emphasized, and the primary components of treatment (including management of medication, increased exercise and activity, and extinction of verbal, vocal, and motor pain behaviors) are detailed.

In medication management, the client is instructed to bring all medications to the pain treatment unit. For several days, the client is allowed to take these medications as needed (within medical prudence) to establish a base line. These medications are then mixed in a "pain cocktail" (the active medications are mixed and delivered in a color- and taste-masking fluid) and delivered to the client at specified intervals and at a total daily strength equivalent to the base line intake. The dosage is then slowly reduced over time. The goal is not necessarily to reach a zero intake level, but rather to withdraw ineffective, dangerous, or iatrogenic drugs and to allow the client to develop alternate pain-coping methods other than medication use.

An increase in activity level and exercise is targeted for change to encourage well behavior that will consequently lead to positive social and behavioral consequences. More frequent exercise and activity may also increase muscle tone and strength and address functional weaknesses specifically related to the pain (compatible with medical and physical limitations). Clients are initially asked to exercise twice daily to their own tolerance level. The exercise is measured in the amount performed (e.g., distance walked or number of flexions) rather than time. Once this base line tolerance level is established, the client is asked to exercise twice daily at a preset amount set slightly below that level. This insures initial success. The amount of exercise is then slowly increased over time and successful performance is systematically praised. Graphic displays of achievements provide further feedback. Complaints during exercise are ignored, and failures are met with readjustments in exercise quotas.

The third major component entails the systematic alteration of the consequences for pain and well behaviors. Treatment staff and family members are taught to ignore systematically verbal, vocal, and motor pain behaviors and to attend to and praise well behaviors. Family involvement promotes generalization of change over time and across settings. Other interventions, such as sensory modulation, biofeedback, and interventions to teach specific social and vocational skills, may be used according to client needs (Fordyce & Steger, 1979).

Contingency management approaches have broad applications in the treatment of chronic pain regardless of the relative contribution of physical pathology to the pain. It utilizes a degree of control that may only be required for clients who have progressed to consistent performance of pain behaviors and whose environment strongly reinforces those behaviors. In those cases in which the progression is less advanced or in which the natural environment is less supportive of pain behaviors, self-management procedures may be sufficient.

Self-Management and Cognitive-Behavioral Interventions. Self-management and cognitive interventions have goals similar to contingency management: the acquisition and performance of cognitive and behavioral skills to cope with pain adaptively. The primary differences among these approaches are that self-management and cognitive strategies place greater responsibility for change on the client, focus more specifically on enhancing clients' sense of personal efficacy with regard to pain, and emphasize the importance of altering clients' perceptions and thinking to effect change (Keefe, 1982; Turk & Genest, 1979).

The first step is to foster a collaborative set and shared conceptualization about the problem. In this approach, treatment is not something that is done to the client, but rather the acquisition by the client of skills relevant to the pain problem. Pain can then be understood, and problem-oriented actions can mitigate the pain. A collaborative set, for example, might be promoted by the following health provider's introduction to the client:

> You have been to several doctors and clinics before you came here, so when you arrived this morning, you probably had some idea of what to expect. At the same time, you might have been wondering whether we would do anything differently here, perhaps hoping that finally something could be done to help. Well, I don't know yet how much assistance we can offer you; finding that out will be our first task. But I do know we do things differently here. Here we don't do things to you or give you things to change your pain. What we will be doing is helping you to use the resources you have to affect your pain. Now you may think you have already tried everything you can to help yourself. And I do know that you indeed want to reduce your pain and do what you can for yourself. What we are going to look for is resources that you may not be aware of and ways of using your abilities in a different manner. We can offer some help for most people, but that help is useful only through your efforts to put it to use. We will want you

> to participate in everything, from learning more about your problem to stages of doing something about it. (Turk et al., 1981, p. 248)

Although there are other possibilities, gate control theory can be used to develop a shared conceptualization of pain and its treatment. The explanation might proceed as follows:

> Pain is a message from the site of injury that is sent to the brain through a mechanism called a gate. The brain interprets the message, but the gate controls what is transmitted to the brain. The gate can be partially or fully open or closed, determining the amount of pain. Various physical, emotional and mental factors control the gate. (Karol, Doerfler, Parker, & Armetrout, 1981, p. 15)

The client can then be shown a list like that illustrated in Table 16-3, and each of the factors can be discussed in more detail.

In contrast to contingency management, a wide variety (or menu) of skills can be taught. The client is an active agent in this process.

TABLE 16-3 Factors That Open and Close the Gate

Open
Physical
- Extent of the injury
- Readiness of the nervous system to send pain signals
- Inappropriate activity level

Emotional stress
- Depression
- Anxiety
- Worry
- Tension
- Anger

Mental factors
- Focusing on the pain
- Boredom due to minimal involvement in life activities
- Nonadaptive attitudes

Close
Physical
- Medication
- Counterstimulation (e.g., heat, massage, acupuncture, or TENS)
- Appropriate activity level

Emotional stability
- Relaxation
- Positive emotions (e.g., happiness or optimism)
- Rest

Mental factors
- Life involvement and interest in activities
- Intense concentration on stimuli other than pain
- Adaptive attitudes

Teaching is accomplished using instructions, modeling, rehearsal, and feedback. Self-control methods, including self-monitoring, stimulus control, competing behaviors, and self-reinforcement, are explicitly included. Skills are selected to address cognitive, affective, behavioral, and psychophysiological aspects of pain, and may include relaxation, self-regulated reduction in medication use, exercise, increased activity, imagery, coping self-verbalizations, alterations in appraisal, and social and vocational skills training. The methods for teaching, practicing, and utilizing these skills in the natural environment follow the guidelines for coping skills training described in Chapter 14. The goal is to develop a flexible set of skills that can be utilized by the client in the natural environment to cope with pain, that promotes a general problem-solving set, and that fosters a sense of control, predictability, and self-efficacy.

Cognitive self-control interventions may be more applicable to verbal, motivated clients who endorse a compensatory model of helping. They may be less applicable to clients whose pain has very strong operant components. Powerful, naturally occurring reinforcement for pain may undermine the effort and motivation required by these interventions. Cognitive self-control programs are clearly applicable for clients who have organically based chronic pain, and may be particularly well suited for the secondary prevention of pain.

Biofeedback and Relaxation Training. As described in Chapter 12, biofeedback and relaxation training are specialized modes of self-control intervention. Via instructions and feedback, clients acquire skills associated with increased awareness and control of physiological functions. The treatment protocols described in Chapter 12 are applicable to pain problems. These procedures have been used as both primary and adjunctive treatments of chronic pain. They have been most frequently used for pain associated with headaches, Raynaud's disease, temporomandibular joint pain, and low back and neck pain (see Ziesat, 1981, for a review). These strategies may also be used to address psychophysiological responses that exacerbate (e.g., muscle spasms) or confound (e.g., gastrointestinal distress) pain. The effectiveness of these procedures as the sole or primary treatment of pain, as described in Chapter 12, is equivocal.

Skills Training. Clients experiencing chronic (and sometimes acute) pain often have deficits in social and vocational skills. These deficits may facilitate the progression to chronic pain or exacerbate the pain once it has reached chronic proportions. Skills deficits may have preceded the onset of pain, may have resulted from the functional limitations imposed by the pain-producing injury, or may reflect the anxiety, depression, and irritability associated with unremitting pain. These deficits reduce the availability of normal sources of reinforcement and consequently increase depression and decrease the performance of well behaviors. It is very important to identify deficits and to provide training to enhance instrumental competence (Keefe, Gil, & Rose, 1986).

The Effectiveness of Cognitive-Behavioral Treatment of Pain

Because a large number of studies have assessed the effectiveness of cognitive-behavioral treatment of pain, only a representative sample can be presented. In an early seminal study, Fordyce et al. (1973) evaluated the application of a contingency management program to thirty-six clients with chronic back pain. The average duration of the pain was seven years, and most clients had had two or more surgeries. After seven weeks of treatment, uptime (not sitting or in bed) was increased 50%. There was a significant reduction in medication use. Exercise increased 100%. There was also a modest reduction in the subjective reports of pain. Follow-up data are not available.

One of the most thorough evaluations has been carried out by Cinciripini and Floreen (1982). One hundred twenty clients whose duration of pain averaged eight years were treated using a combination of contingency management, biofeedback and relaxation training, behavioral group therapy, self-monitoring, contracting, and family therapy. Before and after intervention, vocal, verbal, and motor behaviors, prohealth talk, and assertiveness were observed. Self-reports of pain, medication use, and daily exercise were obtained. Despite the fact that most of the clients were unemployed prior to intervention and nearly half were receiving compensation, treatment was highly successful. After treatment, over 90% of the clients were free of medication. There were substantial reductions in pain behavior and increases in well behavior, physical activity, fitness, and voluntary exertion. At a one-year follow-up, most of the clients had maintained or extended these gains, and 50% of the clients were working.

Gottlieb et al. (1977) used a self-control program with seventy-two clients experiencing chronic pain that was associated with organic damage but resistant to medical treatment. The average duration of the pain was six years, and most clients had had at least two surgeries. The clients were taught self-paced reduction in medication, were engaged in social skills training and group and family therapy, and were given biofeedback training. There was also a specific emphasis on physical therapy and vocational training. The program resulted in significant reductions in pain behaviors and medication use and in increases in activity levels. Of the clients contacted six months after treatment, over 80% were working or in vocational training.

Multimodal cognitive-behavioral interventions appear to be effective in the treatment of persons with chronic pain. However, the evaluative studies of these interventions suffer from a number of methodological flaws. The treatments are not standardized. There is a lack of standardized outcome measures. Often, there is no comparison group of clients who do not receive treatment. To a degree, the extended history of severe pain experienced by these clients mitigates some of these problems. The history of the pain problem provides a powerful base line against which the effects of treatment can be compared. Controlled studies would entail the ethical problem of delaying treatment for some clients. However, there are two areas that particularly need to be addressed. The maintenance of treatment gains has not been clearly established. Data from existing studies suggest that 30 to 70% of clients report continued benefits over a one- to five-year interval after treatment is terminated (Keefe et al., 1986). More effort is required to promote maintenance and systematically to assess the long-term effects of treatment. The second major concern is that outcome is typically evaluated using group averages and relies on the statistical significance of differences between outcome measures from pre- to posttreatment. This approach does not provide information about the variability of clients' responses to treatment and the amount of change relative to normal functioning. Treatment outcome should be assessed using multiple measures to include subjective experiences of pain, pain behavior, medication use, activity and exercise level, and social and vocational adjustment. Social and vocational measures in particular are likely to reflect sustained functional improvement in the natural environment.

Despite these shortcomings, the contribution of cognitive-behavioral approaches to the assessment and treatment of chronic and operant pain is impressive. Progress is being made in remediating what was previously thought to be an intractable, costly source of human suffering. Much remains to be done.

Primary Prevention of Pain

Pain is one result of a number of disease processes (e.g., coronary artery disease, ulcers, and arthritis), traumatic events (e.g., car accidents and gunshot wounds), or contact with destructive physical or chemical agents (e.g., fire, radiation, and poisons). In this sense, the primary prevention of pain entails reducing the probability of disease and injury. This is obviously a very broad topic. We will focus on the prevention of injury and pain due to automobile accidents. The term "accident" is a misnomer, because it suggests that luck or fate plays a major role in the occurrence of these mishaps. Using this perspective, little can be done to prevent such events. However, there are specific agents that cause injury. Contact with these agents is influenced by individual and collective decision making and behavior. In this sense, accidents are not accidental.

In this section, we will review the research on preventing injury due to motor vehicle accidents in a very specific group: young children.

Automobile accidents kill or injure more children than any other pediatric health problem (Christophersen, 1984). The technology for reducing or preventing death and injury is available: child restraint devices, or car seats. A child riding unrestrained in an automobile is sixteen times more likely to be killed or seriously injured in an accident than one who is wearing a restraining device (Scherz, 1982). But only 10 to 15% of children are buckled. How can we increase parents' consistent use of restraints for their children when riding in an automobile? Until passive devices (e.g., air bags) are mandated, we can try to legislate seat belt use for children, engage in public education, or attempt individualized intervention with parents.

Child-passenger safety legislation is relatively inexpensive but has proved to be only modestly effective. Tennessee was one of the first states to pass such a law. Enactment of the law resulted in an increase in the use of child safety belts and seats from 9% to 29%. In a neighboring state, Kentucky, which did not pass such legislation, no comparable increase was found. The Tennessee law was also accompanied by a public education and information program. While effective, it appears that legislation and education alone are not sufficient (Christophersen, 1984).

Individualized preventative programs have also been tried. For example, Christophersen and Sullivan (1982) developed a hospital-based program in which new mothers were given education concerning child restraint, including modeling about how to position and restrain an infant. They were also provided with a car seat. Approximately 70% of the mothers were observed to use car seats for their infants at discharge from the maternity stay, but only 28% were observed to continue their use one month later. Attempts have also been made to get pediatricians to educate and encourage parents in child auto safety. Most pediatricians do not counsel parents in this regard. Systematic multicomponent intervention, including in-hospital education and a written prescription to purchase a car seat, a reminder one month later with a demonstration of correct use, and a reminder two months later, was found to be moderately effective. Use rates on discharge from the hospital were 38% and increased to 58% after the third intervention (Reisenger & Bires, 1980). It appears that health providers need a structure in order to intervene and that parents need multiple interventions to respond.

Most educational approaches use the avoidance of child injury and death to motivate parents to use child seat belts. The probability of such an event is highly remote, easily rationalized, and does not serve as a salient, immediate stimulus for child restraint. In fact, using seat belts often seems to be a hassle. Some immediate positive payoff is needed to motivate parents. Research suggests that children behave better in the car when they are buckled (Christophersen, 1977). This potential reinforcer was used to intervene with parents who did not use child restraints. During one office visit, the behavioral advantages of child restraint were described and a loaner seat was provided. This resulted in the use of child restraints in 62% of the cases immediately after the office visit, 75% six months later, and 37% one year later (Christophersen & Gyulay, 1981).

This brief excursion into the primary prevention of injury and pain provides an example of the tactics and issues relevant to other types of accidents. Primary prevention can focus on either changing individual behavior or altering the exposure to the pathogenic agent via individual or community education and legislation.

PAIN: A SUMMARY

Perhaps more than cancer and heart disease, pain involves an intimate interaction among biochemical, physiological, and psychosocial processes. This is evident in understanding the proximal and distal causes of pain, and in engaging in preventative and clinical interventions for pain-associated disorders. The dualism that is apparent in labeling pain as either real (biological) or not (psychogenic) is not a productive perspective, practically or theoretically. There is a connectedness that is often belied by traditional ways of thinking. This is also true of infectious diseases.

BEHAVIORAL, PSYCHOSOCIAL, AND ENVIRONMENTAL INTERVENTIONS IN INFECTIOUS DISEASES

In Chapter 7, we learned that the germ theory of infectious diseases is inadequate. Bacteria, viruses, and other microorganisms do cause infectious diseases, but psychosocial, environmental, and behavioral variables also play a role by influencing host resistance to and contact with infectious agents. Our individual health-impairing and health-promoting behaviors and collective decisions and actions affect the occurrence of and contact with pathogens. Resistance to disease is complexly determined by a variety of biological, developmental, and psychosocial variables, including diet, drug ingestion, stress, coping skills, and social support. These variables, in interaction with the successful invasion of the body by infectious agents, determine the probability of infectious diseases and may affect recovery from such diseases. Seeking health care in a timely and appropriate fashion is also critical in the prevention and treatment of infections. Health behaviors relevant to infectious diseases include getting immunizations, recognizing and differentiating self-limiting, nonthreatening infections from nonself-limiting, serious infections, and complying with antibiotic and other treatment regimens and recommendations.

In the remainder of this chapter, we will focus on individual and community-based interventions relevant to the prevention, control, and treatment of infectious diseases. More specifically, this will include two topics: prevention and control of infectious diseases and attempts to enhance immune functioning and resistance to disease by stress management.

Prevention and Control of Infectious Diseases

Consider the following problem. You have a bathtub into which water is flowing. You are given a dipper and the task of emptying the tub of water. How would you solve the problem? The common sense solution is to turn off the faucet rather than simply to bail out the water. This is the goal of the prevention and control of infectious and other diseases (Albee, 1983). As described in Chapter 7, the probability of infection depends on the interaction of host and environmental variables. That is, it depends on the availability of the infectious agent in the environment and on the behavior and resistance of the host. Efforts at prevention and control can focus on altering the environment, the host, or both (Runyan, DeVillis, DeVillis, & Hockbaum, 1982).

Let us first consider strategies to alter the environmental availability of infectious agents. This is accomplished by public health programs. Attempts to reduce the occurrence of infectious diseases begins with identifying the incidence of these diseases in the population and then searching for social, demographic, economic, and geographic correlates of the diseases. The classic example is John Snow's (1855) work on cholera in London in the nineteenth century. Snow carefully mapped the geographic distribution of cholera cases and found that they were clustered around a specific water source, the Broad Street pump. He concluded that this water supply was the source of the disease. Often, the specific cause of a disease may not be known, but actions can still be taken to reduce the incidence of the disease. In public health, efforts to prevent or contain disease often entail altering the environment by either direct action or regulation. Snow, for example, simply removed the Broad Street pump. Such efforts often do not focus on individual behavior or worry about personal choice. They entail mandatory restrictions or laws. This is an excellent example of the enlightenment model of helping (see Chapter 1). Although many other specialties in psychology typically focus on the behavior of individuals or small groups, community psychology emphasizes analysis and intervention in a broader ecological context and consequently has much to offer to public health (Runyan et al., 1982).

The second mode of preventing infectious diseases entails altering the host. This may be done by altering individuals' behavior in a manner that reduces their contact with infectious agents or enhances their resistance to those agents. We will examine two such efforts: motivating individuals to get immunizations and encouraging individuals to engage in "safe sex" to control the spread of AIDS.

Immunizations. One obvious way to prevent infectious diseases is to get immunized against these diseases. Immunization consists of the introduction of a weakened form (usually by pretreatment drying or exposure to ultraviolet light) of an infectious agent into the body. This vaccine is not strong enough to cause clinical symptoms of the disease but presents the specific immune system with antigens that elicit the development of memory B- and T-cells. This results in active immunity when exposure to that infectious agent occurs in the natural environment (Spense & Mason, 1987).

Vaccines have been vital to improvements in health. For example, the average number of annual polio cases from 1951 to 1955 was 35,000 compared to 8 cases in 1984. These vaccines have proven effectiveness in preventing once prevalent and dangerous infectious diseases. In most cases, there is little risk of iatrogenic reactions (LaForce, 1987). Partly because of this success, persons have become complacent about getting completely immunized in a timely fashion. For example, 10,000 cases of vaccine-preventable diseases were reported in the United States in 1982 (Center for Disease Control, 1983). Getting immunized involves individual behavior—scheduling and going to a health provider. How can individuals be motivated to get immunizations for themselves and their children?

Public health regulations require proof of immunization for children for entrance into school. But this leaves many vulnerable preschool-age children unprotected. It is not unusual to find 50% or more of these children to be immunization deficient. Further, many adults are not properly immunized. Regulatory interventions are important but not sufficient. Efforts must be made to remind and encourage individuals to get themselves and their children immunized (LaForce, 1987; Yokley & Glenwick, 1984). Several strategies have been used to accomplish this, either alone or in combination: prompting, increased access to immunization services, and monetary or other types of incentives.

Prompting entails sending a postcard or making radio announcements reminding parents to get their children immunized. Written prompts can be form letters or personalized letters, can provide information or make emotional appeals, and can be sent once or several times. Sole reliance on prompts usually results in increased rates of immunization on the order of 10 to 20%, especially if personalized and sent more than once. The combination of multiple prompts and increased access to immunization services has resulted in increased rates of 20 to 30%. The combination of prompts and monetary, lotterylike incentives has resulted in increased rates of immunization between 30 and 40%. These interventions are also relatively economical (Yokley & Glenwick, 1984). A combination of environmental-regulatory and host-behavioral interventions is probably most effective.

Another example in which the prevention and control of infectious disease necessarily entails altering individual behavior is AIDS. Recall from Chapter 7 that the two primary modes of transmission of the HIV AIDS virus are the use of unsterilized hypodermics (most often associated with illicit drug use) and contact with body fluids during intimate sexual interaction. Government agencies, schools, media, and many private groups (e.g., Gay Men's Health Crisis, Mothers of AIDS Patients, and San Francisco AIDS Foundation) have initiated an immense campaign to educate individuals about the nature of AIDS, its transmission, and behavioral means by which contact with the AIDS virus can be minimized or avoided (U.S. Department of Health and Human Services [DHHS], 1986b). The following personal actions have been recommended.

In terms of transmission by hypodermic needles, the message is relatively simple: Do not use intravenous drugs for nonmedical (illegal or recreational) purposes. If such drug use occurs, do not share hypodermic equipment. Dealing with the sexual transmission of AIDS is more complex. Assuming contact with HIV has not occurred via another route, the best absolute way to avoid acquiring the AIDS virus is by sexual abstinence. Abstinence is probably not a realistic recommendation for some adolescents and many adults. The best strategy for sexually active individuals is sexual monogamy for both partners. Again assuming no other route of contact, persons who have been in a relationship in which both partners have been absolutely faithful for the last five to seven years are safe. For those who wish to be sexually active but not monogamous, a number of steps can be taken to reduce the risk of getting AIDS. These strategies, shown in Table 16-4, are often termed "safe sex" (DHHS, 1986a, 1986b).

Educational efforts to control the spread of AIDS must also target individuals who have, with or without their knowledge, the AIDS virus. Responsible behavior by HIV-infected individuals is critical to preventing the spread of AIDS and to their own health. At-risk individuals should get a blood test for AIDS. If the test is positive, the infected individuals should inform their past, current, and future sexual partners. If infected individuals continue to be sexually active, they should engage in the safe sexual practices described above, even when interacting with other infected individuals. They should not donate blood or organs and should not get pregnant. They should seek prompt and regular medical

TABLE 16-4 "Safe Sex": Actions to Reduce Contact with the AIDS Virus

Do not have sex with multiple partners or with persons who have had multiple partners
Avoid sex with persons who have AIDS or a positive blood test for the AIDS virus, or with members of high-risk groups (gay and bisexual men, prostitutes, past or current i.v. drug users, sexual partners of infected persons, persons with hemophilia who received the blood clotting factor before 1985, and persons from Haiti and central Africa)
Use a condom from start to finish during intimate sexual interaction
Avoid sexual practices that injure sensitive body tissues (membranes of the rectum, vagina, penis, and mouth)
Use touching for sexual expression but avoid deep, open-mouth kissing

attention, and inform their health providers of their status (DHHS, 1986a, 1986b).

The educational strategies used to prevent and control the spread of AIDS have primarily utilized the presentation of information in a realistic but nonemotional manner. How successful have they been? For several reasons, this is a difficult question to answer. First, the educational efforts have been relatively recent. Some time must elapse before the current strategies can be evaluated. Second, it is hard to estimate the impact of the educational interventions because AIDS is often asymptomatic and has a long and variable incubation period. Changes in the incidence of AIDS resulting from current education may only be apparent in a few years. But we are not totally blind in this regard. AIDS is not the first serious sexually transmitted disease without a cure that has reached epidemic proportions. In 1941, syphilis caused approximately 14,000 deaths in a United States population of 132 million. Similar to the current AIDS education program, the intervention for syphilis in the 1940s focused on efforts to alter sexual behavior and to encourage the use of prophylactic measures during sexual interaction. At that time, interventions promoting sexual abstinence were not successful, but those encouraging "safe sex" were (Peterman & Curran, 1986). However, there are differences between the syphilis problem in the 1940s and the current AIDS problem. HIV is different in some respects. Persons infected with HIV are chronic carriers and may be unaware they are carriers because the virus can be asymptomatic.

There is some preliminary, tentative evidence that the campaign against AIDS is working. Gay men are reporting changes in their sexual practices, especially a reduction in the number of sexual partners. They also appear to be engaging in "safe sex"; there has been a decrease in pharyngeal and rectal gonorrhea in some male gay groups (Peterman &

Curran, 1986). Continuing assessment over the next few years will be necessary to determine whether the AIDS education campaign is working. Actions in addition to education need to be taken. For example, easy, economical access to confidential testing for AIDS and to the purchase of condoms is important.

Are different, more extreme measures needed to counteract the AIDS epidemic? Several such measures have been suggested: compulsory blood testing for HIV in high-risk populations or as a prerequisite to receiving a marriage license; disclosure of individuals' positive AIDS status to employers, insurance companies, and public health agencies; tracing, informing, and testing the previous sexual partners of persons with AIDS; and identifying individuals with AIDS so that sexual contact with those persons by others can be avoided. Up to this point, these more extreme, mandatory regulations have been avoided in most states (Lewis, 1987). According to current evidence and theories, these extreme measures are either unnecessary or counterproductive dehumanizing infringements on personal rights. For example, quarantining and informing employers are unnecessary because transmission of the virus by casual contact does not occur. Mandatory, nonconfidential testing of high-risk groups may actually discourage rather than encourage the use of testing, thus driving the problem underground. Tracing and informing the past sexual contacts of infected individuals is most beneficial when effective treatment is available.

Prevention and Control of Infectious Diseases: A Summary. It is more useful to close the faucet prior to bailing out the bathtub. Prevention of infectious diseases by altering the environment or host behavior are critical health promotion endeavors. We have reviewed two efforts to prevent infectious disease: motivating individuals to get immunizations and altering individuals' sexual behavior to prevent the spread of AIDS. These and similar preventative interventions complement the discovery and use of curative interventions. Another strategy in the fight against infectious diseases entails enhancing host resistance (or immune functioning) via stress management.

Stress Management and Host Resistance

Stress is one of a number of variables that modulate immune functioning and resistance to disease. Although the stress-immune-disease connection is highly variable, one implication is that it may be possible to enhance immune functioning and resistance to disease by helping high-risk individuals to reduce stress or to cope more effectively. In this section, we will review research that assesses the impact of stress management on immune functioning and host resistance.

Let us begin with a series of classic studies on institutionalized elderly individuals done by Rodin and her colleagues (Langer & Rodin,

1976; Rodin, 1979; Rodin & Langer, 1977). Recall from Chapter 7 that aging individuals may be especially vulnerable biologically because of a decline in immune functioning. They may also experience an increasing number of health problems because of social and environmental challenges accompanying aging: reduction in roles (e.g., retirement or children leaving home), decreased social support (e.g., loss of contact with friends and coworkers), bereavement, a lack of meaningful reference groups and activities, and institutionalization in nursing homes and other facilities. Although aging does not necessarily entail such changes and such changes are not necessarily stressful, aging individuals are at risk.

In the initial study, Rodin and her colleagues (Rodin, 1979) randomly assigned aging individuals in a nursing home to one of two floors. On one floor, the residents were provided with enhanced choice, control and responsibility over their activities, living space, and social relationships. The residents on the other floor were informed that the staff would work very hard to take care of them. There were no differences between the groups in gender, health, and time in the nursing home. Those provided with enhanced choice, control, and responsibility reported and were observed to be happier, more active, more alert, and more involved than their "cared for" counterparts. Those given greater control were also rated as having improved physical health after intervention, whereas the health of the persons from the other floor declined. Eighteen months after the intervention, 15% of the group with enhanced control had died compared to 30% of the residents from the other floor. Thus, a brief, simple intervention to enhance the control of aging individuals had dramatic results.

Does this control have to be real, or is it the perception of control that is important? How are the effects of control on health mediated? To answer these questions, Rodin's group (Rodin, 1979) intervened in a different manner with a similar group of nursing home residents. Residents were assigned to one of three groups. One group received no intervention. A second group was given information asserting that aging does not necessarily result in a decline in health (an educational intervention). A third group was told that physical and adjustive problems were often the result of the environment rather than personal characteristics. The attempt was to attribute problems to environmental circumstances rather than to oneself (a reattribution strategy). The group receiving the reattribution intervention were more sociable, participated in more activities, and were physically healthier relative to those receiving education or no intervention. They also excreted lower amounts of adrenal corticosteroids, or hormones associated with stress. The reduction in corticosteroids suggests that the improved health status of residents receiving the reattribution intervention may have been mediated by neuroendocrine mechanisms.

The third study in the series (Rodin, 1979) attempted a more powerful intervention. Residents in a nursing home were randomly assigned to one of four groups. One group received a self-control and self-instructional intervention focusing on the development and use of coping skills to address stressors commonly experienced by aging individuals (see Chapter 11). A second group was given increased responsibility, control, and choice, like the intervention used in the first study. The two remaining groups were attention placebo (a general discussion of pain-related issues) and assessment control (only administered pre- and post-treatment measurements) groups. The self-control plus self-instructional group engaged in more self-reported coping responses, was more active, and happier, reported less stress, and was better adjusted according to staff ratings than the other three groups. These effects were maintained at a one-year follow-up. Both after the intervention and at follow-up, individuals in the self-control and self-instructional group also excreted lower levels of corticosteroids, which were inversely related to self-reported stress.

This series of studies clearly support the notion that interventions that teach behavioral and cognitive coping skills and enhance control through modification of the environment can have a powerful effect on the psychological and physical health of aging and perhaps other vulnerable populations. The research also provides suggestive evidence that these effects may be in part mediated by the modulation of endocrine and thus immune functioning. This evidence is, however, indirect in that no measures of immune functioning or of immune-related incidence of disease were reported. There are some recent studies that directly assess the impact of stress management on immune functioning. Let us examine two such studies.

In the first study, geriatric residents from an independent living facility were randomly assigned to one of three groups: relaxation training, social support, or no treatment. Relaxation training was taught and practiced in twelve sessions over a month. The social support intervention entailed twelve visits by college students over a month. Before and after these interventions and at a one-month follow-up, the following psychosocial and immune variables were measured: psychological distress, life satisfaction, locus of control, natural killer cell activity, antibody response to herpes simplex I, and T- and B-lymphocyte proliferation to two antigens. Relative to functioning at the pretreatment assessment, individuals in the relaxation group reported reduced distress, showed enhanced natural killer cell activity, and produced less antibody response to the herpes virus (indicating enhanced immune functioning) after the intervention. These changes were not maintained at follow-up, but none of the participants reported use of relaxation after the intervention. There were no significant changes in psychosocial and immune measures in either of the other groups (Kiecolt-Glaser et al.,

1985). The use of relaxation appeared to result in enhanced immune functioning in these aging individuals and, with continued use, may have had positive health benefits. The lack of an effect in the social support intervention is puzzling. Social support typically reduces the impact of stress. It may be that the participants already had sufficient social support or that the visits from college students were not perceived in a positive manner.

A second study by Kiecolt-Glaser et al. (1986) attempted to replicate the immune enhancing effect of relaxation in a different sample. Thirty-four medical school students had blood drawn twice, once one month prior to examinations and once during examinations. Each time blood was drawn, a number of psychosocial and immune variables were measured: psychological distress, loneliness, nutrition, helper versus suppressor T-cell ratio, and natural killer cell activity. After the first blood draw, the students were randomly assigned to either a hypnosis-relaxation group or a no treatment control. Hypnosis/relaxation was taught and practiced in ten sessions over the month. The relaxation group showed no increase in distress during examinations, whereas the control group reported significant elevations in distress. The helper versus suppressor T-cell ratio and natural killer cell activity decreased significantly during examinations, but significantly less so in students in the relaxation group who reported regular use of the coping skill. These immune differences were not due to nutrition. The results again suggest that stress management can enhance both humoral and cellular immunity and perhaps resistance to disease.

The data from these two studies represent the first controlled, empirical evidence that is consistent with anecdotal information and theoretical formulations suggesting that positive emotions, imagery, and similar techniques may enhance health by influencing the effects of the neuroendocrine systems on immune functioning (see, e.g., Cousins, 1976). This is certainly an exciting and intriguing possibility. Such interventions could serve as important complements to other types of preventative and clinical interventions. However, our understanding of the phenomenon and our development of effective stress management interventions to enhance disease resistance have a long way to go. As apparent in the research by Rodin, Kiecolt-Glaser, and their colleagues, we are far from any "magic antistress, disease-resistance bullet." Stress, coping, immune functioning, and resistance to disease are complexly determined. Stress is only one of many variables influencing host resistance. Stress management procedures have not had consistent, uniform effects. For example, relaxation but not social support was effective in Kiecolt-Glaser's work. Interventions modulated some aspects of immune functioning while leaving others unaffected. Further, it is not clear that the immune enhancement effected by these interventions is clinically significant and lasting (Kiecolt-Glaser's research) or, when the results are clinically significant, whether the effect is mediated by alterations in immune functioning (Rodin's research).

These data are congruent with the notion of persons as multilevel systems. What occurs at one level affects and is affected by what occurs at other levels. Even in the prevention and treatment of infectious diseases, the control, support, and reassurance provided by a warm, colleagial relationship as well as by more formal psychosocial and medical interventions are powerful sources of healing.

BEHAVIORAL, PSYCHOSOCIAL, AND ENVIRONMENTAL INTERVENTIONS IN INFECTIOUS DISEASES: A SUMMARY

The prevention and treatment of infectious diseases is not solely a straightforward public health and medical endeavor. Interventions using behavioral principles to alter individuals' behavior and to promote host resistance to infectious agents are important targets of health promotion. The examples used in this chapter by no means exhaust the potential applications and strategies. A number of other infectious and other immune-related diseases, including genital herpes, arthritis, asthma, and allergies, have been addressed in behavioral medicine research. A number of other issues, including promotion of the timely use of medical treatment, compliance with therapeutic regimens, and coping and recovery from infectious and other immune-related diseases, have been targets of behavioral interventions.

Perhaps most exciting is the potential extention of research on psychoneuroimmunology to the prevention and treatment of infectious, autoimmune, and allergic diseases. Realization of this potential will require much additional research. We cannot "sell" stress management and similar types of interventions before they are proven to be effective. These interventions will never be a cure-all for infectious, autoimmune, and allergic diseases. Less "sexy" but probably more immediately productive targets of behavioral and psychosocial interventions focus on altering individual behavior and the environment to prevent the occurrence of infectious diseases, as in the applications in promoting immunizations and controlling the spread of AIDS. Further applications of behavioral principles to health-related behavior and psychoneuroimmunology in the prevention and treatment of disease are considered in the next chapter.

REFERENCES

Albee, G. (1983). The argument for primary prevention. In H. A. Marlowe & R. B. Weinberg (Eds.), *Primary prevention: Fact or fallacy?* 137–149. Tampa: Florida Mental Health Institute.

Aronoff, G. M., & Evans, W. O. (1985). Pharmacological treatment of chronic pain. In G.M. Aronoff (Ed.), *Evaluation and treatment of chronic pain*, 93–114. Baltimore: Urban & Schwarzenberg.

Aronoff, G. M., Wagner, J. M., & Spangler, A. S. (1986). Chemical interventions for pain. *Journal of Consulting and Clinical Psychology, 54*, 769–775.

Beck, A. T., Ward, C. H., Mendelson, M., Mock, J., & Erbaugh, J. (1961). An inventory for measuring depression. *Archives of General Psychiatry, 4*, 561–571.

Bradley, L. A., Prokop, C. K., Gentry, W. D., VanDer Heide, L. H., & Prieto, E. J. (1981). Assessment of chronic pain. In C. K. Prokop & L. A. Bradley (Eds.), *Medical psychology: Contributions to behavioral medicine*, 92–117. New York: Academic Press.

Brena, S. F. (1983). Drugs and pain: Use and misuse. In S. F. Brena & S. L. Chapman (Eds.), *Management of patients with chronic pain*, 66–73. New York: Spectrum.

Center for Disease Control. (1983). Current trends. *Center for Disease Control Morbidity and Mortality Weekly Report, 32*, 770–773.

Christophersen, E. R. (1977). Children's behavior during automobile rides: Do car seats make a difference? *Pediatrics, 60*, 69–74.

Christophersen, E. R. (1984). Preventing injuries to children: A behavioral approach to child passenger safety. In J.D. Matarazzo, S. M. Weiss, J. A. Herd, N. E. Miller, & S. M. Weiss (Eds.), *Behavioral health: A handbook of health enhancement and disease prevention*, 673–685. New York: John Wiley & Sons.

Christophersen, E. R., & Gyulay, J. E. (1981). Parental compliance with car seat usage: A positive approach with long-term follow-up. *Journal of Pediatric Psychology, 6*, 301–312.

Christophersen, E. R., & Sullivan, M. A. (1982). Increasing the protection of newborn infants in cars. *Pediatrics, 70*, 21–25.

Cinciripini, P. M., & Floreen, A. (1982). An evaluation of a behavioral program for chronic pain. *Journal of Behavioral Medicine, 5*, 375–389.

Cousins, N. (1976). Anatomy of an illness (as perceived by the patient). *New England Journal of Medicine, 295*, 1458–1467.

Fordyce, W. E. (1976). *Behavioral methods for chronic pain and illness*. St. Louis: C. V. Mosby.

Fordyce, W. E., Fowler, R. S., Lehmann, J. R., Delateur, B. J., Sand, P.L., & Treishman, R.B. (1973). Operant conditioning in the treatment of chronic pain. *Archives of Physical Medicine and Rehabilitation, 54*, 399–408.

Fordyce, W. E., & Steger, J. C. ((1979). Chronic pain. In O. F. Pomerleau & J. P. Brady (Eds.), *Behavioral medicine: Theory and practice*, 125–154. Baltimore: Williams & Wilkins.

Fox, E. J., & Melzack, R. (1976). Transcutaneous electrical stimulation and acupuncture: Comparison of treatment of low back pain. *Pain, 2*, 141–148.

Gottlieb, H., Leban, C. S., Koller, R., Madorsky, A., Hackersmith, V., Kleeman, M., & Wagner, J. (1977). Comprehensive rehabilitation of patients having chronic low back pain. *Archives of Physical Medicine and Rehabilitation, 58*, 101–108.

Jeans, M. E. (1979). Relief of chronic pain by brief, intense transcutaneous electrical stimulation: A double blind study. In J. J. Bonica & D. Albe-Fessard (Eds.), *Advances in pain research and therapy*. (Vol. 3), 155–173. New York: Raven Press.

Kanton, W. (1984). Depression: Relationship to somatization and chronic medical illness. *Journal of Clinical Psychiatry, 45*, 4–11.

Kantor, T. G. (1984). Peripherally acting analgesics. In M. J. Kuhar & G. W. Pasternack (Eds.), *Analgesics: Neurochemical, behavioral and clinical perspectives*, 244–263. New York: Raven Press.

Karol, R. L., Doerfler, L. A., Parker, J. C., & Armetrout, D. P. (1981). A therapist manual for cognitive-behavioral treatment of chronic pain. *JSAS Catalog of Selected Documents in Psychology, 11*, 15–16 (Ms No. 2205).

Keefe, F. J. (1982). Behavioral assessment and treatment of chronic pain: Current status and future direction. *Journal of Consulting and Clinical Psychology, 50*, 896–911.

Keefe, F. J., & Block, A. R. (1982). Development of an observation method for assessing pain behavior in lower back pain patients. *Behavior Therapy, 13*, 363–375.

Keefe, F. J., Gil, K. M., & Rose, S. C. (1986). Behavioral approaches in multidisciplinary management of chronic pain: Programs and issues. *Clinical Psychology Review, 6*, 87–113.

Kiecolt-Glaser, J. K., Glaser, R., Strain, E. C., Stout, J. C., Tarr, K. L., Holliday, J. E., & Speicher, C. E. (1986). Modulation of cellular immunity in medical students. *Journal of Behavioral Medicine, 9*, 5–21.

Kiecolt-Glaser, J. K., Glaser, R., Williger, D., Stout, D., Messick, G., Sheppard, S., Ricker, D., Romisher, S. C., Brener, W., Bonnell, G., & Donnerberg, R. (1985). Psychosocial enhancement of immunocompetence in a geriatric population. *Health Psychology, 4*, 25–41.

Kremmer, E., Block, A., & Gaylor, M. (1981). Behavioral approaches to chronic pain: The inaccuracy of patient self report measures. *Archives of Physical Medicine and Rehabilitation, 62*, 188–191.

LaForce, F. M. (1987). Immunizations, immunoprophylaxis, and chemoprophylaxis to prevent selected infections. *Journal of the American Medical Association, 257*, 2464–2470.

Langer, E., & Rodin, J. (1976). The effects of choice and enhanced personal responsibility for the aged: A field experiment in an institutional setting. *Journal of Personality and Social Psychology, 34*, 191–198.

LeFebvre, M. F. (1981). Cognitive distortion and cognitive errors in depressed psychiatric and low-back pain. *Journal of Consulting and Clinical Psychology, 49*, 517–525.

Lewis, H. E. (1987). Acquired immunodeficiency syndrome: State legislative activity. *Journal of the American Medical Association, 258*, 2410–2414.

Lindsay, P. G., & Olsen, R. B. (1985). Malprotiline in pain-depression. *Journal of Clinical Psychiatry, 46*, 226–228.

McNairly, S. L., Maruta, T., Ivnik, R. J., Swanson, D., & Ilstrup, D. (1984). Prescription medication dependence and neuropsychologic function. *Pain, 18*, 169–177.

Melzack, R. (1975). The McGill Pain Questionnaire: Major properties and scoring methods. *Pain, 1*, 277–299.

Melzack, R., & Wall, P. D. (1983). *The challenge of pain.* New York: Basic Books.

Peterman, T. A., & Curran, J. W. (1986). Sexual transmission of human immunodeficiency virus. *Journal of the American Medical Association, 256*, 2222–2225.

Reisenger, K. S., & Bires, J. A. (1980). Anticipatory guidance in pediatric practice. *Pediatrics, 66*, 889–892.

Richards, J. S., Nepomuceno, C., Riles, M., & Suer, Z. (1982). Assessing pain behavior: The UAB pain behavior scale. *Pain, 14*, 363–375.

Rodin, J. (1979). Managing the stress of aging: The role of control and coping. In S. Levine & H. Ursin (Eds.), *Coping and health*, 171–202. New York: Plenum Press.

Rodin, J., & Langer, E. (1977). Long-term effects of a control-relevant intervention. *Journal of Personality and Social Psychology, 35*, 897–905.

Rosenstiel, A. K., & Keefe, F. J. (1983). The use of coping strategies in chronic back pain patients: Relationship to patient characteristics and current adjustment. *Pain, 17*, 33–44.

Runyan, C. W., DeVillis, R. F., DeVillis, B. M., & Hockbaum, G.M. (1982). Health psychology and the public health perspective: In search of the pump handle. *Health Psychology, 1*, 169–180.

Scherz, R. G. (1982). Auto safety: The First Ride . . . A Safe Ride campaign. In A. B. Bergman (Ed.), *Preventing childhood injuries: Report of the 12th Ross Round Table on Critical Approaches to Common Pediatric Problems*, 57–63. Columbus, OH: Ross Laboratories.

Snow, J. (1855). *The mode of communication of cholera.* London: Churchill.

Spense, A. P., & Mason, E. B. (1987). *Human anatomy and physiology* (3rd ed.). Menlo Park, CA: Benjamin/Cummings.

Sternbach, R. A. (1973). Psychological aspects of pain and the selection of clients. *Clinical Neurosurgery, 21*, 323–333.
Taylor, P., Hallet, M., & Flaherty, L. (1981). Treatment of osteoarthritis of the knee with transcutaneous electrical nerve stimulation. *Pain, 11*, 233–240.
Turk, D. C., & Genest, M. (1979). Regulation of pain. The application of cognitive and behavioral techniques for prevention and remediation. In P. Kendall & S. Hollon (Eds.), *Cognitive-behavioral interventions: Theory, research and practice*, 287–318. New York: Academic Press.
Turk, D. C., Meichenbaum, D., & Genest, M. (1981). *Pain and behavioral medicine: A cognitive-behavioral perspective*. New York: Guilford.
Turk, D. C., & Rudy, T. E. (1986). Assessment of cognitive factors in chronic pain: A worthwhile enterprise? *Journal of Consulting and Clinical Psychology, 54*, 760–768.
Tursky, B. (1976). Development of a Pain Perception Profile. In M. Weisenberg & B. Tursky (Eds.), *Pain: New perspectives in therapy and research*, 81–99. New York: Plenum Press.
Tursky, B., Jamner, L., & Friedman, R. (1982). The pain perception profile: A psychophysiological approach to the assessment of pain report. *Behavior Therapy, 13*, 376–394.
U.S. Department of Health and Human Services, U.S. Public Health Service. (1986a). *Facts about AIDS*. Washington, DC: U. S. Government Printing Office.
U.S. Department of Health and Human Services, U.S. Public Health Service. (1986b). *Surgeon General's report on Acquired Immune Deficiency Syndrome*. Washington, DC: U.S. Government Printing Office.
Wall, P. D., & Sweet, W. H. (1967). Temporary abolition of pain. *Science, 155*, 108–109.
Ward, N. G., Bloom, V. L., Dworkin, S., Fawcett, J., Narasimhachari, N., & Friedel, R. (1982). Psychobiological markers in coexisting pain and depression. *Journal of Clinical Psychiatry, 43*, 32–38.
Yokley, J. M., & Glenwick, D. S. (1984). Increasing the immunization of preschool children: An evaluation of community interventions. *Journal of Applied Behavior Analysis, 17*, 313–325.
Ziesat, H. A. (1981). Behavioral approaches to the treatment of chronic pain. In C. K. Prokop & L. A. Bradley (Eds.), *Medical psychology: Contributions to behavioral medicine*, 292–307. New York: Academic Press.
Zuckerman, M., & Lubin, B. (1965). *Manual for the Multiple Affect Adjective Checklist*. San Diego: Educational and Industrial Testing Service.

17

Behavioral Health and Medicine: Current Status and Future Directions

INTRODUCTION

The application of behavioral sciences to health and medicine has grown dramatically in the past fifteen years. This book has introduced you to some of these developments. It has described the theories, research, and applications of biomedical and behavioral sciences to health promotion and maintenance, to the understanding of the etiology and course of disease, and to the prevention and treatment of illness. Behavioral health and medicine will continue to grow and mature in the coming decades, providing the opportunity to better understand the relationship of behavior and biology and to effectively promote individuals' health.

In this chapter, the major perspectives and themes characterizing the interdisciplinary field of behavioral health and medicine will be reiterated. The current status of research and application will be summarized and critically evaluated. Finally, future developments and challenges to the field will be described.

CONCEPTUAL ISSUES IN BEHAVIORAL HEALTH AND MEDICINE

Paradigms Revisited: How to See the Forest for the Trees

Behavioral health and medicine utilize theories, research, and principles from a number of disciplines and professions and apply that information to a wide variety of problems in a number of settings. It involves a mixture of psychology, sociology, physiology, genetics, pharmacology, and other fields of study. It requires some working knowledge of topics ranging from neuroanatomy, neurophysiology, and neurochemistry to cognitive processing, emotional expression, and social ecology. It focuses on such diverse topics as alcohol and tobacco use, exercise, client-clinician communication, stress and immunization, and on such diverse health problems as heart disease, cancer, infections, and pain. It deals with individuals and groups of varying characteristics in diverse settings. Such a broad range of goals, targets, methods, settings, and principles is very challenging and sometimes confusing.

How can we gain some perspective? How can we see the forest for the trees? The discussion of paradigms in the first chapter and the continuing references to those paradigms throughout the book were efforts to provide such a perspective. The development and use of such a perspective are critical to an understanding of behavioral health and medicine and to the growth and maturity of the field. The systems perspective asserts that the multiple levels of analysis, from the molecular to the ecological, used by biomedical and behavioral scientists and practitioners are not incompatible. One level of analysis is not more valid or useful than the others. In fact, all of these seemingly disparate pieces are connected and interactive. The nexus of biology and behavior is the focal point in behavioral health and medicine. Basic research in this field entails delineating the reciprocal relationships between biology and behavior. Applied research and service entail manipulating either biology or behavior to change the other.

The systems perspective also asserts that persons are sensitive, active organisms. They plan, learn, act, and adapt to maintain biobehavioral homeostasis. Preventative and clinical interventions to alter health-behavior relationships are most effective when the sensitive, active characteristics are recognized and utilized rather than ignored. The compensatory model of helping describes such an approach to intervention. In the compensatory model, the client-health provider relationship is characterized by collaboration and shared decision making. Both parties are responsible for finding solutions to problems. These paradigms provide guidelines concerning the methods, data, and solutions that are relevant to problems addressed by behavioral health and medicine.

BIOBEHAVIORAL RELATIONSHIPS: VARIATIONS ON THREE THEMES

The relationship between behavior and biology was heuristically organized around three themes: health-impairing and health-promoting habits, illness-related decisions and actions, and the psychophysiological effects of stress. Health-impairing and health-promoting habits have a direct impact on health by introducing substances into the body or by using the body in a manner that alters biological functioning. Smoking, alcohol consumption, exercise, seat belt use, sexual activity, and immunization are some examples of these behaviors. In conjunction with a number of biological, environmental, and genetic factors, these behaviors determine our risk for disease. Illness-related decisions and actions also have a direct effect on biological functioning. They refer to the recognition and interpretation of physical symptoms, to actions in response to those symptoms (e.g., self-care and medical treatment), to communication and interaction with health providers, and to adherence to treatment recommendations. Engaging in these behaviors in a timely and appropriate fashion importantly affects recovery from disease.

Stress refers to the indirect, psychophysiological effects of thinking, emotions, and behavior on biological functioning. Via the nervous, endocrine, and immune systems, our appraisal of the environment, our ability to adapt to challenges, and our style of effecting goal-directed behavior can profoundly influence host resistance and susceptibility to disease. Disease and its diagnosis and treatment also present challenges to which we must adapt. Our ability to cope with such challenges strongly affects our recovery and adjustment.

The role of these three biobehavioral mechanisms in the etiology and course of four prevalent and serious classes of disorders were considered: heart disease, cancer, infectious diseases, and pain. In each case, psychosocial and behavioral processes directly contribute to the development, expression, and course of the disorder. Biobehavioral mechanisms play similarly important roles in a host of other health problems not detailed in this book, such as high blood pressure, stroke, diabetes, ulcers, asthma, and arthritis.

Preventative and Clinical Applications

Although the relationship of health and disease to behavior is an intriguing theoretical and research problem, knowledge concerning this relationship also has important practical applications. Modification of behavior provides a powerful means to promote health and to prevent and treat disease in a manner that complements biomedical interventions. We spent considerable time and effort describing techniques to modify health-related behaviors: operant and respondent conditioning, self-control, modeling and rehearsal, cognitive and self-instructional procedures, and biofeedback and relaxation. We … that these behavior-modification strategies can be used effectively to alter a wide range of overt behaviors and covert psychological and psychophysiological processes revelant to health and disease.

The application of these cognitive-behavioral techniques to health issues has a number of advantageous characteristics. First, the procedures are clearly delineated so that they can be taught to a variety of health professionals and used in a reliable fashion to effect change in target behaviors. Second, the targets of change are overt, objectively specified behaviors so that the efficacy of the interventions can be reliably and validly assessed. Third, cognitive-behavioral procedures promote the flexible approach to intervention required by the diversity of clients, settings, and problems encountered in behavioral health and medicine. Finally, these methods of changing behavior promote client responsibility, initiative, and involvement congruent with self-regulation and the compensatory model of helping.

Cognitive-behavioral intervention focuses on promoting health by modifying psychosocial, environmental, and behavioral variables. It is not necessarily the most important and certainly not the sole modality of intervention. Health promotion and disease prevention and treatment necessitate the use of a number of other types of intervention, including biomedical, community-ecological, and legal-regulatory measures. The challenge is to integrate these various modalities in a manner that is both effective and efficient.

CURRENT STATUS AND FUTURE DIRECTIONS IN BEHAVIORAL HEALTH AND MEDICINE

Health Behavior

Health-impairing and health-promoting behavior has become a major focus of health interventions in the past twenty years, partly as a result of the reduced risk of acute, infectious diseases and the increased incidence of chronic diseases like heart disease and cancer. It is now commonly accepted that health behaviors such as tobacco and alcohol consumption, lack of exercise, and unhealthy dietary practices are major risk factors for chronic diseases. However, our understanding of the relationship between health behaviors and disease risk is incomplete. The strength of the behavior-disease relationship is not always clear, and the interaction of behavioral (e.g., high fat diet) with other risk factors (e.g., genetic contributions of blood cholesterol levels) has not been clearly specified. This makes it difficult to know which of multiple behaviors to target and how to combine biomedical and behavioral interventions to reduce the risk for disease (Kaplan, 1984).

Our understanding of the determinants of health habits is also far from complete. It appears that a complex array of physiological, psychosocial, developmental, and environmental variables influence health behaviors. To further complicate matters, the role of these variables appears to vary according to the individual and the health habit being considered. Basic research is required to identify these multiple determinants in order to know which combination of variables needs to be manipulated to alter health behaviors.

A number of cognitive-behavioral strategies have been used to modify health habits with varying degrees of success. We are just approaching the point of being able to effect clinically significant change in some of these habits. The development of more effective health habit interventions requires progress in several directions. First, we must develop programs that prevent the development of destructive habits and promote the development of healthy ones. This will require "user friendly," developmentally appropriate, widely applicable educational and motivational programs for use in school and home settings. Second, interventions to alter already established health habits must be further modified so that change is maintained and so that the programs can be effectively delivered in the media or in community settings such as the work place and the school. Third, these interventions must be economically efficient as well as clinically effective. Fourth, we must seek ways to integrate biomedical and behavioral strategies to alter health habits. The combination of several intervention modalities may be more effective than any one alone.

The modification of health habits is an area that offers a genuine opportunity for growth and for a significant contribution to health care. The cost of health care has been escalating rapidly over the last twenty-five years. In 1960, Americans spent 5.3% of the gross national product on health care. Currently, this figure is approaching 11%, or over 400 billion dollars annually (Easterbrook, 1987, Jan. 26; U.S. Bureau of the Census, 1985). Most of this expenditure is on clinical, after-the-fact medicine. This increase in health care expenditures cannot be sustained, and thus there is increasing pressure to prevent disease. The importance of primary prevention is also evident in the health objectives for 1990 offered by the Department of Health and Human Services (Harris, 1980; see also Table 17-1).

The Management of Stress

Research on stress and its management has progressed substantially since Selye's (1956) seminal work thirty years ago. In particular, we have a relatively good understanding of the cognitive, personal, and situational variables related to stress. Recent research has also identified the importance of social support as a modulator of stress. In contrast, we lack substantive knowledge about how persons cope with stress in the natural environment and the characteristics of effective coping

TABLE 17-1 Health Objectives for America in 1990

Health prevention
Control of high blood pressure
Improved family planning
Enhancement of maternal and infant health
Promotion of immunization
Reduction in sexually transmitted diseases
Health protection
Control of toxic agents
Enhanced occupational safety
Prevention of accidents
Enhanced dental health
Improved surveillance and control of infectious disease
Health promotion
Reduction in tobacco use
Reduction in the misuse and abuse of alcohol
Enhanced nutrition
Enhanced physical fitness and exercise
Reduction in stress
Reduction in violent behavior

strategies. A better understanding of coping processes is required to teach effective stress management strategies to individuals. The relationship between the impact of stress and its temporal parameters (duration and timing) is also not clearly understood. Are acute and chronic stress equally debilitating? Is stress more problematic at some periods during one's life than others? Prospective, longitudinal studies are required to answer these questions and to delineate the role of stress in the etiology of disease.

Our understanding of the psychophysiological mechanisms by which stress affects our health has grown substantially. However, the neural, endocrine, and immune mechanisms by which stress influences biological functioning are complex. Physiologists and immunologists are only beginning to untangle how each of these systems works and how they are reciprocally related. Research on brain neurochemistry, neuroendocrinology, and psychoneuroimmunology has strong implications for biobehavioral interventions. The physiological correlates of stress are highly variable, depending on a number of psychosocial parameters (e.g., the timing and duration of stress and the availability of control and coping responses) as well as biological factors (e.g., genetics, age, and gender). Understanding the relationships among these multiple variables will challenge us for decades to come.

Stress management has become a "hot" topic as individuals are seeking ways to improve their health. Many legitimate and effective programs are available (e.g., Meichenbaum, 1985), but there are also many "quack" programs purporting to be effective without sufficient evidence to support those claims. Individuals and corporations are spending money on these sometimes exotic and bizarre stress management programs. The lack of results may sour the public's acceptance and utilization of legitimate programs. The baby may be thrown out with the bath water.

In the future, stress management methods may be more frequently applied to prevent physical and psychological problems in at-risk groups (e.g., the elderly, children, and workers in high-stress occupations). Stress management may also be increasingly used as one facet of health promotion and disease prevention in the work place. The health effectiveness and cost benefits of such programs must be documented in terms of reduced absenteeism, reduced health care utilization, and increased productivity. The programs must be flexible enough to address a wide clientele, but specific enough to address differences in the developmental level and setting characteristics of the groups being targeted. The long-term maintenance and effectiveness of these programs must also be documented.

The application of stress management procedures to specific diseases is in some cases more advanced. Targets of these programs include coping with serious diagnostic communications, preparing for aversive diagnostic and treatment procedures, coping with the side effects of medication, and managing the multiple challenges posed by chronic illness. For example, stress management programs have been applied to individuals with cancer, heart disease, diabetes, and epilepsy. These interventions are often quite cost effective, reducing hospitalization time and demands on staff and preventing the recurrence of serious clinical episodes. However, many of these programs target only one or a few of the sources of stress associated with disease. Expansion of these programs to provide a broader range of coordinated services is needed to address the multiple challenges faced by individuals with acute and chronic diseases, injuries, and disabilities. These services should address problems experienced by these clients from the time of the onset of the condition through treatment and rehabilitation. Pain centers and hospices may serve as models for these programs.

Another recent trend is the use of professionally led and lay self-help groups to foster individuals' ability to cope with disease or disability (Tyler, 1980). The utility of the social, emotional, and informational resources available from such groups has not been clearly established. In some cases, the effects may be destructive rather than constructive. The careful development, implementation, and evaluation of these programs are needed before their efficacy can be assessed.

Utilization of Health Care Services

Biomedical and behavioral interventions are effective only if used in a timely and appropriate fashion. Many persons who are not ill seek services, and many who are seriously ill delay seeking treatment or fail to access the health care system at all. We are only just beginning to understand how persons recognize and interpret their symptoms and how they respond to remediate those symptoms. Without more knowledge about these processes, our educational efforts to encourage accurate symptom perception (including the surveillance of asymptomatic problems like high blood pressure) and to promote effective responses to symptoms (self-care, or professional care) are at best going to be modestly effective. Programs promoting accurate recognition and appropriate action could be very cost effective. They would reduce unneeded utilization of services and the increased costs due to delay in seeking treatment for serious problems.

Another set of issues arises once individuals access the health care system. Effective client-health provider communication is a prerequisite to good health care. It facilitates accurate diagnosis, reduces the stress associated with diagnosis, medical procedures, and hospitalization, and promotes adherence. This "art" of medicine can be taught. Health professionals can learn to communicate in an effective, caring manner. It may also be useful to teach clients how to communicate more effectively with clinicians. This emphasis on communication is congruent with the increasing consumerism shown by clients, and may be important in dealing with the rapid escalation in malpractice litigation. In 1973, an annual average of three claims was made for every one hundred physicians. In 1983, this figure rose to twenty claims per one hundred physicians. Malpractice premiums tripled from 1981 to 1985 (Easterbrook, 1987, Jan. 26). Solutions to the malpractice problem will probably require legal and statutory remedies, but it may also be addressed by the development of a collaborative, realistic, mutually informed client-health provider relationship.

The final issue in health care utilization is adherence. Adherence is a problem in cognitive-behavioral as well as biomedical interventions. Some progress has been made in understanding the determinants of adherence, and some modestly effective interventions have been made to promote better adherence. But this problem is by no means solved.

SUMMARY

The field of behavioral health and medicine has grown dramatically during the past two decades. It has already made substantial contributions to health care. But it is still in its early stages of development. To continue to develop and to realize its potential, biomedical and behavioral scientists must continue basic research on the relationships between biology and behavior. This study of the dynamic interplay between the mind and body is one important foundation on which effective interventions to promote health and to fight disease are built. An equal effort is required to develop and implement effective educational and clinical programs. These programs must be rigorously evaluated in terms of their impact on health and their cost effectiveness.

The continuing growth and success of behavioral health and medicine require a close working relationship between biomedical and behavioral scientists and practitioners. Behavioral scientists and clinicians are the new kids on the health care block. They have to demonstrate convincingly a working knowledge of biomedical sciences and procedures. They must provide evidence that behavioral interventions are effective and compatible with biomedical procedures. The true potential of behavioral health and medicine will only be realized by interdisciplinary understanding, training, and collaboration.

REFERENCES

Easterbrook, G. (1987, January 26). The revolution in medicine. *Newsweek,* pp. 40–74.

Harris, R. P. (1980). *Promoting health—Preventing disease: Objectives for the nation.* Washington, DC, U.S. Government Printing Office.

Kaplan, R. M. (1984). The connection between clinical health promotion and health status. *American Psychologist, 39,* 755–765.

Meichenbaum, D. H. (1985). *Stress management training.* New York: Plenum Press.

Seyle, H. (1956). *The stress of life.* New York: McGraw-Hill.

Tyler, L. (1980). The next 20 years. *Counseling Psychology, 8,* 19–21.

U.S. Bureau of the Census. (1985). *Statistical abstracts of the United States: 1984.* Washington, DC: U.S. Government Printing Office.

Name Index

Abraham, S., 35
Adler, N., 147, 149, 150
Akil, H., 196
Albee, G., 278
Alexander, P., 172
Allen, R., 80
Anand, B., 258
Andersen, R., 52, 53
Antonovsky, A., 105
Apley, J., 202, 208
Argyle, M., 311
Arnoff, G., 361
Asterita, M., 79, 85, 86, 87
Audy, J., 105
Ax, A., 87

Bacon, C., 184
Baldanado, A., 162, 163
Bandura, A., 30, 101, 231, 234, 310
Barofsky, I., 345, 346
Basmajian, J., 271, 274
Beck, A., 108, 250, 369
Becker, M., 53, 60
Beecher, H., 191, 192, 198, 199
Bell, C., 342
Benson, H., 277
Berkman, L., 77, 121
Bernstein, D., 275, 277
Bibace, R., 28
Birk, L., 259
Blackburn, H., 331
Blair, L., 6
Blanchard, E., 270, 271
Blumenthal, J., 128
Bolstad, O., 244
Bootzin, R., 243
Borkovec, T., 275, 277
Bovjberg, D., 147
Boyd, W., 161
Bradley, L., 368, 369
Brandt-Rauf, P., 99
Brenna, S., 362
Bresler, D., 188
Brickman, P., 3, 19, 20, 21
Bridbord, K., 168
Bringham, T., 29

Brownell, K., 35, 37, 41, 247, 289, 291, 293, 296
Burish, T., 179, 323, 351, 352
Burnham, M., 122
Butensky, A., 127

Cannon, T., 196
Cannon, W., 66, 101
Caplan, R., 60
Carey, M., 351, 352
Carey, R., 183
Carmody, T., 339
Carver, C., 101, 103, 105, 336
Casey, K., 190, 194, 195
Cassem, N., 131, 132, 133, 134
Chesney, N., 125, 127, 336
Chrisman, N., 52, 53
Christophersen, E., 377, 378
Cipriani, P., 375
Clark, M., 188
Clark, R., 162
Clymer, R., 54
Coates, T., 295, 329, 332
Cobb, S., 77
Cohen, F., 72, 77, 78, 80, 90
Cohen, J., 128
Cornfield, D., 148
Costa, P., 51
Cousins, N., 92, 386
Craig, K., 197, 202
Craun, A., 344
Cromwell, R., 133, 338
Croog, S., 135

Davidson, G., 30, 277, 279
Davidson, P., 200
Davis, M., 58, 312
De Long, R., 200, 308
De Longis, A., 69
Dembroski, T., 67
Depue, R., 90
Derogatis, A., 184, 350, 354
Di Matteo, M., 56
Di Nicola, D., 56, 58
Dingle, J., 11
Dishman, R., 41, 42, 292
Doehrman, S., 133
Dohrenwend, B., 68, 120
Doll, R., 168, 169
Douglas, R., 156
Dunbar, J., 60, 300, 301
Dunkel-Schetter, C., 183
D'Zurilla, T., 250

Easterbrook, G., 398
Edwards, J., 184
Eisenberg, J., 163, 164
Eisenthal, S., 299
Eisler, R., 311
Engel, G., 2, 3, 12, 13, 120
Epstein, L., 339
Evans, A., 151
Evans, R., 288
Everly, G., 312, 313

Fabrega, H., 15
Farquhar, J., 19, 233, 289, 296, 330
Feldman, J., 11
Ferarre, N., 73
Folkman, S., 68, 69, 71, 72, 74, 308
Fordyce, W., 53, 190, 203, 206, 207, 208, 209, 368, 371, 372
Fowler, J., 323
Fox, B., 162, 163, 168, 170, 171, 173, 176, 178, 181, 182, 184
Fox, E., 363
Frankenhauser, M., 89
Frankl, V., 72
Franks, C., 286
Freeman, L., 259
Friedman, H., 56
Friedman, N., 122, 123, 125, 128, 129, 334, 335

Garrity, T., 133
Gatchel, R., 262, 271
Genest, M., 91, 316, 365, 369, 372
Gentry, W., 131, 132, 133
Glaser, R., 152
Glasgow, R., 286, 288
Glass, D., 122, 123, 129
Goldfried, M., 22, 250, 309
Goode, E., 29
Gorczynski, R., 148
Gordon, W., 345, 347, 348
Gottlieb, H., 365, 368, 375
Greenfield, N., 152
Grinker, R., 68
Gross, A., 323
Gruen, W., 338
Guyton, A., 101

Hackett, T., 131, 132, 133, 134
Hagen, R., 35

Haley, J., 30
Hall, D., 344
Hallsten, A., 230
Hann, N., 13, 21, 77
Hardy, A., 155, 156
Harris, J., 351
Harris, R., 395
Hartmann, D., 308
Haskell, W., 41
Hassett, J., 262
Hayes, S., 313
Haynes, R., 57, 60, 299, 300, 302
Haynes, S., 137
Head, J., 339
Heberman, B., 172
Heinrich, R., 348, 349
Henderson, B., 164
Higgins, I., 341
Hiller, K., 311
Hirschi, J., 35
Hitt, C., 39
Hodgson, R., 35, 36
Holmes, T., 68
Holroyd, K., 68, 87
Hughes, G., 287, 289
Hunter, E., 73

Irwin, J., 145, 146, 149, 150

Jacobs, C., 348
Jacobs, S., 72
Janis, I., 30, 36, 53, 76
Jarvik, M., 43
Jay, S., 352, 353
Jeans, M., 363
Jemmot, J., 68, 99, 145, 149, 150, 171
Jenkins, C., 120, 121, 122, 125, 128
Johnson, J., 13
Jordan, M., 27
Joseph, J., 158

Kalish, H., 228
Kamiya, J., 260
Kanfer, F., 198, 237, 239, 244, 308
Kannel, W., 116, 118
Kanner, A., 51
Kanton, W., 365
Kantor, T., 361, 362
Kaplan, R., 394
Karol, T., 374
Karusa, J., 22
Kasl, S., 151, 331
Kazdin, A., 215, 216, 218, 230, 238, 279
Keefe, F., 364, 365, 368, 370, 372, 374, 376
Keesey, R., 35
Kendall, P., 318, 319, 337
Keys, A., 119
Kiecolt-Glaser, J., 152, 380
Kirscht, J., 53, 58, 59, 60
Klein, R., 133
Klopfer, B., 199
Knowles, J., 10
Koenig, P., 188
Koplan, J., 118
Koshland, D., 143
Kozlowski, L., 285
Krantz, D., 25
Kremmer, E., 368
Kristeller, J., 30, 56
Kubler-Ross, E., 13
Kuhn, T., 2

Lacey, B., 87
Lachman, S., 229
La Force, E., 380
Lando, H., 287
Lang, P., 258
Lange, A., 311
Langer, E., 30, 73, 318, 384
Lau, R., 50, 52
Lazarus, R., 68, 69, 70, 71, 72, 74, 90, 178, 184, 308
Le Bow, M., 35, 36, 37
Le Febvre, M., 369
Leopold, R., 181
Leventhal, H., 42, 50, 51, 54, 58, 61, 71, 87, 101, 179, 201, 246, 283, 286, 289, 299, 300, 331
Levine, J., 196
Levine, S., 70
Levy, S., 174, 176, 177
Lewinsohn, P., 108
Lewis, H., 383
Ley, P., 7, 56, 58, 61, 299
Lichtenstein, E., 283, 284, 286, 288
Lichtman, R., 183
Lilienfield, A., 340, 341, 343
Lindeman, E., 68, 319
Lindsay, P., 362
Lindsley, D., 258
Lipsitt, L., 320
Lloyd, R., 145, 146
Locke, S., 68, 99, 141, 143, 145, 149, 150, 171
Lyles, J., 351

Maccoby, N., 233, 289, 330
Mages, N., 180, 181
Mahoney, M., 30, 237, 238, 244, 249
Marin, S., 158
Marlat, G., 29, 247
Martin, S., 156, 158
Mason, E., 142, 143, 144
Mason, J., 67, 87, 380
Masters, J., 318
Masur, F., 301
Matarazzo, J., 2, 4, 256, 283, 339
Mathews, K., 127
Mayer, J., 33, 35, 37
McAlister, A., 331
McFall, R., 250
McIntosh, J., 176, 177
McKenna, R., 36
McNairly, S., 362
Mechanic, D., 74
Meichenbaum, D., 76, 90, 91, 199, 250, 251, 307, 316, 365, 396
Melamed, B., 21, 233, 318
Melzack, R., 190, 192, 193, 196, 363, 366, 367
Mermelstein, R., 288
Meyer, A., 330
Meyer, D., 61
Meyerowitz, B., 183, 345
Miller, D., 161, 162, 166, 169
Miller, J., 6
Miller, J.G., 14
Miller, N., 90, 183, 260, 263, 271
Miller, T., 183
Miller, W., 73
Milsum, J., 105
Minuchin, S., 323
Moos, R., 318, 323
Morrison, T., 171
Morrow, G., 351
Moss, A., 131, 132
Murphy, L., 89
Mushin, J., 200

Nadich, M., 296
Nathan, P., 296
Nelson, R., 308
Nerenz, D., 77, 179, 180, 201
Nessman, D., 339
Newberry, B., 165, 171, 175
Newman, V., 39
Norton, J., 140
Nucholls, C., 69

Obrist, P., 67, 87, 261
Ockene, J., 288
O'Leary, K., 249
Oldridge, N., 292
Olton, D., 261, 271
Osler, W., 122

Parkes, C., 72, 247
Patel, C., 265
Paulley, J., 188
Peck, A., 180
Pennybaker, J., 49, 50, 61, 122, 176
Pepper, E., 271
Peterman, T., 155, 156, 383
Petrie, A., 200
Pinkerton, S., 227, 229
Polivy, J., 34, 36
Pomerleau, O., 214, 287, 296
Poste, G., 162
Powell, D., 287
Pranulis, M., 133
Prehn, R., 172
Premack, D., 215
Pumphrey, J., 182

Rabkin, J., 68
Rachman, D., 11, 13
Ray, O., 196, 289
Redd, W., 179, 351
Reese, E., 218
Reisenger, K., 377
Reiser, D., 15
Ribsal, P., 292
Richards, J., 368
Roark, G., 151
Robbins, L., 32
Rodin, J., 27, 29, 30, 36, 59, 67, 73, 318, 384, 385
Rogers, M., 146, 171
Rogertine, G., 184
Rose, M., 323
Rosenman, R., 122, 123, 125, 127, 128, 129
Rosenstiel, R., 369
Rosenthal, T., 234
Roskies, E., 333
Ross, R., 129
Rozin, P., 39
Rugh, J., 274
Runyan, C., 379

Sackett, D., 11, 58
Safer, M., 52, 53

Sarason, I., 69, 308
Schacter, S., 72, 284
Schag, C., 345, 348, 349
Schwarz, G., 110, 214, 273, 277, 279
Seligman, M., 73
Selye, H., 66, 74, 87, 395
Shapiro, A., 198
Shapiro, D., 103, 116, 260, 261, 277
Sheldon, H., 97, 154, 155
Shellenberger, R., 273
Silverberg, E., 184
Singer, J., 77
Sklar, L., 13, 172, 183
Smith, D., 156
Smith, G., 148
Snow, J., 379
Snyder, J., 52, 132, 225, 323
Snyder, S., 196
Somers, H., 7, 8
Spense, A., 142, 143, 144, 380
Spiegel, D., 347
Starr, C., 144
Stephenson, H., 176
Sternbach, R., 201, 206, 207, 369
Stokes, J., 114, 117, 118, 119
Stone, G., 29
Strauss, L., 344
Straw, M., 290
Stuart, R., 30, 290
Stunkard, A., 34, 35, 290, 295
Suinn, R., 127
Suls, J., 78
Surwitt, R., 116, 120, 130, 261, 323
Symmington, G., 67
Szaz, T., 19, 21, 22

Tanig, M., 68
Taylor, S., 183, 347, 363
Telch, C., 348, 349
Temoshok, L., 176, 184
Thoreson, C., 309, 335
Tjoe, S., 131
Trotta, P., 344
Tsai, S., 114
Turk, D., 57, 91, 182, 199, 202, 203, 316, 320, 323, 353, 365, 369, 370, 372, 373
Turskey, B., 271, 366
Tyler, L., 397

Wadden, T., 293
Walker, K., 5, 7
Wall, P., 192, 193, 196, 198, 363
Ward, N., 362
Warner, K., 289
Weinberg, J., 73
Weiner, H., 109
Weiss, J., 67, 283
Weissenberg, M., 200
Weissman, A., 77, 174, 176, 345
Wernick, R., 319
White, L., 271
White, R., 30
Wilder, R., 151
Williams, R., 97, 122, 127, 128, 131, 135
Wills, T., 21
Wilson, G., 249, 286, 289, 290, 291
Wing, R., 322, 323
Wolf, H., 87, 199
Wolpe, J., 229
Woods, S., 51
Woody, E., 35
Worden, J., 174, 176
Wortman, C., 78, 346, 347
Wrubel, J., 72

Yalom, I., 347
Yokley, J., 380, 381

Zegans, L., 109
Ziesat, H., 374
Zifferblatt, S., 61, 296
Zola, I., 11
Zuckerman, M., 308, 309
Zyzanski, S., 121

Subject Index

Accidents
  behavior and, 31–32
  causes of, 31–32
  deaths and, 31–32
  models of helping and, 20–21
  prevention of, 376–378
  trauma and, 98
Adaptation
  cancer and, 182–184
  stress and, 89–92
Adherence
  client–health provider interaction and, 58–59
  definition of, 57–58
  enhancement of, 297–302
  illness representation and, 61–62
  importance of, 10–11, 58
  natural environment and, 59–60
  physiology and, 60–61
  treatment of heart disease and, 132–135, 338–339
Aging
  cancer and, 169–170
  heart disease and, 119–120
  immune functioning and, 145, 152
  nursing homes and, 318, 384–386
  stress and, 73
  stress management and, 385–386
Alcohol
  cancer and, 167–168
  health consequences of, 9
  legislation and, 29
  prevention of disease and, 10
  misuse, treatment of, 29–30
Animism
  definition of, 5
  history of medicine and, 5–6
Appraisal
  coping and, 76
  pain and, 197–199, 369–370
  personality and, 72–73
  physiological arousal and, 87–88
  situational effects on, 73–74
  stress and, 70–72
  time demands and, 311–313

Arthritis
  immune system and, 145
  incidence of, 188
  pain and, 188
Assessment
  biofeedback and, 265–268
  cancer and, 345–346
  cognitive interventions and, 249–252
  operant interventions and, 218–219
  pain and, 366–370
  self-control programs and, 239–242
  stress management and, 308–309
  type A behavior and, 123–125
Atherosclerosis
  blood pressure and, 118
  diet and, 115–118
  exercise and, 118–119
  heart disease and, 115–117, 329–330
  stress and, 120
  type A behavior and, 127, 333–336
AIDS
  cancer and, 170
  causes of, 107–108, 154–155
  coping with, 157–158
  definition of, 154–155
  prevention of, 381–383
  symptoms of, 155
  transmission of, 155–156, 381–383
  treatment of, 156–157
Aspirin, 361, 363
Autonomic nervous system
  biofeedback and, 260–263
  cardiovascular system and, 114–115
  functions of, 80–82
  heart disease and, 120, 128–129
  immune system and, 145–146
  physiology of, 80–83
  stress and, 66–67, 79–82
  type A behavior and, 129

Biofeedback
  chemotherapy side effects and, 351
  clinical applications of, 263–265
  clinical procedures of, 265–270
  description of, 259–261
  effectiveness of, 270–273
  equipment, 261–263
  mechanisms of, 273–274
  pain treatment and, 374
Biomedical paradigm
  description, 2–3
  evaluation of, 8–14
  health-impairing behavior and, 26–27
  history of, 5–6
  pain and, 189–190
Blood pressure
  biofeedback and, 263–265
  deaths and, 33
  exercise and, 41
  heart disease and, 118, 130, 329
  regulation of, 102–103
  symptom recognition and, 10–11
Breast self-examination, 343–345

Cancer
  AIDS and, 170
  behavior and, 31–32, 164–169
  causes of, 31–32
  chemotherapy and, 178–179
  deaths and, 9, 31–32
  definition of, 162
  diagnosis of, 176–177
  fear of, 161, 180–182
  host resistance and, 169–171
  immune system and, 142–144, 171–173
  incidence of, 162–163
  pain and, 182–183, 352–353
  physiology of, 164–166
  prevention of, 330–334
  psychosocial assessment and, 345–346
  radiation therapy and, 179
  recurrence of, 181–182
  rehabilitation after, 180–181
  self-help groups and, 347–348
  social support and, 183–184
  surgery and, 177–178
  symptom recognition and, 174–175, 343
Carcinogens
  prevention of cancer and, 341–343
  types of, 164–169
Chronic illness
  adherence and, 302
  challenges of, 90–91
  coping and, 320–323
  symptom representation of, 50–51, 313–314
Cognitive therapy
  description of, 236–237, 248–249
  modification of type A behavior and, 333–336
  pain and, 353, 372–376

procedures in, 249–255
self-instruction and, 253–255
stress management and, 313–314, 318–319
Communication of health provider and client
adherence and, 58–59, 299–300
cancer and, 177–182, 345–348
diagnosis and, 54–57
importance of, 6–8
influence in, 54–57
providing information and, 314–316
self control and, 234
stress and, 89–91
Community interventions
AIDS and, 381–383
cancer and, 341
exercise and, 295–296
health enhancement and education and, 255–256
heart disease and, 329–333
infectious diseases and, 379–383
nutrition and, 295–306
smoking and, 289
Compensatory model of helping
description of, 20–21
evaluation of, 21–22
health-impairing behavior and, 30–31
health provider–client communication and, 56–57
Conditioning, classical (respondent)
applications of medical problems and, 229–231
chemotherapy for cancer and, 179
definition of, 227
immune system and, 147–148
pain and, 207–210
physiological responses and, 260–261
principles of, 227–229
Conditioning, operant
applications to medical problems and, 218–225
diabetes and, 225–227
pain and, 201–203, 207–210
pain treatment and, 371–372, 375–376
physiological responses and, 260–261
principles of, 214–219
Control
cancer and, 176–184, 345–348
health provider communication and, 56
host resistance and, 383–387
importance of, 29–30
information and, 314–316
models of helping and, 56–57
pain and, 198
recovery from heart disease and, 132–135
stress and, 67, 73
Coping. *See also* Stress management
aversive medical procedures and, 318–320
cancer and, 174–184, 245–354
cardiac catheterization and, 337
definition of, 75
determinants of, 78
heart disease and, 132–135
infectious diseases and, 157–158
physiological arousal patterns and, 87–88
social support and, 77–78
types of, 75–77
Coping skills training. *See* Stress management

Diabetes
behavior and, 31–32
causes of, 31–32, 107–108
coping and, 320–323
deaths due to, 9, 31–32
exercise and, 41
social support and, 323
treatment of, 225–227
Diagnosis
AIDS and, 155–156
cancer and, 176–177
health provider–client communication and, 54–56
heart disease and, 337
pain and, 190–192
Diet. *See* Nutrition, obesity and
Disease
behavior and, 25
biomedical paradigm and, 3
definition of, 96–97
etiology of, 8–9
prevention of, 10, 395–396
recognition of, 11–12
stress and, 89–91
systems paradigm and, 15–19, 100–105, 107–111
Dualism
definition of, 5–6
psychogenic pain and, 206–207

Emotions
AIDS and, 158
cancer and, 161–162, 176–182, 343
chemotherapy side effects and, 351–352
classical conditioning and, 228–229
coping and, 75–77
disease and, 6–8
heart disease and, 121, 132–134
illness actions and, 51–52
illness threats and, 90–91
pain and, 200–201, 205–210, 364–365, 368–369
relaxation and, 278–279
symptom recognition and, 50–51
tranquilizers and, 110–111
Endocrine system
cancer and, 168–169, 172
functions of, 83–86
immune system and, 84–86, 145–147
physiology of, 83–86
stress and, 66–67, 83–86
type A behavior and, 128–129
Endorphins
chronic pain and, 210
function in pain modulation and, 195–196
Enlightenment model of helping
description of, 19–20
evaluation of, 20–21
health-impairing behavior and, 29–30
Etiology of disease
causes of, 31–32, 107–110
shifts in history, 8–9
stress and, 89–90
Exercise
benefits of, 41
determinants of, 41
enhancement of, 240–245, 292
heart disease and, 118–119, 134–135
obesity and, 41
pain treatment and, 371–374

Flooding, 229
Folk medicine, 52
Food preferences
alteration of, 282–295
cancer and, 167
determinants of, 39–40
heart disease and, 116–118

Gate control theory of pain
description of, 192–195
pain treatment and, 373
General adaptation syndrome, 66–67
Germ theory, 141

Headaches, 265–270
Health
definition of, 96–97
systems paradigm and, 100–107, 110–111
Health care utilization
AIDS and, 157–158
cancer and, 163
cost of, 395
importance of, 10–11, 397–398
pain and, 188
timing of, 297–298
Health-impairing behavior
AIDS and, 155–156, 381–383
biomedical paradigm and, 26–27
cancer and, 164–169, 341–345
causes of death and, 31–32
compensatory model of helping and, 30–31
determinants of, 27–28
enlightenment model of helping and, 29–30
heart disease and, 116–118
importance of, 25–26, 393–395
infectious disease and, 153–154
medical model of helping and, 28–29
modification of, 283–297
moral model of helping and, 29–30
stress and, 91–92
systems paradigm and, 27–28
Heart disease
behavior and, 31–32
blood pressure and, 118
causes of, 31–32, 116–130
cholesterol and, 116–117
deaths due to, 9, 31–32, 113–114
definition of, 115–116
eating and, 31
exercise and, 41
incidence of, 113
physiology of, 114–116
prevention of, 329–336
recognition of, 130–133
recovery from, 132–135
smoking and, 42, 118
social support and, 121–122
stress and, 120–121

systems conceptualization of, 15–18
treatment of, 336–340
type A behavior and, 122–129
Heredity
cancer and, 164, 169–171
heart disease and, 119
role in health and disease, 97–98
types of disease and, 97–98
Homeostasis
disease and, 107–110
health and, 100–107
Host resistance
aging and, 384–386
cancer and, 169–171
definition of, 141
infectious diseases and, 148–150
stress and, 383–386

Illness actions
cancer and, 174–176
determinants of, 52–54
heart disease and, 130–132
types of, 51–52
Immune system
AIDS and, 154–155
cancer and, 142–143, 171–172
chemotherapy and, 179
conditioning of, 147–148
endocrine system and, 84–86, 145–147
infectious diseases and, 99–100, 141–145, 151–152
nervous system and, 145–147
nonspecific, 142
resistance to disease and, 148–151
specific, 142–145
stress and, 84–86, 385–386
Infectious diseases
AIDS and, 155–156
causes of, 99–100
coping with, 157–158
germ theory and, 141
health-impairing behaviors and, 153–154
immune system and, 141–151
prevention of, 378–383
transmission of, 153–154

Legislation
AIDS and, 381, 383
alcohol and, 29–30
carcinogens and, 168–169
health-impairing behavior and, 28–30
immunizations and, 380
safety belts and, 20, 376–377
smoking and, 289, 342

Malingering
medical model of helping and, 4
pain and, 190–192, 209, 371–374
Materialism
definition of, 2–3
history of medicine and, 5–6
Medical model of helping
description of, 3–4, 20
evaluation of, 8–14, 21
health-impairing behavior and, 28–29
health provider–client communication and, 56–57
history of, 6–7
relationship to biomedical paradigm, 4–5
Modeling
applications to medical problems, 233–234
breast self-examination and, 344
definition of, 231
pain and, 202, 208
principles of, 231–233
stress management and, 253–254, 309–310, 318–319
Mononucleosis
definition of, 151
stress and, 151–152
Moral model of helping
description of, 19–20
evaluation of, 19–21
health-impairing behavior and, 29–30

Narcotic analgesics
cancer and, 182, 352
endorphins and, 195–197
pain treatment and, 361–363
Nutrition
basic dietary constituents and, 37–39
cancer and, 167–168, 350
disease and, 38–39
healthy diet and, 39–40
heart disease and, 118, 134–135, 330–332
immune system functioning and, 145, 149
modification of, 292–294
obesity and, 37–39

Obesity
behavior and, 33–34, 37
biology of, 34–35
cancer and, 170
causes of, 33–34
emotions and, 35–36
exercise and, 41
relationship to disease, 31–33
social relationships and, 36–37
treatment of, 240–247, 290–292
Observational learning. *See* Modeling

Pain
acute, 204–205
appraisal and, 197–198
aversive medical procedures and, 318–320
behavioral expression of, 201–203
cancer and, 181–182, 352–353
chronic, 205–206
definition of, 189
endorphins and, 195–197
gate control theory of, 192–195
heart disease and, 115–116
incidence of, 188
measurement of, 366–370
mood and, 200–201
operant and respondent, 207–210
personality and, 200
physiology of, 192–197
placebo and, 198–200
prevention of, 364–366
psychogenic, 206–207
specificity theory of, 190–192
Pain treatment
assessment and, 366–370
biofeedback and, 263–273
cognitive-behavioral programs and, 370–376
definitive, 204–205, 360
drugs and, 361–363
sensory control and, 363–364
symptomatic, 204–205, 360–361
Paradigm
biomedical, 2–3, 5–6
compensatory model of helping, 20–21
disease and, 107–110
enlightenment model of helping, 19–20
evaluation of, 8–14, 21–22
health and, 100–107
medical model of helping and, 3–8
moral model of helping and, 19
nature of, 1–2, 392
systems, 14–17, 100–110, 392
Placebo
biofeedback and, 271–272
definition of, 198
information and, 13
medication and, 339
pain and, 198–200
Poisons
disease and, 99
cancer and, 170
Preparation for medical procedures
burn treatment, 318–320
bone marrow aspiration, 353
cardiac catheterization, 337
cancer chemotherapy, 178–179
dental work, 229–230
endoscopy, 251–255
general principles of, 318–320
information and, 314–316
radiation therapy, 180
surgery, 177–178, 233–234, 319
Prepared childbirth
compensatory model of helping and, 21
pain and, 201
relaxation and, 278
stress and, 91
Prevention of disease
cancer and, 166–169, 340–344
causes of disease and, 31–33
exercise and, 292, 295–296
food preferences and, 292–296
heart disease and, 329–336
infectious diseases and, 378–383
pain and, 364–366, 376–378
rationale for, 110–111, 327–328, 393–394
smoking and, 288–289
targets of, 10, 395–396
weight control and, 290–292, 295–296
Psychoneuroimmunology
definition of, 141
immune system conditioning and, 147–148
immune system and stress and, 148–151
stress and, 150–153, 387–388

Reductionism
definition of, 2–3
history of medicine and, 5–6
Reinforcement

adherence and, 58–60, 301–302
biofeedback and, 259–261
health-impairing behavior and, 27–44
illness actions and, 49–53
immunizations and, 380–381
implementing in clinical practice, 219–224
nutrition and, 293
pain and, 202–203, 207–210
pain treatment and, 371–376
principles of, 214–219
seat-belt use and, 377–378
self, 244–245
smoking modification and, 284–285
Relapse
dieting and, 36, 290–292
prevention of, 247–248
smoking and, 43, 287–288
Relaxation training
chemotherapy side effects and, 351–355
clinical applications of, 278–279, 349
effects of, 277–278
host resistance and, 383–387
meditation, 277
modification of type A behavior and, 333–336
pain treatment and, 374
progressive muscle relaxation, 274–277
self-control and, 245–246

Self-care
cancer and, 181
definition of, 51–52
diabetes and, 225–226
heart disease and, 131
immunizations and, 380–381
Self-control
applications of, 238
description of, 236–238
development of, 237–238
eating and, 240–245, 290–292
exercise and, 240–245, 292
evaluation of clinical applications of, 246–248
food preferences and, 292–295
pain treatment and, 372–374
physiology and, 258–259
procedures in, 238–246
smoking and, 284–288
Self-help groups, 347–348
Self-observation
adherence and, 301
cognitive therapy and, 249–250
nutrition and, 293
pain treatment and, 366–369
self-control and, 239–241
time management and, 312
Self-regulation. *See also* Self control
disease and, 107–110
health and, 105–107
negative feedback and, 101–105
Smoking
cancer and, 42, 166–168, 341–342
cessation programs for, 283–288
costs of, 42
determinants of, 42–44
development of, 42–43
disease and, 9–10
heart disease and, 42, 118, 134–135, 329–330
physician warnings and, 286
prevention of, 288–289, 330
Social skills
biofeedback and, 268–269
pain treatment and, 374–375
stress and, 311
training of, 311, 316–317
Social support
adherence and, 59–60
cancer and, 182–184, 347–348
definition of, 77
diabetes and, 323
heart disease and, 121–122, 131–132
health and, 77–78
host resistance and, 383–387
stress management and, 316–317
Specificity theory of pain, 190–192
Stimulus control
adherence and, 298–302
dieting and, 243
health-impairing behavior and, 27–28, 33–34
illness actions and, 51–53
immunizations and, 380–381
nutrition and, 293
operant conditioning and, 217–218
respondent conditioning and, 227–228
seat-belt use and, 377–378
self-control and, 243–244
smoking and, 285
Stress
appraisal and, 70–75

Stress (*Cont.*)
autonomic nervous system and, 66–67, 79–82
behavior and, 69–70
biology of, 66–68
cancer and, 171–173
coping and, 75–78
definition of, 65–71
disease and, 89–91, 395–397
endocrine system and, 83–86
environment and, 68–69
health-impairing behavior and, 91–92
heart disease and, 120–121, 132–135
immune system and, 148–151, 171–173, 385–386
process of, 88–89
social support and, 77–78
systems paradigm and, 70, 74
Stress management
aging and, 385
aversive medical procedures and, 318–320
cancer and, 348–353
chronic disease and, 320–323
cognitions and, 253–255, 313–314
environment and, 317–318
heart disease and, 336–338
host resistance and, 384–387
procedural guidelines for, 307–310
providing information and, 314–316
social skills training and, 311
social support and, 316–317
time management and, 311–313
type A behavior and, 333–336
Symptom interpretation by individuals
active nature of, 50
adherence and, 60–61
determinants of, 50–51
dimensions of, 50
emotional arousal and, 51
heart disease and, 130–133
pain and, 189
Symptom recognition by individuals
body perception and, 49–50
cancer and, 174–175
determinants of, 49–50
heart disease and, 130–133
importance of, 48–49
Systematic desensitization
description of, 229–230
chemotherapy side effects and, 351–353
Systems paradigm
description of, 14–17
disease and, 100–105, 107–110
health and, 100–107
intervention and, 110–111
pain and, 203–204

Time management, 311–313
Trauma
accidents and, 376–378
definition of, 98
Type A behavior
assessment of, 123–125
definition of, 122–123
development of, 127–128
heart disease and, 122–129
modification of, 333–336
psychophysiology of, 127–129

Utilization of health care. *See* Health care utilization

Vaccinations. *See* Self-care
Vascular system, 102–103, 114–115

Weight control. *See* Nutrition; obesity
White blood cells. *See* Immune system